Yonce / Personal

THE PSYCHOLOGY
OF COMMUNICATION DISORDERS
IN INDIVIDUALS
AND THEIR FAMILIES

THE PSYCHOLOGY OF COMMUNICATION DISORDERS IN INDIVIDUALS AND THEIR FAMILIES

Walter J. Rollin

Professor, Communicative Disorders in Special Education
San Francisco State University

Prentice-Hall, Inc., Englewood Cliffs, New Jersey 07632

Library of Congress Cataloging-in-Publication Data

Rollin, Walter J.
  The psychology of communication disorders in
individuals and their families.

  Includes bibliographies and index.
  1. Communicative disorders—Psychological
aspects. 2. Communicative disorders—Patients—
Family relationships. I. Title.
RC423.R65 1987   616.85′5   86–30564
ISBN 0–13–732561–4

Cover design: Ben Santora
Manufacturing buyer: Harry P. Baisley

We gratefully acknowledge use of the following material:
Pages 2–5.   From J.C. Hansen, R.R. Stevic, and R.W. Warner, Jr. *Counseling: Theory and Process*, Third Edition. Copyright © 1982 by Allyn and Bacon, Inc. Used with permission.
Page 21. From O. Backus. The study of psychological processes in speech therapists. In D.A. Barbara. *Psychological and Psychiatric Aspects of Speech and Hearing*. Springfield, Ill.: Chas C. Thomas, 1960. Courtesy of Charles C. Thomas, Publisher, Springfield, Illinois.
Pages 43–44, 115–116. Adapted with permission of The Free Press, a Division of Macmillan, Inc. from *Handbook of Stress: Theoretical and Clinical Aspects*, edited by Leo Goldberger and Shlomo Breznitz. Copyright © 1982 by The Free Press.
Pages 45, 68. Jon Eisenson. *Adult Aphasia*. Copyright © 1984, pp. 236–238. Reprinted by permission of Prentice-Hall, Englewood Cliffs, New Jersey.

This book can be made available to businesses, industry, organizations,
associations, and mail order catalogers at substantial discounts
when ordered in quantity. For more information, contact:
    Prentice-Hall, Inc.
    Special Sales Department
    College Division
    Englewood Cliffs, N.J. 07632
    (201) 592-2863

Printed in the United States of America

10 9 8 7 6 5 4 3 2 1

ISBN 0-13-732561-4   01

Prentice-Hall International (UK) Limited, *London*
Prentice-Hall of Australia Pty. Limited, *Sydney*
Prentice-Hall Canada Inc., *Toronto*
Prentice-Hall Hispanoamericana, S.A., *Mexico*
Prentice-Hall of India Private Limited, *New Delhi*
Prentice-Hall of Japan, Inc., *Tokyo*
Prentice-Hall of Southeast Asia Pte. Ltd., *Singapore*
Editora Prentice-Hall do Brasil, Ltda., *Rio de Janeiro*

I dedicate this book to Jon Eisenson—
teacher, mentor, colleague, and friend—
whose thoughts and ideas expressed more than thirty years ago
inspired me finally to write this book.

In memory of my father
and mother, who cared.

CONTENTS

PREFACE

This book was written for two major reasons. One was to share with the reader the current state of knowledge regarding the psychological and social dynamics of the communicatively disordered population with whom we work. Second was to present counseling strategies that the reader might use to assist that population in coping more successfully with emotional factors accompanying these disorders.

During the course of my investigations into the psychological processes that constitute the various disorders, I was intrigued by the extent of contributions made by many other diverse academic disciplines, including linguistics, neurology, psychiatry, psychology, sociology, laryngology, and social psychology. It was a formidable challenge to try to bring them all together in order to establish a common frame of reference for fully understanding the needs of the communicatively disordered individual. I hope I have made a start in that direction. Even then it was plainly clear that subjective clinical data far exceeded the rigors of empirical evidence, in terms of quantity at best. The questions are certainly there for the asking and I attempted to raise some research issues in several chapters.

An even greater challenge was posed by the myriad counseling theories and therapies available to us as counseling speech-language-hearing professionals. I attempted, therefore, to establish a counseling base upon which counseling strategies could evolve for each of the various disorders. Although some overlapping was unavoidable, I believe also it was an essential factor toward reinforcing my discussion of the counseling processes common to the remediation of each of the disorders. In this regard, my intention was essentially to describe the counseling process as necessary for the development of the ideal client-therapist relationship in communicative disorders therapy.

For those who desire or require comprehensive descriptions of various counseling approaches, I have provided a substantial list of pertinent references. I discuss my own counseling approach for each of the disorders in an essentially generic fashion, as it was my intention only to introduce basic concepts and processes.

I wrote this book with consideration for several different groups of readers. For those readers at the undergraduate level it is an opportunity to arouse interest in generic psychodynamic processes associated with the major communication disorders and stimulate further reading and investigation. It will probably be most helpful if this group reads each chapter in sequential order so that a gradual understanding of psychotherapeutic processes can emerge and thus better prepare these readers for the impact of Chapter 9.

Those who are now in graduate studies should also benefit from the above, but beyond that as well. It is hoped that interest in developing counseling skills will be enhanced and that at the same time the reader will be inspired to challenge the many premises raised by myself and other authorities cited throughout the text.

For practicing professionals, regardless of work setting, it is hoped that a greater clarification of the counseling boundaries in speech-language pathology and audiology is accomplished. Whether a clinical researcher or research clinician, such a reader will be provoked into either solidifying previously held assumptions and beliefs, modifying them, or questioning even further the premises made throughout the book. No doubt my text should force the recognition of what it may mean for counseling to continue to be neglected as an intervention strategy among our more traditional ones.

There is a final group of professionals for whom I have written this book. They are the wide variety of practicing psychotherapists, many of whom I have known personally and professionally through the years, and who, because of their unfamiliarity with the complex dynamics of the communicatively disordered population, encouraged me "to get it all on paper."

There were several tangential topics I was tempted to explore. These were touched upon only generally. One of them concerns our evaluation of the therapy we do. There is very little we do to evaluate the outcome of our therapeutic interventions beyond superficial measurable linguistic units of discourse. Less is known of how our clients change and to what degree, particularly in regard to interpersonal communicative behavior. Hopefully, others will take up this challenge.

Although I may not have gotten it all on paper to provide the definitive answers to all of the issues raised, I hope I have at least pointed in the direction for our profession to come to terms with all that is implied in the title of this book. The guidelines are there in order for readers, so inclined, to follow so that they may formulate their own counseling model and develop approaches unique to their own personal and professional needs and the special needs of their clients.

ACKNOWLEDGMENTS

I would not have been able to write this book without the kind permission given by the many publishers and authors for material quoted and paraphrased and without the direct and indirect contributions of communicatively disordered individuals and their families.

I am very grateful also to my graduate students, namely, Nancy TeSelle, Deborah Van Atta, Adele Ghio, Julie Hutchinson, Maria Pagengella, and Cathay Gunn, who often served as highly critical referees of the ideas and concepts I shared with them throughout the writing of the book and who also provoked me positively with ideas of their own.

I would like to especially thank Nancy TeSelle for her extraordinary skill and intelligence in critiquing, editing, and typing the entire volume. Her word processing skill certainly facilitated the constant modifications, omissions, substitutions, and additions I needed to make throughout its preparation.

I am indebted also to my children—Todd, Brad, Hannah, and Sarah—who were certain from the beginning that I would complete the task and who reinforced each milestone with praise and joy.

It would have been nearly impossible to undertake and complete this task without the loving support and encouragement given by my wife, Bonnie, who not only inspired me to keep going, but who also refrained from sharing her own professional critiquing until I had completed the entire text. I myself could never have been so patient.

The meeting of two personalities is like the contact of two chemical substances: if there is any reaction, both are transformed.

Carl Jung, *Modern Man in Search of a Soul*

THE PSYCHOLOGY
OF COMMUNICATION DISORDERS
IN INDIVIDUALS
AND THEIR FAMILIES

1

BASIC COUNSELING THEORY
AND PRACTICES

INTRODUCTION

To many speech-language pathologists and audiologists the term *counseling* or *psychotherapy* elicits an automatic negative response, probably due in part to attitudes that have been inculcated during the sixty-year life of the speech-language-hearing-profession. Until the 1950s, therapeutic practices were essentially characterized by symptom-based strategies with scant attention given to the dynamics of the client-therapist interpersonal relationship. Although therapists and such major authorities as Van Riper, Perkins, and Johnson were now beginning to regard the value in attending to the interpersonal communicative needs of their clients, on a different front therapists were adopting behavioral models to remove or modify speech-language "deficits." Ironically, although most professionals acknowledged then, and still do, the importance of treating the whole person, in practice this has seldom been the case. As Backus (1960) forewarned in her timeless essay more than twenty-five years ago:

> The great risk now appears to be that the increasing numbers of people entering the field, the greatly expanded body of knowledge, together with the

1

growing prestige of the profession—will produce an increasing dedication to subject matter and to the profession (I—It) rather than dedication to the person (I—Thou). Such a trend would inevitably bring serious consequences to clients, therapists, and to the profession. (p. 525)

Backus does not deny the value of using our knowledge of the various mechanisms of speech, language, and hearing principles of therapy to bring about communicative change, but she does insist that by the nature of what we do as therapists we enter into relationships with our clients. We would add that as speech-language-hearing therapists, we cannot not relate. Because of this reality it is appropriate to try to understand better the psychological processes underlying relationships in the therapeutic environment.

We admit that differentiating psychological processes directly related to speech-language-hearing issues from deep-seated psychopathologies (which indeed fall outside the realm of our chief professional interests) may at times be difficult to ascertain. We believe, though, that it is possible to establish counseling guidelines that speech-language-hearing professionals can follow in the treatment of their clients. To do so, it will be necessary for us to discuss first the relation of psychotherapy to counseling.

RELATION OF PSYCHOTHERAPY TO COUNSELING

If we were merely to define counseling lexically as meaning "advise, recommend, guide, and exchange ideas and opinions," there would be no reason for attempting to relate the term to psychotherapy. Then, as speech-language-hearing therapists, our task would be simple, in that we would have no further responsibility to our clients than to impart to them the store of knowledge, expertise, and good sense with which presumably we have been trained. If, on the other hand, we are to define counseling more realistically in its connotative form, we must say that counseling is a dynamic process that involves a complex interaction between and among people. To insist that such professionals as the lawyer, vocational counselor, high school counselor, family physician, and speech-language-hearing professional adhere only to imparting information to their clients would be naive, indeed, as communication (and who should know better than us?) involves an active and reactive interrelationship between helper (counselor) and helpee (client). Furthermore, we need to recognize that because informational content and people obviously vary from profession to profession, the quality, degree, and nature of the counseling interrelationship will differ as well.

It is important to define psychotherapy first and then examine it more closely. By lexical definition, psychotherapy is the psychological treatment of mental, emotional, and nervous disorders. Taken on the more abstract level, interpretations and applications of the process have been made by differing schools of thought and by varied helping professionals, such as psychiatrists, clinical psychologists, clinical social workers, and family and child therapists. Intrinsic to psychotherapy, regardless of the school or the helping profession, is the idea that the interrelational process between client and therapist determines the ultimate outcome of therapy. The complexity of the process is dependent not only on the theoretical orientation but also on the nature, severity, and degree of the disorder. (For further appreciation of the extensive range of disorders, the reader is referred to the DSM-III criteria established by the American Psychiatric Association [1980].) Although the psychotherapeutic professions still abide by nosological criteria and rules (disease classification), they recognize the vast diversity of people who are troubled by the demands and complexity of life in the twentieth century. We no longer compartmentalize all those who suffer emotionally into vacuous categories of "neurotic," "maladjusted," or "abnormal." For this reason, our task in differentiating between psychotherapy and counseling is more challenging and difficult.

Viewing Counseling and Psychotherapy on a Continuum

In attempting to differentiate between counseling and psychotherapy, it would appear obvious for us to consider these processes along a continuum, but this is not as simple as it might seem. Hansen, Stevic, and Warner (1977) reviewed several writers in the field who attempted to differentiate counseling from psychotherapy along a continuum. One group views the continuum in terms of degrees of normalcy versus neuroses, and other writers view the continuum in terms of process, or the manner in which the counselor or psychotherapist works with clients. Hansen, Stevic, and Warner point out that because people vary in their ability to deal with role problems in their environment or with deep-seated intrapersonal conflicts, it would be better to consider the degree to which, or the intensity with which, people suffer from their problems. We would agree with such an analysis in that it helps us to avoid the use of labels to categorize individuals and instead urges us to focus on how individuals uniquely cope with their difficulties.

As we see it, the counselor would work with individuals who are essentially able to function in their daily living but who are troubled by either internal or external circumstances that interfere with maximal functioning. Contrarily, the psychotherapist would work with individuals who are devastated by either internal or external circumstances, be it a role conflict, deep-seated psychopathology, or both, and who need to restructure their personalities in order to function maximally. That is, these are individuals who may be profoundly affected by an adverse circumstance in their lives, regardless of neurosis per se.

One further differentiating feature justifying either counseling or psychotherapeutic intervention is that of the therapeutic relationship itself.

We believe that psychotherapy requires an intense and complex relationship between therapist and client in which the relationship becomes the essential process for change. The therapeutic relationship in counseling is also intrinsic to helping the individual learn new means of coping with and adjusting to life circumstances, and, although dynamic, it is not the only factor responsible for change.

We recognize that the distinctions we have made between counseling and psychotherapy are not always precise and that by the nature of any therapeutic process, overlapping is certain to occur. Nonetheless, as we will see further on, it is possible to establish boundaries, allowing the speech-language-hearing therapist to function effectively, securely, and ethically as counselor during the therapeutic process. At this point, though, we need to illustrate the major distinctive elements of psychotherapy and counseling.

Distinctive Elements of Psychotherapy

Typically, the psychotherapist focuses on intrapersonal conflicts characterized by anxieties, depression, guilt, and ambivalences that, although real to the individual, may have little basis in objective reality. The psychotherapist is concerned with the following questions about the client's personality:

1. What has been its course of development?
2. What factors have impeded its growth?
3. What factors are impeding its growth now?

With the medical model as a referent, the psychotherapist views the individual as sick and requiring major reductions in psychopathological behavior. (It should be noted, however, that in the last twenty years several schools of psychotherapy have developed that lean toward a so-called well model with which the individual is not viewed as sick but as behaviorally dysfunctional.) Regardless of theory, the psychotherapeutic process is characterized by either classical approaches or blended procedures, such as depth psychoanalysis, cognitive-emotional psychotherapy, behavior modification psychotherapy, and biological process psychotherapy.

In essence, psychotherapy consists of the reorganization and reinterpretation of destructive elements of conflict within the personality.

Distinctive Elements of Counseling

The essential task of the counselor is to help individuals work toward an understanding of themselves in order to learn new ways of coping with and adjusting to life situations. There is no necessity for individuals to restructure or reorganize their personality in order to cope with marital difficulties, change careers, or eliminate stress associated with vocal abuse—unless, of course, such individuals are guided by deep-rooted psychopathological conflicts. Indeed, such individuals would require the psychotherapeutic intervention discussed earlier. But we are concerned now with the individual whose problems relate directly to role definition—that is, difficulty in adapting a particular role to a particular life situation (the divorced father, the stuttering child, the single-parent mother).

The counseling process is characteristically supportive, insight-reeducative, and usually short term. It is used to help individuals make practical changes in their lives without modifying established personality patterns. Represented by distinctive and blended schools of thought, counseling is based on a well model and employs procedures not unlike those of psychotherapy. These would include cognitive-emotional counseling, client-centered counseling, behavior modification counseling, and informational-educational counseling. Let us now consider these various theories in depth, toward developing a model we may apply in our work with the communicatively impaired who require counseling assistance.

MAJOR COUNSELING THEORIES

The Self Theory or Client-Centered Approach of Carl Rogers

Probably the most influential figure in the field of counseling has been Carl Rogers, whose first book, *Counseling and Psychotherapy* (published in 1942), has served as the seminal source for counseling theory practices as they have evolved over forty years. Rogers, in his ever-growing wisdom, has modified his theory, consistent with the dramatic changes that have taken place in all aspects of society. From his earliest statement in 1942 that "the self is a basic factor in the formation of personality and the determination of behavior" to his thesis in 1959 that the self is "the organized, consistent conceptual Gestalt composed of characteristics of the 'I' or 'me' and the perceptions of the relationships of the 'I' or 'me' to others and to various aspects of life, together with the value attached to these perceptions" (p. 20), Rogers views change in the client to be the direct result of the dynamic way in which the client and therapist experience their relationship. According to Rogers, the structure of personality is based on three major elements, which he describes as the phenomenal field, the organism, and the self.

The phenomenal field, the organism, and the self According to Rogers (1951), people are always in the center of an ever-changing phenomenal field that is continuously being experienced either consciously or unconsciously. How we respond depends on how we perceive reality, whether it be internal or external. That is, when our perception of reality changes, so do our reactions.

As might be illustrated in speech-language therapy, if an aphasic client perceives his or her disability as the only reality, then it is that on which the client remains focused and to that which the client negatively reacts. If, on the other hand, the client perceives his or her remaining assets as the reality, there is greater likelihood of more positive reactions. We do not wish to imply that an either/or perception is desirable because the client must also perceive the reality of the desirability. If the client can perceive both realities, then his or her reactions are more likely to result in positive change.

Rogers considers the organism to be the total individual who acts as a complete, organized system in which modification of any part of that system produces changes in any other part or parts. The organism consists of all the thoughts, behaviors, feelings, and physical attributes that constitute the individual.

As humans, we never function in separate parts but holistically or as a total entity in order to have our needs expressed or satisfied. In order to achieve self-actualization or dynamic and continuous growth, Rogers clearly advises us that it does not occur without struggle and pain. It is always easier to maintain the status quo or take the pathway of least resistance. As we will see in our discussion of stuttering, it is very difficult to relinquish that with which we have been familiar. Conversely, the organism desires to develop as fully as possible without the constraint of external controls. But positive change can take place only by altering our perception of reality and not our reaction to it. Rogers implies that the more we are willing to become aware of our reactions, and symbolize them consciously, the more likely we are to grow positively.

Rogers's most important principle is that of the self. As an individual strives for self-actualization, that person must differentiate and discriminate the objects of his or her feelings and perceptions—personal environment, experiences, the self, and the interrelationships of these. In doing so, the individual becomes less fixed and more open to his or her perceptions or, stated differently, the individual's experiences are more accurately symbolized. The person comes to understand the incongruity between certain of his or her experiences and the personal concept of self. Feelings that in the past have been denied to awareness or distorted in awareness are experienced more fully, resulting in a reorganization of the self-concept. As the self-structure continues to reorganize, the concept of self becomes more congruent with the individual's experience, with the self now including experiences that previously would have been too threatening to recognize or acknowledge (Rogers 1959).

In their discussion of the self, Avila and Purkey (1977) provide evidence to support the thesis that human behavior is not determined so much by life situations per se as "by the individual's perception of the situation (p. 56). Thus it is particularly important to recognize that there may be a discrepancy between the actual reality and the way the individual perceives that reality. The relationship between the two realities is dynamic, however, and influenced by the complex interrelationships among the individual's experiences, life environment, and unique human constitutional factors.

In summary, the personality evolves around the self, which is the nucleus. As the organism interacts with its environment, the self develops. In doing so, the values of other people are either integrated or distorted. Phenomenologically, the organism integrates experiences that are consistent with the concept of the self. If the experiences are inconsistent, they are perceived as threats. Of crucial importance to self-concept is that it is always in process and, as a function of its dynamic interaction with the phenomenal field, changes and grows.

It is obvious that although each of us is unique in fulfilling the values necessary for self-actualization, our basic needs are essentially similar. Rogers hypothesizes that each individual has the ability and the capacity to settle personal conflicts through the enhancement of his or her own value system as well as through the collective value system (Rogers 1959, 1961).

Having examined Rogers's basic self theory of personality, we can now appropriately consider how his principles may be understood in the context of our work with the communicatively disordered individual.

Application to the communicatively disordered We have already noted that an aphasic client may focus on the disability to the exclusion of other aspects within his or her phenomenal field. For this client and for others with different communicative disorders, how they perceive their subjective realities is dependent on the nature and quality of their interrelated past experiences. Included among these are parenting, socializing, and physical environment. We would further add such inherent factors as native intelligence and constitutional predilections that contribute to our uniqueness as individuals. Each of us, then, as do the communicatively disordered, responds every waking moment to those figures or significant perceptual elements that stand out from the ground or the entire perceptual environment. Because the phenomenal field includes perceptual experiences that are both internal and external to the individual, the communicatively disordered person may either react to the critical comments made by others, or to his or her own displeasure with the disorder, or to both. Thus that person's particular perception becomes fixed within his or her personal phenomenal field.

We have also pointed out Rogers's belief that the organism acts in a total way to the phenomenal field, and that changing any aspect of the organized system will bring about changes in other aspects. Thus the communicatively disordered individual who fixates only on the disorder aspect of his or her person will tend to view that as representing the totality of his or her organismic nature. It is, therefore, difficult for this person to recognize within the personal phenomenal field the potential for changing not only attitudes about the disorder but also the opportunity for developing more positive attitudes regarding other parts of himself or herself. Of chief importance, however, is that the potential does exist because the organism is constantly striving "to expand, extend, develop, mature" (Rogers 1961, p. 351). It entails, however, the opportunity, the motivation, the will, and the courage to become more fully aware of self-being and self-functioning. As part of this process, which has been described as self-actualization, the communicatively disordered individual must be helped to recognize that, regardless of the disorder, he or she is worthy; that the person has the capability and potential not only to modify or elminate the disorder but also to remove the contaminating, destructive, and limited perceptions of other aspects of his or her life. In sum, the individual need not continue to symbolize all significant experiences in terms of only the disorder itself.

A Behavioral Theory

We shall now look at behavioral theory—considered by many to be antithetical to Rogers's self theory model—and how it may serve as a counseling strategy for the communicatively disordered.

B. F. Skinner (1953), the chief proponent of behavioral theory, believes that human behavior is determined essentially by the environment and that the way humans react is in response to external events that occur around them. The basic assumption underscoring behavioral theory is that behavior is learned when that behavior is followed by an event in the environment that brings satisfaction to the individual. The probability of that behavior being repeated is thereby increased. The satisfaction to the individual may be brought about by events either external or internal to the individual. An example of Skinner's assumption is the infant who babbles. Through maturation and perhaps external influences, the infant discovers pleasure by babbling, and it is therefore rewarding. The probability for that behavior to recur is increased. Thus operant conditioning occurs as a result of a specific behavioral event, the behavior shaped by the consequences of the environmental events that follow. In this way babbling is reinforced, paving the way for higher levels of speech development.

Most learning theorists would contend that learning can also occur through imitation or by identifying with the model copied, without the necessity of receiving a reward. In citing the work of Bandura (1962, 1965, 1969), Hansen, Stevic, and Warner (1977) indicate that through the observation by one individual of another individual's response, vicarious learning is possible. They add, however, that actual reinforcement may be necessary for the observer's performance of the behavior.

A learning theory position   We have already seen that behavior operates to produce the reinforcement. Each is dependent or contingent on the other. That is, behavior that is rewarded or given positive reinforcement can be increased in frequency or maintained, whereas behavior that is punished by the removal of positive reinforcers or the addition of negative reinforcers can be extinguished or decreased in frequency.

Establishment of new behaviors is dependent on the immediacy of the reward. New behavior may be extinguished if a reward is terminated abruptly or if infrequently presented. Partial reinforcement, however, or a schedule of reinforcement, may help to maintain behavior once it has been learned. According to Hansen, Stevic, and Warner (1977), reinforcement schedules consist of "ratio reinforcement" and "interval reinforcement." For the former, a reward is given after a certain number of responses have occurred. For interval reinforcement, a proper amount of time must pass for a reward to be given. "In most cases, people who have been exposed to either of the intermittent schedules will retain the learned responses longer than if they had been on a continuous schedule" (p. 167).

Hansen, Stevic, and Warner further describe how we develop more complex behaviors through the processes of extinction, generalization, discrimination, shaping, and mediating.

EXTINCTION

Our ability to change our behavior continuously is dependent on the frequency of the intermittent reinforcement and our own recognition of what is appropriate to any one stage of our development. In order to grow from child to adulthood, reinforcement of earlier behavior is withheld so that the behavior will decrease and eventually be eliminated.

GENERALIZATION

A second important principle of learning is that of generalization. In essence, a stimulus that is accompanied by a reinforcement produces a particular response, but it also transfers to other stimuli as well. It is important for the two stimuli to be related in some way, however, if the response is to recur. We are familiar with the child who vocalizes when the mother appears and who transfers the same response when the father appears. Without generalization, it would be difficult to explain the rapid development of language during the early formative years.

DISCRIMINATION

Our uniqueness no doubt results partly from the way we generalize but also from the way we learn to discriminate between situations or events. Thus we also make small changes in behavior when exposed to similar situations. "The law of discrimination states that the relationships between stimuli and responses that have been generated through the process of generalization may be broken down separately" (p. 168). Through the interaction of extinction and reinforcement, the appropriate response to a stimulus is reinforced, whereas an inappropriate response to a similar event is not reinforced. The infant learns early to respond similarly to both parents but differently to strangers because the stimulus given is most likely different.

SHAPING

"Shaping is the process of moving from simple behaviors which are approximations of the final behavior to a final complex behavior" (p. 168). It is a process in which specific behaviors that come close to the desired behavior are reinforced. Any extraneous behaviors receive no reinforcement. It is crucial that at each level of the process, successive approximations of the behavior are expected before any reinforcement is provided. Infants apparently learn this process as they move through the highly complex evolution of speech and language development. Parents tend to reinforce those sounds and words that approximate the desired final product and typically do not reinforce those behaviors that remain static. How parents seem to know when to recognize the appropriateness at each level of development is unclear and not our purpose to discuss at this time. Similarly, we do not know if the infant makes adjustments of vocal and verbal behavior by responding to its own internal time clock of appropriateness. Certainly as we develop we reinforce ourselves for behaviors that are rewarding, but just when this begins is also uncertain.

MEDIATING

As humans, we distinguish ourselves from other animals by our ability to develop mediating responses that permit us consciously to plan, evaluate, and react to our environment through the use of language and symbolization. With this capacity we learn to use our reasoning process to label stimuli and "mediate their effects." In citing Skinner (1971), Hansen, Stevic, and Warner very clearly acknowledge that as humans we have the ability not only to mediate the effects of environmental events but also the ability to become aware of that capacity.

As a direct result of Skinner's formulation we have seen the emergence during the last two decades of counseling and psychotherapeutic strategies based on behavioral principles. It is, therefore, appropriate for us now to consider how these principles may be applied generally in counseling the communicatively disordered.

Application to the communicatively disordered   Mowrer (1977) has made one of the most important contributions to our understanding of how behavioral strategies can be employed in counseling the communicatively disordered. Citing Menacker (1976), Mowrer emphasizes the importance of the client being an active participant along with the therapist in removing barriers to more effective communicative interaction with others. Both work together to achieve favorable environmental conditions conducive to positive behavioral change. The process is essentially directive rather than reflective, which is characteristic of self theory. Mowrer describes it as an empirical-rational approach; it is assumed from the beginning that the client will derive the greatest benefit "from an instructional, highly directive attack on the problem" (p. 131). Use of the intellect is key to desired change.

From the individual who desires a more effective way to manage the voice to the individual who is plagued by severe disfluency, the counseling process is a learning situation in which the client is helped to define the specific behaviors that contribute to the difficulty. The goals of counseling must be stated in specific terms and therapy directed toward one specific concern at a time. Thus, if loud vocalization is seen as a behavior that must be extinguished, the counselor and client work together to reinforce vocal intensity that is more hygienic and balanced. That this may not occur immediately is apparent from our discussion of shaping and therefore any close approximation to the desired goal is to be rewarded through either counselor affirmation or client self-realization. In essence, the client is helped to develop whatever system of self-management is deemed appropriate in order for that person to control his or her communicative destiny.

The Rational-Emotive Therapy Model

The fundamental assumption behind Albert Ellis's rational-emotive therapy (RET) model is that we essentially control our own destinies as long as we believe in and act on the values that are important and significant to us. A corollary to this assumption is the position that most emotional disturbance is a function of basic irrational beliefs that are "self-defeating and absurd." Ellis believes that we can learn to use RET as a self-help tool and through the process discover our irrational beliefs and learn the "use of the logico-empirical methods of scientific inquiry: questioning, debating, challenging, and disputing of irrational beliefs. The purpose of the process is to induce the person to recognize the absurdity of his beliefs, to relinquish them, and to adopt new, more adaptive ones" (Ellis and Grieger 1977, p. 3).

The ABCs of RET   It is Ellis's contention that whenever an "activating experience or activating event" (*A*) occurs and is followed by an "emotional and/or behavioral consequence" (*C*), we have two major choices of thinking or beliefs: either rational or irrational (*B*). Say, for example, that you have written a paper based on original research, and the study is rejected by the editor of the journal to which it has been submitted. You are now at point *A*. You react to the experience with an emotional and/or behavioral consequence (*C*), which follows almost immediately. The irrational response would be the belief that *A* caused *C* and you conclude that your study wasn't worthwhile to begin with, that your research and writing abilities are poor, and that the editor was uncaring in doing this to you. A more rational or reasonable response would be to acknowledge that you are displeased with what happened and frustrated after all the work you have put in, but then to do something realistic in order to prevent the event from happening again. This might include obtaining a critical evaluation of the paper and/or submitting the study to another journal.

Ellis (1962) contends that it is not events that upset us but rather our view of events. He lists many central illogical beliefs that are common to Western thought and that contribute to neuroses. Several of these are summarized as follows:

1. It is of the utmost importance for an adult to be approved or loved by nearly everyone for virtually everything that adult does.
2. One should be completely competent, adequate, and achieving in everything one does.
3. Certain people are evil, bad, or wicked and therefore should be blamed severely and punished for their transgressions.
4. It is horrible, terrible, and catastrophic when things do not progress the way one would like.
5. Human unhappiness is caused by external events and we have minimal or no ability to control our sadness or eliminate those negative feelings.
6. If anything should be dangerous or scary, we should be overwhelmed with and distressed about it.
7. It is simpler to avoid confronting life's difficulties and our responsibilities than to take on more rewarding modes of self-discipline.
8. Past events in our lives determine our present behavior; they always have and cannot be changed.
9. Difficulties in life should not exist, and people and events should be different from the way they are; also, it is catastrophic if the perfect solutions to the grim realities of life are not immediately discovered.
10. We should be very concerned and upset by other people's problems and difficulties.
11. Maximum human happiness can be achieved by inertia and inaction or by passively and uncommittedly "enjoying oneself."

These are only a few of the 259 central self-defeating irrational ideas Ellis has collected. He contends, however, that although such beliefs exist in virtually all of us, in varying degrees, some individuals are likely to behave more irrationally than others.

The three Ds of RET   Because RET is essentially a "logico-empirical method of scientific questioning," according to Ellis, we must have an internal "debate" with ourselves regarding our rational and irrational beliefs. The method further involves "discriminating" between the negative and positive aspects of our behaviors and differentiating between the myths we tell ourselves and reality-based logical conclusions. It means acknowledging our inconsistencies and contradictions in our thinking and behaving. Crucial to the process is the necessity for "defining" the terms we use to describe our behaviors, resulting in finer differentiations. In referring to the principles of general semantics, Ellis reminds us that we must avoid overgeneralizations, labeling, and inexact descriptions of events and our own behaviors if we are to pursue a logical life course.

The counseling process   Like Rogers and other representative figures of the humanistic school of psychotherapy, Ellis (1962) believes that "one of the main functions of psychotherapy is to enhance the individual's self-respect (or 'ego strength,' 'self-confidence,' 'self-esteem,' 'feeling of self-worth,' or 'sense of identity') so that he may thereby solve the problem of self-evaluation" (p. 99–100). Ellis emphasizes the importance of understanding the way in which the client sees his or her own world and considers the client's behavior from the client's point of view. The therapist must refrain from getting immersed in the client's irrational belief system or behavior and must instead strip away the illogical ideas that are the basis of the client's anxieties and self-deceptions. Although Ellis recognizes the importance of being supportive and empathic and allowing the free expression of feelings, the therapist must also be confrontive, directive, and persuasive if the client is to be channeled into a more rational mode of thinking and, therefore, behaving (Ellis, 1962).

In summarizing Ellis's cognitive counseling approach, Hansen, Stevic, and Warner (1977) describe it as a teaching process in which the client is helped to recognize the "shoulds, oughts, and musts" that dominate his or her thought processes (p. 208). Like the teacher, the therapist provides access to such teaching tools as books, articles, tape and video recordings, and films and filmstrips. RET is described as a process to modify the individual's basic value system. The following are among the techniques used:

1. Role playing to demonstrate to the client his or her irrational ideas
2. Modeling to demonstrate to the client more rational ways of behaving
3. Unconditional acceptance and humor to demonstrate to the client that he or she is accepted as a person despite the absurdity of his or her beliefs.

Although RET is considered essentially a learning process, Ellis also believes that there is a powerful biological element or predisposing innate tendencies that contribute to our belief systems and behaviors. That we may never behave completely rationally is not as essential as our being persistent and conscientious in moving in that direction.

Cognitively counseling with the communicatively disordered   It would appear that RET can readily be applied to the self-defeating cognitive processes of various communicatively disordered individuals. Not unlike the more traditional behavioral approach with the communicative disorder described earlier, RET could be applied as both an educational and a counseling tool to modify or eliminate the irrational beliefs that contribute to the quality and severity of some communicative disorders.

It is of some significance that Ellis should base several important aspects of his theory on the postulates of general semantics, among whose pioneers was Wendell Johnson, one of the most prolific authorities on stuttering behavior in the twentieth century. Johnson (1946, 1959) and one of his students, Dean Williams (1957), developed strategies that essentially attacked the *"linguistic insanities"* (italics my own) and irrational behaviors that appeared to perpetuate stuttering behaviors and maintain the self-effacing and self-destructive attitudes of stutterers. The work of more recent proponents of a cognitive-behavioral approach to the treatment of stuttering, such as that of Rubin and Culatta (1971), Shames, Egolf, and Rhodes (1969), and Goldberg (1981), is discussed in Chapter 4.

Use of RET in counseling the vocal abuser and/or misuser would appear appropriate because abuse or misuse of the voice can be eliminated by a conscious and rational decision to use the voice in a different manner. The speech-language pathologist is the obvious professional to educate and counsel the client toward that end. Those who view vocal personality as an important dimension of continued vocal mismanagement (Cooper 1973) could readily apply RET principles with a voice client, combining an objective analysis of the actual vocal possibilities with a rational acceptance of that person's vocal self-image.

We will presently see how behavioral and self theory principles may be reconciled in the development of a counseling model for the communicatively disordered.

DEVELOPING AN APPROPRIATE COUNSELING MODEL FOR THE COMMUNICATIVELY DISORDERED

Development of a counseling model for use by speech-language-hearing professionals must consider not only the practical realities of the special needs of the client but also those elements of counseling theory that may be readily applied regardless of type of communicative disorder.

The Essential Similarities Among Theories

Even the mildly interested reader of counseling theory would immediately recognize marked differences among the theories dictated by the various schools. But because actual practices of counselors representing these schools bring them much closer together, we prefer to discuss the similarities in the counseling process. Implicit in our assumption is that counselors are human beings first and, regardless of professional orientation, are nonetheless subject to the often mysterious forces that underlie their own personality processes and behaviors. (We will explore these issues in chapter 9.) Among the processes of counseling, we will consider the goals of counseling, the client–therapist relationship, and the techniques of therapy.

The goals of counseling   Fundamental to all counseling approaches is the common agreement that counseling is structured to facilitate changes in the client's behavior. Though self theory counselors tend to be concerned with modifying and reorganizing the *total* behavioral or structural pattern of the individual's personality, and behavioral counselors more concerned with altering *specific* counterproductive behavior patterns, both groups recognize the significance of etiological factors that underlie all behaviors. Neither school, however, dwells solely on etiology, as changing present and future behaviors is deemed most important.

Common as well is the reduction of depression, anxiety, guilt, anger, and frustration while discovering new ways to cope successfully with life. Though differences emerge in terms of degree, the self-actualization, positive self-regard, and person-in-process concepts of the self theory are certainly compatible with the self-acceptance, self-direction, and choice-making concepts of rational-emotive theory and other behavioral approaches.

The process of counseling   In the self theory approach, the client is given total freedom to express feelings. Regardless of the feelings expressed, they are accepted unconditionally by the counselor, and the client learns to examine those feelings and experience them in an objective manner. The client discovers the incongruity between distorted perceptions of experience and concept of self. As experiences are more objectively examined, the client begins to reorganize concepts of the self, thereby leading toward congruency between both. As the client begins to take more responsibility for his or her behavior, the possibilities for positive change are increased. The client soon realizes the limitless opportunities for taking charge of his or her life while minimizing the effects that external events, situations, and people have had on him or her. The client now more readily adapts to new and changing life circumstances with positive feelings of worthiness and infinite capabilities for growth.

Scales to measure objectively the dynamic aspects of the counseling process related to self theory have been developed by Carkhuff (1969 a, b, 1971, 1977). A major extension of self theory, Carkhuff's model includes not only the need for client self-exploration and self-understanding but also the need for client action. Understanding alone without action is seen as essentially unproductive. Carkhuff's research appears to represent an attempt to shift self theory toward a position in which the counseling process can be more effectively objectified as is characteristic of behavioral therapy. Moreover, his eclectic position reminds us of the action-oriented position of rational-emotive theory.

In rational-emotive therapy, the client is also given the opportunity to express personal feelings and attitudes. Whereas other behaviorists would be more concerned with changing specific attitudes, sufficient opportunities are provided to express feelings as well. RET views the client as capable of making rational decisions based on his or her own thought processes. Although this may appear to differ from self theory in that the latter emphasizes a working through of feelings toward self-realization, RET allows clients to discover the irrational attitudes that have interfered with their mental health. They, too, are helped to recognize the incongruities between their irrational attitudes and the realities of their self-potential. As in self theory counseling, clients learn that it becomes unnecessary to continue to blame external issues or events on their maladaptive behavior and that they have the power and choice to make whatever decisions in their lives are deemed rational and necessary.

Although more traditional behavioral counseling emphasizes and uses reinforcement and shaping schedules, with greater attention given to behavioral changes rather than attitudinal change, the actual process does not differ that much. In RET, the self-perpetuating irrational attitudes and behaviors are attacked and ultimately extinguished, though behaviors may not be changed immediately. Clients certainly differ with regard to their own time line for change and with the gradual withering away of self-defeating indoctrinations.

We recognize that although many significant distinctions may be made among the various behavioral approaches and even more between them and the self theory approach, in terms of therapeutic process, they all share in common, but to differing degrees, the importance of insight. Hansen, Stevic and Warner (1977) note its necessity if behavior is to change. That is, before any change can be expected, clients must know *why*. The major difference, of course, is that in RET and other behavioral approaches, rational thinking is employed, whereas in self theory, an affective or emotional mode constitutes the therapeutic process.

The client—counselor relationship   Probably the most important attribute of self theory therapy is the dynamic interplay of client and counselor. Crucial to this process is the counselor's belief that the client has the ability to cope successfully with all those experiences that are brought into conscious awareness. A further assumption is that the counselor must feel totally non-judgmental toward and empathic with the client and his or her thought structure. Thus, an atmosphere is established whereby the client can perceive that same unconditional positive regard and empathic understanding. As these conditions are initiated through the two persons being in contact, the client feels freer to express feelings verbally and/or motorically. What is most important now is the ability of the counselor to reflect back to the client those feelings expressed. We do not mean a mere restatement of content but an expression of authentic understanding that is manifest in the counselor's speech, voice, bodily movement, and other metalinguistic forms.

As we noted earlier, the client soon begins to express feelings that refer more to the self rather than to the nonself or to the feelings and attitudes of others. In doing so, the client differentiates and discriminates the objects of these feelings and perceptions. They include the environment, other people, perception of self, and experiences and how all of these are interrelated. The more able the client becomes in receiving the empathic feedback from the counselor, the less threatened he or she feels in revealing previously feared material. As the client's feelings of vulnerability and anxiety diminish, the therapeutic relationship becomes more congruent, resulting in greater self-regard and more positive changes in behavior (Rogers, 1951).

Although RET and other behavioral approaches are not primarily interested in motivating clients to express feelings per se, they are concerned with learning about their clients and the feelings and attitudes that perpetuate their self-defeating behavior. Like self theory, RET emphasizes the importance of an effective client–counselor relationship and the engendering of trust by the client in the counselor. Behavioral counselors recognize the importance of being authentic, genuine, and honest with their clients and of avoiding coldness, aloofness, and self-righteousness.

Also involved is the creation of a therapeutic atmosphere in which the client feels accepted and recognized as a person who has the potential for change. That it is the behavioral pattern and not the person that is to be changed constitutes the key motivating factor. Through the interplay of client and counselor by means of verbalization, as in self theory, the counseling process occurs. As we shall discuss later, this has significant implications for those who are communicatively impaired and for counselors who must skillfully modify their usual methods regardless of theoretical orientation.

RET and other behavioral approaches rely more on "teaching" clients new attitudes and behaviors, including the use of confrontation. Self theory advocates respond more to expressions of affect and share the belief that clients must perceive and evaluate the relationship of external events to their internal needs.

The research literature clearly indicates marked differences among the various approaches to counseling, but it also demonstrates significant similarities, particularly in actual practice. Truax (1966) studied and analyzed a hyperactive child successfully counseled by Carl Rogers, who differentially reinforced specific classes of the client's responses. In a later study (1968) Truax's clients were more motivated to explore their feelings when authenticity, empathy, and nonpossessive warmth were used as reinforcers. Staples et al. (1975) had clients rate their behavior therapists and found them to be as warm and to score higher on the dimension of accurate empathy than did traditional therapists. Anderson, Douds, and Carkhuff

(1967) examined forty counseling interviews in which effective use of confrontation contributed to the positive dynamics of therapy, regardless of the counselor's behavioral or self theory orientation.

It is readily apparent that although theory may separate out distinguishing features among the behavioral, rational-emotive, and self theory schools of thought, in actual practice these distinctions tend to dissipate. We believe it has been far more important, then, to give greater attention to the similarities as we now move toward their applicability in counseling the communicatively impaired.

What Is and What Is Not Applicable in Counseling the Communicatively Disordered

In the Preface and in the introduction to this chapter we have stated the overall value of and the necessity for interacting with communicatively disordered clients on an interpersonal level. This implies a counseling relationship. The justification for such a relationship with many such individuals has already been well documented by Mowrer (1977) and Luterman (1984), among others, and needs no further elaboration here.

We believe, however, that before we can substantiate the efficacy of counseling, and which approach is appropriate to use with which communicatively disordered persons, we need to discuss those factors that warrant the use of counseling and those that do not. Bear in mind, however, that these factors are not mutually exclusive and that the uniqueness of the individual disorder, counselor, and clinical circumstance will often dictate a course not initially indicated. Our discussion will consider the contrasting principles generally, thereby serving as an introduction to our analysis of and application to the pertinent disorders presented in later chapters.

Origin of the disorder   The decison to intervene psychotherapeutically[1] cannot be determined solely by etiology. Just as communicative disorders that are psychogenic in origin may not necessarily require psychotherapeutic intervention by the speech-language pathologist or audiologist neither may communicative disorders that etiologically are genetic, neurogenic, or otherwise organic require such intervention.

As speech-language pathologists and audiologists, we place great value on our assessment and case history—taking procedures in order not only to differentiate among etiologies but also to determine which specific aspects of communication performance are impaired, which are variable, and which are intact. Based on these determinants we plan our pertinent treatment strategies. Because our assessment also informs us of the factors that in the past maintained or continue to maintain the disorder, we consider their

---

[1]The use of the term *psychotherapy* shall henceforth be used contextually and synonymously with the term *counseling* where the two tend to overlap.

significance also in the overall treatment plan. What do these premises suggest, and where do they lead us?

First, it is obvious that, theoretically at least, we generally regard each individual uniquely, albeit with a tendency toward some generalization and comparison with others. We further view the individual holistically (at least we say we do) and profess the desire to treat the person and not the disorder. If this is so, and if we are to act consistently with our philosophical and theoretical beliefs, our decision to intervene psychotherapeutically should be based on specific indicators regardless of etiology or disorder. The specific indicators are as follows:

1. *Present environmental stress related to organicity:* We would include the wide range of neurological, neuromuscular, oral-maxillary-facial-laryngeal, and physiological disorders, which either congenitally or adventitiously create stress for the individual.

2. *Previous physical disability:* The physical disabilities described above are not apparently present, but these individuals persist in their perception that they are.

3. *Previous environmental stress:* As above, and with the continuous or intermittent pressures that the individual experienced earlier but that no longer exist in objective reality.

4. *Present environmental stress:* Here we refer to the continuous or intermittent pressures of varying degrees from family members, peers, school, job, and so on, related or unrelated to speech-language-hearing, with which the child or adult must cope.

5. *Nondescript stress:* The individual cannot identify or describe any external pressures but is stressed by continuous or intermittent undefined self-actuated pressures.

6. *Persistent abuse or misuse of the mechanism for speech and language:* These would include the articulatory, respiratory, phonatory, and resonatory functions. The individual denies any reason for the persistence of the disorder.

It is important that we recognize the obvious overlapping among these etiological correlates and that any one could be considered with any other. We further note that each may vary in quality and degree. We also recognize that individuals differ in how they respond to the multidimensional forces in their environment. Finally, we should take caution that we relate the causative factors to disorders of communication.

It should be apparent that maladaptive behaviors aside from clearly discernible speech-language-hearing disorders will result from the factors just described. With that understanding, we now turn our attention to how the speech-language-pathologist and audiologist as counselors decide to intervene psychotherapeutically.

Dealing with related issues The major determining factor that must guide us along the counseling path is the establishiment of a definitive relationship between the client's disordered communication and maladaptive psychological behavior and/or interpersonal maladjustment. This is not as simple as it appears. One obvious consideration is the motivation of the client. Assuming we have established the connection, does it follow that the client will follow suit? Not necessarily, if the client's agenda does not include psychological probing. Besides, can we assume that psychotherapeutic intervention is appropriate at the time, regardless of verifiable cause-effect relationships and client motivation? No, not if the major overriding element, such as the disorder itself, demands our traditional speech-language therapy intervention.

Secondly, we must remember that the initital referral was made for speech-language therapy and not for psychotherapy. This consideration takes on greater significance in the case of young clients whose parents must participate in the speech-language therapy process. Can we expect them to share in a psychotherapeutic approach that may involve probing into their possibly dysfunctional family life?

The reader may now be wondering why we should complicate our professional duties and not adhere to the practices in which we have been traditionally trained. Perhaps this is true, but we might then do our clients an injustice in not providing them the best we truly have to offer in terms of a total organismic approach to communication competence.

Let us, therefore, identify several guidelines we may use in facilitating our decision to intervene psychotherapeutically, assuming that the disorder is related in part at least to psychological issues and recognizing as well the difficulties involved. We should take caution, however, to refrain from doing so if we have any doubt as to that decision.

1. Determine, indirectly, the extent to which environmental influences impinge on the perpetuation of the disorder. Such influences may be revealed during the gradual developing therapeutic relationship.
2. Be sensitive to overt client disclosure of troubled feelings and attitudes about self and/or toward others.
3. Be alert to undisclosed indicators of emotional distress as revealed through physical illness, moodiness, anxiety, or depression in the client.
4. With respect to children in particular, be sensitive to those who are hyperactive, withdrawn, passive, uncooperative, disruptive, inconsiderate, sad, hostile, undisciplined, angry, demanding, rejecting, or fearful.
5. Be cognizant of the child client's relationship to the parents and to siblings in terms of mutual disrespect, uncaring, negative verbal or nonverbal communication, and other inappropriate interactions.
6. Recognize excessive parental concern, anxiety, depression, defensiveness, denial, rejection, self-effacement, or inappropriate affect.

Our list is certainly not exhaustive, and we must be cautious not to overinterpret but rather to describe to the best of our ability those behaviors that are apparent in the client, parents, and significant others. We must also be mindful of the fact that the behaviors we have described, in and of themselves, are not necessarily contributory to, or manifestations of, the communicative disorder. Only if we gather together all of the clues that are available to us can we then decide an appropriate course of action.

Going beyond related issues When there is no apparent link between the communicative disorder and the client's emotional disturbance or dysfunctional psychological behavior, it is generally wise for the speech-language pathologist or audiologist to refrain from intervening psychotherapeutically. This rule, though obvious and more clearly justified than in the previous section, nonetheless presents some difficulty. Two major questions emerge.

First, can we be certain that there is no underlying connection, and in our avoidance or ignorance of that fact may we not then be practicing somewhat shortsightedly? Second, how do we cope with the client who insists on using us and the relationship to ventilate feelings about self and other life issues unrelated to the disorder? The latter question should not be difficult for the self-assured, sensitive, and empathic therapist who can gently guide the client back to the initially referred complaint. But do all of us have the necessary competence to do that effectively? We shall address this issue later. The answer to the first question is somewhat implied in our answer to the second one. But it demands even greater scrutiny. In any case, our task is even more complex when we work with children and with the parents involved.

Speech-language therapy is by its very nature interpersonal, unless of course we hold the belief that it is only necessary to treat the disorder. Even so, we are still in a relationship with our clients whether we admit it or not. As Backus (1960) has so clearly stated:

> In the field of speech disorders we are exhibiting conflicting attitudes regarding a decision to reckon squarely with psychological pressures in human behavior. We are interested and at the same time we are afraid, both for the professional and for personal reasons. There is a threat professionally because we are not prepared in this area; and personally, as our own anxiety is stirred. Since most of us have been well integrated enough to pursue successfully our educational aims and to engage productively in professional work, it may be inferred that we have rather well-developed defenses against anxiety; hence the conflicting attitudes show up less as overt anxiety than as responses of defensiveness against the idea of delving into unconscious processes. There are the commonly heard responses which reflect irritation and then attempt to belittle the idea: "Why does he always have to go around poking around in other people's insides?" "Why on earth must you make everything psychological?" The defense may take the form of an extreme position in either direction: on the one hand, a pseudo-positive position of intellectualizing about psychological processes, talking about them in clients with studied casualness; on the other hand, an out-and-out negative position, that no one but psychiatrists should be concerned with the depths of human existence.
>
> The latter attitude is easily recognized as being discrepant when we consider that of necessity we deal with unconscious processes in ourselves and others,

both personally and professionally. Our own emotional responses to others together with the ways in which we deal with their behavior, have an impact on them for good or ill. These constitute our own private system of "psychotherapeutic" measures, whether we are aware of them as being that or not. So it is not a question of whether we will use psychological tools or not, but rather of the extent to which the psychological tools we are using are in accord with those broad principles which promote or hinder growth." (p. 507–508)

Determining the need for referral   It is clear that the emotional needs of our clients demand that we develop our intellectual and personal abilities so that we may make appropriate clinical decisions. Although the task may be a formidable one, and not always successively carried out, if we can at least attempt to ascertain what is and what is not appropriate and in our professional domain, our decision to refer to other mental health professionals will be more apparent.

If we are unable to determine how to proceed, it would be appropriate to consult with other colleagues who might help us. We might also decide that we can help our clients through traditional symptomatic therapy regardless of their emotional needs. Whatever our course of action, we will need to defend the decision that is made.

An Eclectic Approach to Counseling the Communicatively Disordered

Earlier, we described several essential similarities among the self theory, behavioral, and rational-emotive approaches to counseling. We also acknowledged that although intrinsic differences existed as well, in actual practice there appears to be a natural merger. With this in mind, we wish to take an eclectic position in presenting a counseling approach to be used with the communicatively disordered that is systematic, practical, and realistic.

There are those who view eclecticism as a somewhat amorphous process akin to grab-bagging indiscriminately bits of techniques from the widest array of therapeutic schools of thought. We prefer to view eclecticism differently. As Robinson (1965) has indicated, the eclectic counselor is one who critically scrutinizes different theories, borrowing concepts that are both valid and testable, and then blends them into a consistent approach. The counselor is then free to use that which is applicable to a particular client and dispense with that which is not. The obvious implication is that all psychotherapeutic relationships are unique and therefore different. Hood (1974), in discussing the client–therapist relationship in communication therapy, declares: "There are quite possibly as many approaches to the clinical management of communicative disorders as there are therapists who have ventured forth into the arena. Much of whatever skill we possess results from our unique ability to recreate the form to meet a wide variety of clinical cases" (p. 46).

We certainly do not advocate the simplistic utilization of ideas taken from several positions without integrating them, or endorse the counselor for whom theory has no relevance. Counseling is too complex a process to be conducted in hodgepodge fashion or to be treated unidimensionally from one rigid viewpoint. We need to consider, then, how an eclectic approach can best be employed in counseling the communicatively disordered client.

Counseling as relationship   Those of us who have chosen the helping profession of communicative disorders as a lifelong career have frequently been admonished that "we should not get too involved with our clients." If we stop to consider that admonishment, we might raise several pertinent questions:

1. What is meant by "involved"?
2. Must we avoid a relationship with our clients?
3. Are we essentially teachers rather than therapists?
4. What is communication therapy without therapist–client communication?

In response to the first question, we understand it to mean that we must refrain from becoming "emotionally" involved with our clients—that is, we must prevent our personal feelings from impinging upon our client. Our answer is that few of us can escape being affected emotionally when we respond to the needs of others. What is of utmost importance, however, is that we learn to distinguish those feelings that belong to us from those that belong to our clients. Empathizing with our clients is quite different from identifying with them. The not infrequent occurrence of burnout in the helping professions is, we believe, due in part to our inability to distance our own emotional integrity from that of our clients.

Not too long ago the author was treating a young woman with bilateral vocal nodules. Although the nodules had been surgically excised, her hoarse voice persisted. During the course of symptomatic voice therapy and vocal hygiene counseling, she began to express her intense dislike of her voice, Apparently the feelings were long-standing. One day she asked me, "Will you get into my feelings?" I replied, "No, but I'll help you get into yours." What was most important is that she understood exactly what I meant, whereupon the path toward reconciling her feelings with a more balanced and effective use of her voice was cleared. A revealing footnote to this case was a comment she made toward the close of our final session: "You know, I was always afraid to get into psychotherapy because it meant getting too involved with a complete stranger. But what's been so strange about these last six months of therapy is that I have been involved, and yet I haven't. Do you know what I mean?" Although a verbal response may have been unnecessary, I replied, "Yes, and in a sense it's been the same for me."

Our answer to the second question is that we cannot help but relate whenever we come in contact with another person. It is unlikely that any one of us in the communication profession would disagree. Yet the difficulty arises when we attempt to define the process by which we relate and entrap ourselves in analyzing, intellectualizing, and classifying.

Kennedy (1977), in a book written for the "nonprofessional counselor," focuses clearly on the meaning of relationship when he states:

> Relationship is something many presume to understand even when they do not. It is also something many persons understand quite well even though they never think about it at all. Being able to be in relationship to others unselfconsciously is, in fact, a sign of good psychological health. People become friends or fall in love without necessarily describing their experience in psychological terms; it is something that is more in the nature of doing rather than theorizing. Being in relationship for these persons demands response rather than a philosophical statement." (p. 27)

The field of communicative disorders fortunately has progressed to the point where many of us, including those who practice strictly traditional symptomatic strategies, are less likely actively to do something to our clients. We would, rather, enter into a reciprocal relationship whereby both therapist and client share the responsibility for effecting communicative change.

In answer to the third question, we believe that therapy is teaching, but in the most dynamic sense of the word, whether we are counseling or eliminating /w/ for /r/ substitutions. It does not consist of two people sitting opposite each other separated by a table or desk, but of two people alongside each other attempting to solve a common problem. Therapy is learning as well, for both client and therapist, in that it is also a sharing of information whereby neither person has more power than the other. Though the knowledge may differ, we have as much to learn about our clients as they do from us. Thus, relieved of the burden of having to come up with all the answers, we are free to experience something very different with our clients. Certainly that may include the painful feelings and frustrations of our clients. And if we begin to understand our work as sharing instead of performing, we are less likely to feel intellectually and emotionally pressured and more likely to experience greater self-confidence, more excitement with our clients' progress, and a distinct feeling of having contributed something of value in both our lives and theirs.

We are not suggesting that what we have just described is necessarily easy, but neither are our personal relationships. They too have their highs and lows like the relationships with our clients, and we must therefore be prepared to cope with all of the unexpected therapeutic situations in which we find ourselves. This brings us to question four.

By definition, the communicative interaction we have with our clients is the essence of what the field of communicative disorders is all about and at the core of the counseling process. Those of us who have taught in communicative disorder programs are familiar with students who, when confronted with a new and perhaps minimally verbal client, exclaim in panic, "But I don't know what to say to him." As teachers and clinical supervisors, we must admit that spoon-feeding simplistic directives to those students will do little to enhance their relationship with clients and will not assist them in developing greater competence or confidence in using their therapeutic skills. It is better that we ask the student, first, what exactly he or she is anxious about and, second, what is being disclosed by the client's nonverbal communication. Helping the student to be responsive to the nonverbal aspects of communication and having that same student verbalize what he or she already knows about the client will put the necessary responsibility on the student attempting to initiate a meaningful therapeutic relationship.

Knowing ourselves in the relationship   Probably one of the most difficult aspects in all of our personal relationships is to be fully aware of what we are, who we are, and what we are feeling when in the presence of others. Kennedy (1977) describes it as the "willingness to listen to what is taking place within ourselves" (p. 6). It means relinquishing for a time our own personal attitudes and ideas so that we can attend fully to the other person. It means opening ourselves to our clients so that they will be less afraid to share the thoughts, ideas, and feelings that trouble them. Rogers has described this as the "unconditional regard" we must have for them. Similarly, Ellis has described it as fostering the individual's self-esteem or sense of identity.

In this way we are enabled to learn as much as possible about our client and to formulate an objective but not insensitive impression of that person. As the relationship continues, there is a reciprocal flow of communication involving feelings and ideas in which not only the client grows but the therapist as well.

TRANSFERENCE

An important aspect of the client–therapist relationship is the transference phenomenon, which Freud found to be necessary if therapy was to have a successful outcome. Because we are not concerned, however, with deep psychoanalytic therapy, we prefer to discuss it in the context of Rogerian therapy and the cognitive-emotive approach of Ellis.

Brammer (1973) described transference as the emergence of feelings in the client that get directed at the counselor. These feelings range broadly from admiration and affection to anger and rejection. According to Brammer, such a phenomenon is not uncommon "in all human relationships where feelings once felt toward someone close to us are now projected to the immediate helper" (p. 65). They emerge as the client attempts to cope with unresolved and unrecognized attitudes toward love objects and authority figures. Therapists must not misinterpret these as feelings their clients are having toward them as individuals. A naive therapist will certainly complicate the therapeutic relationship if he or she responds personally to these feelings. Rogers (1951) advises that transference be handled similarly to other attitudes expressed by the client—that is, by understanding and accepting—thereby guiding the client to perceive those feelings as natural but having nothing to do with the therapist.

The following excerpt from a clinical interview with a stuttering client illustrates transference:

CLIENT: I kept thinking about what you said about my avoidance of speaking situations last time.

THERAPIST: I get a sense you were preoccupied with it?

CLIENT: Yeah, but it was like your voice was always there, telling me that I needed to focus on what I was afraid of.

THERAPIST: Like somehow, I must have made a very distinct impression on you?

CLIENT: That right! The way my father was always telling me to speak more slowly when I was a kid.

THERAPIST: Then you've been feeling like that same child again?

CLIENT: In a way, but that's ridiculous because you're not my father.

This protocol suggests that the rapport established between the therapist and client has provoked considerable feelings that the client is assigning to his therapist. It is as if the therapist has become somewhat of a father figure for the client, yet at the same time he is denying the impact of his aroused feelings.

Ellis and other cognitive-behavioral therapists are not concerned with transference per se. Ellis views it essentially as an irrational belief that the client needs the therapist's approval and without it is unable to accept himself or herself. Consistent with the rational-emotive approach, the therapist distances and separates personally from this projection. We wonder, though, if in actual practice this is indeed possible, particularly when we consider the concept of countertransference.

COUNTERTRANSFERENCE

Opposite to transference is countertransference, which consists of feelings that the therapist has toward the client, based on personal past experiences or external events. These feelings are likely to become activated when the client is transferring, but may also occur independent of the client's projections. (We discuss this further in Chapter 9.) The important element to understand about countertransference is that it describes something about ourselves. Whether that consists of feelings of powerful attraction or antipathy to our client, it reveals aspects of ourselves, of our own value systems, and therefore we must be conscious of it before we can move ahead therapeutically.

Ellis does not believe the countertransference can take place in rational-emotive therapy because the therapeutic relationship is essentially cognitive and not emotional in nature. We do not believe this. Even for symptomatically oriented speech-language and hearing professionals, it is not unusual for us to fall prey to the psychodynamic events being experienced by client and therapist. They are just as likely to occur while teaching language to a five-year-old child as while helping an aphasic individual retrieve language. We do not wish to imply that in such cases we should attempt to analyze or interpret these feelings to our clients or manipulate their life relationships, but only to recognize and understand them so that they do not contaminate the ongoing traditional therapy.

The following is an excerpt from a clinical interview with the same client discussed earlier in which countertransference occurs:

THERAPIST: I get the feeling that you're holding yourself back from that job interview, because you feel you'll fail.

CLIENT: It's not that; it's just that I don't feel ready for it.

THERAPIST: Or that you don't feel you're good enough for the job?

CLIENT: Maybe that's it. But I feel like I'm being pushed into it.

THERAPIST: By me?

CLIENT: Well, that's part of it.

This excerpt suggests a very subtle inclination by the therapist to want more for the client that the client can handle at the moment. What is difficult for the therapist is to separate his own expectations for the client from those that the client is uncertain of in himself. The question for the therapist is: Do I want him to do it for me, or do I want him to do it for himself?

Brammer and Shostrom (1968) provide us with specific guidelines to handle transference in our counseling relationships and to keep it from developing into a deep transference relationship.

1. The usual technique for resolving transference is one of simple acceptance that permits the client to live out his projected feelings and to feel free in the interview.

2. The counselor may ask clarifying questions about the forms of anxiety which the client seems to be manifesting.

3. The counselor may reflect the client's feeling level.

4. A stronger technique will exist when the counselor interprets the transference feeling directly. An interpretation involves communicating information to the client that he has not already stated himself and which therefore may be rejected.

5. The counselor may focus on what is going on presently with the client's feelings rather than on why he is having these feelings.

6. Frequently, calling attention to feelings causes the client to react in the opposite manner; therefore, a counselor may want to call attention to negative but not to the positive transference.

7. The counselor may test the idea that the client is projecting feelings by asking him to reverse the projection and encourage repetition until the client feels that the statement represents what he is really feeling.

8. The counselor may interpret transference feelings as an expression of "being deficiency" in which the client is seeking environmental support rather than viewing the feeling as a transference from the past to the counselor.

9. The last suggestion is that the counselor may refer the client to a coun-

selor more qualified to give intensive psychotherapy when their relationship develops to an intensity which is beyond the competence of the counselor. (pp. 267–268)

Active listening and understanding   One of the most fundamental principles we must learn while training for the field of communicative disorders is the ability to listen objectively to our clients' speech and language patterns. While the emphasis has been on the "how" of communicating, less focus has been placed on "what" is being communicated. This unbalanced approach restricts our ability to understand fully the communicatively disordered person, unless of course we are only interested in the disorder. But can we really separate the disorder from the person? It is doubtful that many of us would reply affirmatively to the question.

We maintain, therefore, that if we are to be consistent with our belief in the necessity of treating the total individual, we must attend to the entire communicative process of that person. In so doing, we not only help our clients learn to manage their communicative abilities more effectively but we as well learn to be more competent as helpers. In a very real sense, our clients become our teachers, and what we allow ourselves to learn from them could well be applicable in dealing with other clients. No academic course can teach us as well.

But learning to listen actively to our clients is not accomplished faultlessly. Who among us would deny that we sometimes make mistakes in our therapy? We all recognize that "to err is human," but we would add that "to err is professional" as well. Frustrating, annoying, and sometimes painful as that might be, we have the potential for learning much from the mistakes we make as long as we can tolerate them within ourselves. The rational-emotive therapist who must dispel the perfectionistic attitudes of the client would most likely agree that the same would be necessary for himself or herself should the client be listened to incorrectly. The self theory therapist would also readily take responsibility for inaccurate active listening and, should the client be misunderstood, take action to understand that client better. Let us examine a case in point.

Mrs. B is the fifty-five-year-old wife of a mildly aphasic client. She complains of her husband's lack of attempts at communicating.

MRS. B: I don't understand. I try to get him to talk to me—I know he can—but he just seems to be thinking of something else when I talk to him. It's like he really doesn't want to be with me but I know that isn't so.

THERAPIST: It sounds like you really need nurturing from your husband.

MRS. B: (looks at therapist quizzically) No. That's not it at all. I feel frustrated because I hear him talk to his friends on the telephone, and if we're to have any kind of relationship we need to communicate with each other.

It is obvious that Mrs. B is trying to communicate her frustration about her and her husband's relationship. She doesn't know what to do about it, and is genuinely concerned. The therapist's response is an interpretation and not based on what the client has actually communicated. It is as if the therapist is putting the burden on his client rather than listening to her frustration and her search for a more meaningful relationship with her husband. In a very real sense the client is helping the therapist to understand.

The reader may wonder how and why the therapist has responded to the client in this way. We submit that the therapist is tuned in to something else not immediately present. Perhaps it is a projection on the therapist's part or expectations of what the wife's problem should be. He appears to have a different agenda than that of the client. The therapist obviously does not have sufficient evidence to make a judgment based on the information given. Not only must the therapist listen to the client more attentively, but he must also listen to himself more actively. Thus a more appropriate response by the therapist would have been something like the following:

THERAPIST: It's so confusing for you, yet you know his difficulty really has nothing to do with the affection he feels for you. It's just that you don't want him to cut himself off from you even though he has difficulty in communicating.

An effective way to learn how we listen is to audio- or videotape a full counseling session so that we may sit back and objectify what is really happening. This is difficult to do because it means learning something about ourselves we may not care to acknowledge. But if we are to be effective change agents, we must be prepared to accept the errors we make, learn from them, and in a sense let the client help us.

One of the difficulties novice therapists, and perhaps a few professional ones, frequently have is not only listening actively but understanding what their clients are communicating. Instead of focusing on the feeling state being expressed, they attend only to the content or the problem being communicated. Our concerns as counseling speech-language pathologists and audiologists are not to solve the client's problem per se but to try and understand the feeling state that underlies the problem. Naturally if the client is struggling to adjust to the output of a hearing aid, it is incumbent on the audiologist to provide the necessary informative guidelines. But if that same client complains of difficulty in adjusting to wearing an aid—embarrassment, feelings of inadequacy—the counseling therapist must be prepared to switch gears and reflect back to the client those feelings the audiologist is experiencing from that person.

This is what is meant by being in relationship to the client—putting oneself into the same life space as the client and remaining totally open to receive whatever the client has to offer, without judging the adequacy, effectiveness, or emotionality of the message. Putting oneself in the place of the client, to experience vicariously what the client may be suffering, is not always easy. Certainly we would not wish to trade places, and yet we must somehow allow ourselves that sense of "what it must feel like," recognizing our own vulnerabilities. In doing so, we clear our own feelings and thoughts of subjectivity and prepare, more or less, an open slate for the client to bounce feelings off of or, as the case may be, to scribble upon. Because by its nature a relationship is reciprocal, the therapist is now free to offer himself or herself uncontaminated by egoistic or absolute "professional edicts." In essence, we are speaking about being authentic, and, if we are, the greater the likelihood for our clients to feel authenticated as well.

The values of the therapist and client and not the technique   We have attempted to identify active listening as fundamental to the ongoing client−therapist relationship and a major determinant toward the enhanced well-being of the client. Having done so, we wish to make clear that active listening is a process and not a technique. That is, it is not dependent on a rigid set of rules that must be followed in an exact fashion with each and every client. On the contrary, it is a transaction that occurs between two people and subject to the distinctive nature of each clinical relationship. It further implies that the therapist must be the determining factor in the dynamic way in which he or she responds to the client.

It is not our intention to imply that technique has no place in counseling. We merely maintain that it should not be the focus of what we do or an end in and of itself, but a flexible guide that makes the clinical relationship viable.

Avila, Combs, and Purkey (1977) review several studies that support the thesis that it is the clinical interrelationship and not representative techniques of the various schools that contribute most to helping. They contend that effective and ineffective helpers cannot be distinguished on the basis of the methods they use but rather in the way they perceive themselves and others and the authenticity with which they relate to the client.

GUIDELINES FOR FACILITATING THE COUNSELING RELATIONSHIP

We propose a series of general guidelines that speech-language-hearing professionals might pursue in facilitating the counseling relationship with their clients. Consistent with the suggested eclectic position, we have included several aspects of self theory, behavioral, and rational-emotive approaches that lend themselves to appropriate blending. The reader should be aware that the selection of any one or combination of these principles will be determined by the unique circumstances of each clinical relationship.

1. *Developing the appropriate attitudes necessary for active listening.* This implies being open to the client's expression of feelings and thoughts and trusting that the client has the capacity to work through problems and the capacity to solve them. Although such feelings and thoughts may not necessarily be consistent with the therapist's perception of reality, they nonetheless represent the client's own way of struggling with his or her own perception of reality. It further implies the viewing of the client as separate from the therapist as a person. McKay, Davis, and Fanning (1983) list several ways in which active listening may be facilitated. Although their book is directed toward everyone, their suggestions are applicable for the counseling speech-language-hearing professional. Their list includes the use of paraphrasing and clarifying and providing feedback to the client. Total listening implies listening with empathy, openness, and awareness. It implies the necessity for the therapist to check out with the client the accuracy with which the communicative message is being perceived. Nothing should be assumed or taken for granted, and if the therapist has any doubt, questioning should be pursued in order to understand what is being communicated and how it is being communicated.

2. *Viewing the client as a person.* As speech-language-hearing therapists, it is necessary for us to separate the disorder from the person, in the sense that the disorder is only one part of the total behavior of the client and does not represent the person. Our perspective, then, must avoid such categorical labels as "stutterer" or "aphasic" to identify these persons. In this way we can better respect the total integrity of the individual while attending to the dysfunctional behaviors as they are manifested. Respecting the integrity of the individual demands our attention to the following therapist attitudes: (a) respecting the client's need to conceal self-threatening emotional material; (b) being open to and accepting of emotional material the client feels a need to express; (c) responding to the client rather than making a good response; and (d) responding to the client nonjudgmentally.

3. *Being aware of the obstacles to active listening.* Because clients are helped through what they experience in their relationship with their therapists, barriers erected to interfere with that knowledge must be brought to conscious awareness. Such barriers would include personal insecurities regarding clinical competency, personal feelings activated by the client's communicative material, and attending to content issues rather than the client's affectual state being communicated. McKay, Davis, and Fanning (1983) describe twelve blocks that interfere with the therapist's ability to listen effectively. They are identified as (a) comparing the client to oneself; (b) mind reading based on intuition, hunches, and attempting to figure out what the client is *really* thinking and feeling; (c) rehearsing how to respond for the client; (d) filtering out some messages from others; (e) judging statements and behaviors before all the information is available; (f) daydreaming; (g) identifying with the client; (h) advising and not attending to

the feelings being communicated; (i) sparring, which includes arguing and debating with the client; (j) being right and rejecting criticism; (k) derailing by avoiding the discomfort or anxiety provoked by the client; and (l) placating (pp. 16–19).

4. *Viewing ourselves realistically.* Our own self-understanding as therapists can significantly affect the interpersonal transactions that take place in therapy and contribute to the success of the relationship. It implies the self-recognition of the following needs: (a) the need to be liked or appreciated by our client; (b) the need to be perfect or successful in everything we do; and (c) the need to have all the knowledge and answers that are possible to have. Obviously, to have these kinds of expectations for ourselves places an impossible burden on our attempts to relate freely to our clients.

Our own struggles as therapists and as human beings require that we strive to accept our limitations, know that we may not necessarily be liked by all our clients, and understand that we may not succeed with all of them. To do otherwise is to present an unreal model to our clients that would be impossible for them to emulate and, further, places an inordinate amount of stress on ourselves. Our goal, then, is to be authentic to ourselves and our clients so that we may be freer to enhance the interpersonal relationship.

5. *Valuing client choice.* The notion that we must do something to our clients in order to facilitate real change is self-aggrandizement, which takes away from clients the opportunity to use their own potential for change and growth. We are merely agents who provide opportunities, possibilities, and means by which clients can choose to move in a more positive direction for themselves. We must also be prepared to allow them to struggle with their resistances, uncertainties, and indecisions, yet at the same time gently guide them toward the goal they have chosen for themselves. This, obviously, is not always a simple task when we stop to consider the difficulties we all have in life's choice-making decisions. To do otherwise is to project what we think is best for ourselves on to the other person and thereby deprive them of their own values. That the attained goal may not always be consistent with our own expectations is the reality we must learn to accept as helping professionals.

6. *Using client–therapist contracting.* The use of contracts between client and therapist in counseling and psychotherapy is not new. It consists of a negotiated agreement between both parties in which desired behavioral changes are specified. Clients are taught to analyze and modify their own behaviors (Mahoney and Thoresen 1974; Derisi and Butz 1975). Based on the original cognitive stuttering therapy formulations of Rubin and Culatta (1973), Shames and Florence (1980) and Goldberg (1981) introduced the practice of contracts in stuttering therapy.

Contracting allows the therapist and client to decide jointly what goals and expectations are desired, with a clear and objective statement of what the requirements are. It also consists of an agreement regarding the degree to which a certain behavior will result in a positive consequence. Opportunities must also be provided to scale downward any expectations or goals the client may not choose to pursue during a particular period of time. Of key importance is setting goals that the client can realistically achieve. Failure to follow through with mutually agreed-upon behavior must be openly discussed so that the client takes full responsibility for his or her choice in not having done so (Hansen, Stevic, and Warner 1977).

7. *Using confrontation.* Confrontation by the therapist is necessary when an incongruency occurs in the following ways: (a) a discrepancy between verbal and nonverbal messages; (b) an inconsistency between communication and action; (c) discrepancies among a series of messages; (d) variances among statements and feelings; and (e) irrational modes of thinking and behavior.

Here, again, it is necessary for the clinician to use caution in bringing discrepancies out in the open. We may not be certain if the client is unaware of them or is consciously behaving in such a manner as a means to resist exploring certain material. The key is to share with the client the difficulty the therapist is having in understanding the discrepant event. This should be done without judgment, but the client must take the responsibility for clarifying exactly what was intended in the message communicated.

Carkhuff and Berenson (1967) describe the use of confrontation on a continuum:

> . . . from a light challenge to a direct collision between the therapist and client. It constitutes a challenge to the client to mobilize his resources to take another step toward deeper self-recognition or constructive action in his own behalf. Frequently it will precipitate a crisis that disturbs at least temporarily the client's personal and social equilibrium. Again crises are viewed as a series of self-confrontations. Confrontation is a vehicle that ultimately translates awareness and insight into action, directionality, wholeness, and meaning in the client's life. A life without confrontation is directionless, passive, and impotent. (p. 172)

Although the counseling speech-language-hearing professional may be somewhat skeptical and uncertain about using confrontation, we would point out that as long as the therapist is clear in his or her own mind about what may be ambiguous in communicative messages from clients, and does not communicate from a place of self-involvement, confrontation can be a useful tool in aiding clients to become integrated with their own experience.

8. *Acknowledging the value of therapist self-disclosure.* Self-disclosure is essentially the sharing of personal information of the self with others. It is obvious that self-disclosure by the client is a necessary condition for the successful consummation of therapy. First defined by Jourard (1958), self-disclosure has been determined to be effective and important for the therapist also. (Jourard & Jaffe, 1970) Although classical psychoanalytic theory strongly opposes its use by the psychoanalyst in depth therapy, some of

the counseling literature appears to defend its use. Apparently, there is a reciprocal effect in the client—therapist relationship in that clients are more likely to increase self-disclosure when their therapists do (Weiner 1978).

Unfortunately, there are no definitive guidelines the speech-language-hearing professional can follow in determining its use, but we do suggest that it is appropriate when there is a mature partnership between client and therapist and when no transference or countertransference is occurring. At best, it can be most useful when the therapist can share personal or professional experiences that relate directly to the client's communicative disorder. It has been found to be most helpful when counseling parents of communicatively disordered children or families of brain-injured adults who require specific information about the disorder and/or speech-language-hearing development in general. Therapists must also trust their own mature judgment, and when in any doubt about sharing, *not* self-disclose.

9. *Blending symptomatic strategies with counseling.* The role of the speech-language-hearing counselor differs significantly from the role of the typical counselor in the management of therapy. We consider it unwise to focus on the client's emotional struggles unless (a) the client clearly indicates a desire to do so; (b) use of symptomatic strategies is being blocked by covert or overt emotional resistance; or (c) the client requires information necessary for the successful execution of speech-language-hearing therapy. If the therapist is unable to obtain a clear perspective of whether or not to proceed with counseling, it might be necessary to assess with the client the appropriateness of doing so. If clinical rapport has already been established, it is unlikely for the client to be particularly threatened. But if so, the therapist can then refrain from any further excursions into emotional probing without risk to the relationship. Once there is mutual agreement, however, it is legitimate for the therapist to incorporate both strategies within and among therapy sessions. Such an approach is useful during the formulation, putting into practice, and appraisal of therapy contracts, but it is certainly applicable in less structured clinical environments as well.

Most knowledgeable therapists are keenly aware of inherent emotional components in most of the symptomatic strategies they use. Not only are clients emotionally affected by the techniques they experience but also by the means with which they are introduced. Most often, encouragement and empathic support are sufficient to neutralize any negative attitudes or responses that may be incurred. Naturally, if such behaviors persist, the therapist must patiently and genuinely deal with them with the client.

10. *Attending to body language and paralinguistic cues.* We have already described how we cannot not communicate with others. As speech-language pathologists and audiologists we must be sensitive to and aware of the way our clients communicate through body movements and gestures (kinesics). It is generally believed by most writers that body language accounts for more than 50 percent of a message's impact. For this reason it is especially important for us to attend closely to the facial expressions, gestures, and posturing

of our clients, as these will reveal information that cannot be derived from the verbal message alone.

It is particularly important that as communication experts we must also critically attend to the use of vocal components of speech (paralanguage), which includes articulation, phonation, resonation, timing, and rhythm as they relate to the message being conveyed. Those of us who protest that "we know all that" should not confuse our vast knowledge of the mechanics of such components with the necessary knowledge of what the mechanics mean and how they are meant.

Paralinguistic cues refer to the intonational, prosodic, inflectional, and melodic features that are characterized by pitch, length, and loudness, as well as by such vocal qualities as breathiness, thinness, hoarseness, and whining. These cues, along with body language, provide us with the fine nuances of our clients' communication that are frequently incongruent with the actual words spoken. They also bring to our awareness the actual feeling state of our clients before their own consciousness of it.

Perhaps that which we tend to assign to subjective and unscientific intuitive judgments are phenomena that can be objectively described and scientifically measured. Several important writers on the subject have already made such significant attempts, among them Birdwhistell (1970), Grinder and Bandler (1976), and Labov and Fanshel (1977).

CONCLUSION

In this chapter we have drawn on the many valuable contributions to the fields of counseling and psychotherapy and have begun to apply eclectically the theories and processes to our work with communicatively disordered persons. Those readers who desire a more thorough background on the many significant issues raised are referred to the extensive bibliography in this chapter.

It should be noted further that the counseling guidelines presented apply to children as well, and that although several aspects may not be appropriate for each or every case, we must assume that the therapist will judge selectively. We also did not distinguish between counseling the communicatively disordered client and counseling the spouse, parents, and other family members. Obviously, the astute therapist would be able to apply appropriately the principles discussed to the individual situation and circumstances presented. Subsequent chapters address these concerns and answer many of the specific questions that have been raised here.

REFERENCES

AVILA, D. L., COMBS, A. W., and PURKEY, W. W. (Eds.) *The Helping Relationship Sourcebook.* 2nd ed. Boston: Allyn & Bacon, 1977.

AVILA, D. L., and PURKEY, W. Self-theory and behaviorism: A rapproachment. In D. L. Avila, A. W. Combs and W. W. Purkey (Eds.), *The Helping Relationship Sourcebook*, 2nd ed. Boston: Allyn & Bacon, 1977.

American Psychiatric Association Task Force on Nomenclature and Statistics. *Diagnostic and Statistical Manual of Mental Disorders*, 3rd ed. Washington, D.C.: American Psychiatric Association, 1980.

ANDERSON, S., DOUDS, J. and CARKHUFF, R. R. The effects of confrontation by high and low functioning therapists. Unpublished research. Amherst: University of Massachusetts, 1967.

BACKUS, O. The study of psychological processes in speech therapists. In D. A. Barbara (Ed.), *Psychological and Psychiatric Aspects of Speech and Hearing*. Springfield, Ill. Chas. C Thomas, 1960.

BANDURA, A. *Principles of Behavior Modification*. New York: Holt, Rinehart & Winston, 1969.

———. Behavioral modification through modeling procedures. In L. Krasner, and L. Ullmann (Eds.), *Research in Behavior Modification*. New York: Holt, Rinehart & Winston, 1965.

———. Social learning through imitation. In M. Jones (Ed.), *Nebraska Symposium on Motivation, 1962*. Lincoln: University of Nebraska Press, 1962.

BIRDWHISTELL, R. L. *Kinesics and Context: Essays on Body Communication*. Philadelphia: University of Pennsylvania Press, 1970.

BRAMMER, L. M. *The Helping Relationship: Process and Skills*. Englewood Cliffs, N.J.: Prentice-Hall, 1973.

BRAMMER, L. M., and SHOSTROM, E. *Therapeutic Psychology*. Englewood Cliffs, N.J.: Prentice-Hall, 1968.

CARKHUFF, R. R. *The Art of Helping*. Amherst, Mass.: Human Resource Development Press, 1977.

———. Helping and human relations: A brief guide for training lay helpers. *Journal of Research and Development in Education*, 4(2) (1971), 17–27.

———. *Helping and Human Relations: A Primer for Lay and Professional Helpers*, Vol. 1: *Selection and Training*. New York: Holt, Rinehart & Winston, 1969a.

———. *Helping and Human Relations: A Primer for Lay and Professional Helpers*, Vol. 2: *Practice and Research*. New York: Holt, Rinehart & Winston, 1969b.

CARKHUFF, R. R., and BERENSON, B. G. *Beyond Counseling and Therapy*. New York: Holt, Rinehart & Winston, 1967.

COOPER, E. *Modern Techniques of Vocal Rehabilitation*. Springfield, Ill.: Chas. C Thomas, 1973.

DERISI, W. J., and BUTZ, G. *Writing Behavioral Contracts: A Case Simulation Manual*. Champaign, Ill. Research Press, 1975.

ELLIS, A. *Reason and Emotion in Psychotherapy*. New York: Lyle Stuart, 1962.

ELLIS, A., and GRIEGER, R. *Handbook of Rational-Emotive Therapy*. New York: Springer-Verlag, 1977.

GOLDBERG, S. A. *Behavioral Cognitive Stuttering Therapy*. Tigard, Oreg.: C. C. Publications, 1981.

GRINDER, J., and BANDLER, R. *The Structure of Magic II*. Palo Alto, Calif.: Science and Behavior Books, 1976.

HANSEN, J. C., STEVIC, R. R., and WARNER, R. W. Jr. *Counseling: Theory and Process*, 2nd ed. Boston: Allyn & Bacon, 1977.

HOOD, S. B. Clinicians and therapy. In L. L. Emerick, and S. B. Hood (Eds.), *The Client-Clinician Relationship*. Springfield, Ill.: Chas. C Thomas, 1974.

JOHNSON, W. *People in Quandaries*. New York: Harper & Row, 1946.

JOHNSON, W., and associates. *The Onset of Stuttering*. Minneapolis: University of Minneapolis Press, 1959.

JOURARD, S. M. Personality Adjustment: An Approach Through the Study of Healthy Personality. New York: MacMillan, 1958.

JOURARD, S. M., and JAFFE, P. E. Influence of an interviewer's disclosure on the self-disclosing behavior of interviewees. *Journal of Counseling*, 17 (1970), 252–257.

KENNEDY, E. *On Becoming a Counselor: A Basic Guide for Non-Professional Counselors*. New York: Seabury, 1977.

LABOV, W., and FANSHEL, D. *Therapeutic Discourse Psychotherapy as Conversation*. New York: Academic Press, 1977.

LUTERMAN, D. M. *Counseling the Communicatively Disordered and Their Families.* Waltham, Mass.: Little, Brown, 1984.

MCKAY, M., DAVIS, M., and FANNING, P. *Messages: The Communication Book.* Oakland, Calif.:New Harbinger Publications, 1983.

MAHONEY, M. J., and THORESEN, C. E. *Self-Control: Power to the Person.* Monterey, Calif.: Brooks/Cole, 1974.

MENACKER, J. Toward a theory of activist guidance. *Personnel and Guidance Training,* 54 (1976), 318–321.

MOWRER, D. E. *Methods of Modifying Speech Behaviors: Learning Theory in Speech Pathology.* Columbus, Ohio: Chas. Merrill, 1977.

PAYNE-JOHNSON, J. C. Family intervention for inner-city populations. ASHA, 24(1) (January 1982), 33–34.

ROBINSON, F. P. Counseling orientations and labels. *Journal of Counseling Psychology,* 12, (1965), 338.

ROGERS, C. R. *On Becoming a Person: A Therapist's View of Psychotherapy.* Boston: Houghton Mifflin 1961.

———. A theory of therapy, personality, and interpersonal relationships, as developed in the client-centered framework. In S. Koch (Ed.), *Psychology: A Study of a Science,* Vol. 3: *Formulations of the Person and the Social Context.* New York: McGraw-Hill, 1959.

———. *Client-Centered Therapy: Its Current Practice, Implications and Theory.* Boston: Houghton Mifflin, 1951.

———. *Counseling and Psychotherapy.* Boston: Houghton Mifflin, 1942.

RUBIN, H., and CULATTA, R. A program for the initial stages of fluency therapy. *Journal of Speech and Hearing Research,* 18 (1973), 556–668.

———. A point of view about stuttering. *ASHA,* (July 1971), 380–384.

SHAMES, G. H., EGOLF, D. B., and RHODES, R. C. Experimental programs in stuttering therapy. *Journal of Speech and Hearing Disorders,* 34 (1969), 30–47.

SHAMES, G. H., and FLORENCE, C. L. *Stutter-Free Speech.* Columbus, Ohio: Chas. C. Merrill, 1980.

SKINNER, B. F. *Beyond Freedom and Dignity.* New York: Knopf, 1971.

———. *Science and Human Behavior.* New York: Free Press, 1953.

STAPLES, F. R., SLOANE, B., WHIPPLE, K., CRISTOL, H. H., and YORKSTON, N. J. Differences between behavior therapists and psychotherapists. *Archives of General Psychiatry,* 32 (1975), 1515– 1522.

TAYLOR, J. S. Public school speech-language certification standards: Are they standard? ASHA, 22(3) (March 1980), 159–165.

TRUAX, C. B. Therapist interpersonal reinforcement of client self-exploration and therapeutic outcome in group psychotherapy. *Journal of Counseling Psychology,* 15 (1968), 225–231.

———. Reinforcement and nonreinforcement in Rogerian psychotherapy. *Journal of Abnormal and Social Psychology,* 71 (1966), 1–9.

WEINER, M. F. *Therapist Disclosure: The Use of Self in Psychotherapy.* Boston: Butterworths, 1978.

WILLIAMS, D. A point of view about stuttering. *Journal of Speech and Hearing Disorders,* 22 (1957), 390–397.

2

PSYCHOLOGICAL CONSIDERATIONS OF APHASIC ADULTS AND THEIR FAMILIES

INTRODUCTION

The field of aphasiology has long recognized the traumatic and devastating impact on the family and on the individual who has suffered a cerebral vascular accident. The neurological, physical, physiological, and linguistic effects have been and are being investigated by neurologists, psychiatrists, neuropsychologists, speech-language pathologists, and psycholinguists, among others. Considerably less attention has been given to the study of the etiology, nature of, and treatment for adult aphasia from the perspective of psychological dynamics. Unfortunately, the research has often been characterized by the methodological problems associated with descriptive studies. The experimental studies have also suffered from difficulties with population variances, measurements of personality behavior, and well-meaning speculative conclusions. Nevertheless, it is hoped that readers will consider the intrinsic values to be gained from much of the research and thus add to their knowledge and understanding of the real world of aphasia.

We have chosen to confine our discussion to psychological aspects with only tangential references to purely neurological, cognitive-linguistic correlates, and assessment and typical treatment procedures. In doing so, we can better explore the many psychosocial dimensions, from the psychogenesis of aphasia through the personality and behavioral changes, and the psychotherapeutic treatment strategies.

PSYCHOGENESIS OF CEREBRAL VASCULAR DISEASE

During the last twenty years medicine and medical science have gradually begun to consider the multiple elements—invasive, genetic, and psychosocial—that combined can change the human organism and create an internal environment conducive to pathological alterations. Our discussion will first center on the psychogenetic aspects, namely, psychosocial stress. This we define as a psychophysical reaction characterized by agitation and/or physiological changes in response to provoking environmental stimuli.

Stress as the Hidden Precursor

Zegans (1982), in reviewing the literature on psychosocial stress, describes its occurrence "in response to those conditions that threaten the human mechanism for achieving security, bonding, status, meaning, intimacy and optimal arousal. Anticipation of the loss of these basic needs produces not only compensatory behaviors but emotional and physiological reactions as well" (pp. 136–137). As a special organismic state, it could affect changes in bodily functions conducive to disease, if intense or chronic enough. Engels (1975) cautions us, however, to view stress as a factor that can trigger an array of organismic reactions. A few of these could contribute to illness, whereas others may lead to healthy, adaptive behavior and personal growth. (The reader wishing to obtain a basic orientation to the term is referred to the exemplary work of Selye [1966], who describes stress as a general adaptation syndrome.)

Zegans presents us with overwhelming "anatomical, physiological, and neurochemical evidence that cognitive-affective responses to stress can alter the functioning of those vital hypothalamic-pituitary pathways that modulate endocrine, autonomic, and immune processes" (p. 150), setting the stage for disease onset. We are asked to consider the complex interplay of physical, social, and behavioral factors, taking into account psychological responses to environmental stress, changes in developmental functioning, intrapsychic conflict, and faulty coping mechanisms.

The relationship of cardiovascular disease and the Type A behavior pattern—"excessive drive, aggressiveness, ambition, involvement in competitive activities, frequent vocational deadlines, and enhanced sense of time urgency"—has been well documented (Jenkins, Rosenman, and Friedman 1968; Jenkins 1976). There has also been some suggestion that hostility and anger are strongly related to coronary atherosclerosis. Virtually no stress research has been done, however, on the possible relationship of coronary behavior patterns to hypertension and cerebral vascular disease, according to Holt (1982). He suggests, in his discussion of occupational stress and disease, that although stroke is a frequent cause of death, it often occurs after retirement and therefore at a late age.

According to National Health Interview surveys of the National Center for Health Statistics published by the U.S. Department of Health, Education and Welfare in 1974, 1983, and 1984, the prevalence of cerebral vascular disease (CVD) was 1,869,000 cases in 1981 as compared to 1,534,000 in 1972. The incidence rate per 1000 persons age 55 to 65 in 1972 was 11.5 whereas the incidence rate for the same age range in 1981 was 13.0, an increase of 1.5 per 1000 persons. The studies revealed that the incidence rate among those sixty-five years and older in 1972 was 48.2, whereas in 1981 it was 45.4, a decrease of 2.8. Although no changing trend was evident when both years were compared, it is apparent that CVD is not always related to old age. Premature arteriosclerotic disease, a major etiological correlate, would have to be explained in terms of indigenous factors other than the aging process alone.

We suggest that because the relationship between stress and hypertension has already been established, we cannot ignore the possible connection between stress and CVD. Sahs, Hartman, and Aronson (1976) refer to hypertension as a major cause of nonembolic cerebral infarctions, which would include thrombosis and hemorrhage. Evans (1983) cautions us, however, that his findings with British stroke victims revealed an inconsistent relationship between high blood pressure (hypertension) and risk of stroke in the elderly. Evans adds, however, that there is a close relationship between high blood pressure and stroke among younger adults.

Individual and Family Life Factors

Our current understanding of the risk factors associated with cardiovascular disease has led us to identify those factors that relate to cerebral vascular disease. These include high serum cholesterol, smoking, obesity, and drugs. The frequent use of mood-altering drugs has been found to be a major contributor to stroke, which might help explain its growing incidence among the forty-five-year and under population.

Because no longitudinal studies, like the Framingham study on cardiovascular disease (Kannel and Gordon 1974), have been conducted, we can only speculate on the significance of individual and family life factors and how these relate to hypertension or high blood pressure. In doing so we must bear in mind that the Type A behavior pattern does not equate with personality and emotional factors per se. It is the interplay of certain behaviors and emotional responses with the environment that is most important. The Psychiatric Epidemiology Research Interview Life Events Scale developed by Dohrenwend et al. (1982) has been a major contribution to the measurement of stressful life events. Although the authors admit to the scale's technical weaknesses, it is nonetheless methodologically rigorous. Among the major stressful circumstances studied were physical exhaustion from illness or injury, loss of social support, and fateful negative events.

With respect to cerebral vascular infarction, we identify some related and other social stressors that could be described similarly with obvious overlapping assumed.

1. *Being married:* divorce, separation, death of a spouse, marital conflict
2. *Job:* loss of, change of, greater responsibilities, fewer responsibilities, forced or unforced retirement
3. *Finances:* diminished, increased
4. *Parenting:* rejection by, conflicts with, children
5. *Aging and illness:* depression and/or anxiety associated with

It is apparent from the extensive research on stress that a simple combination of reported stressful events is insufficient to account for incipient disease processes. A more fruitful approach for researchers would be to look at the role of particular combinations of events within specified periods of time and relate these to individual constitutional and personality factors.

We believe, however, that the dynamic way or the style with which the organism, effectively or ineffectively, copes with stress will determine, in part, vulnerability to certain disease processes. This is not to suggest that specific traumatic events like the death of a spouse would not induce a high degree of stress in the significant other, but it is *how* that person adapts to that stress which is of crucial concern.

Specific Behavioral Indicators and Measures for Prevention

Regardless of the uncertainties about stress-induced hypertension and resultant cerebral infarction, it is important to consider what specific behavior indicators, if any, would move us to predict such infarctions. Frequently, before a massive CVA, the individual may suffer a little or minor stroke that does not seriously handicap the person or get brought to the attention of others. Such a stroke is a temporary disruption of the blood supply to the brain, commonly known as a transient ischemic attack, or TIA. It may be characterized by a temporary drooping of the corner of the mouth, brief tingling or numbness in an arm or leg, transient blurring or loss of vision, dizziness, or temporary disturbance of speech. The author has interviewed countless numbers of family members following a full-blown CVA who report the following uncharacteristic psychosocial changes to have occurred during the months or weeks previous to the trauma:

1. *Atypical moodiness and depression,* characterized by withdrawal and noncommunicative behavior

2. *Anxiety and tension*, characterized by sudden bursts of anger, agitation, restless-ness, and frustration over minor or major life matters
3. *Preoccupation with insignificant details or objects*, characterized by staring off into space or contemplating such innocuous objects as a bowl of artificial fruit
4. *Short-term memory loss*, characterized by not remembering such events as the drive home from work or a visit to a friend
5. *Flatness of affect*, characterized by masklike expressions, phlegmatism, inaction, or unresponsiveness to others

Conceivably such behavioral indicators may be related to the incidence of one or several TIAs and thus need to be brought to the attention of a physician. What is significant, however, is that these behavioral changes may occur in conjunction with the stress-inducing life events previously dis-cussed. Because a TIA may be a warning signal of an imminent thrombosis, the latter can be avoided through anticoagulant medication, change of diet to lessen the amount of fat, weight reduction, or carotid endarectomy as determined by X-ray. We would further suggest, through physician referral hopefully, that the individual seek out counseling or, if marital and family stress appear to be present, family therapy.

Of course we cannot conclude with certainty that there is a direct relationship between life stressors and the onset of TIAs. But until more definitive evidence is forthcoming, we need at least to consider the possibility of a relationship between the two.

PSYCHOSOCIAL FACTORS SUBSEQUENT TO CEREBRAL VASCULAR DISEASE

The neurological, physical, physiological, and psycholinguistic changes pro-duced by a cerebral vascular accident have been well documented by empiri-cal and clinical research conducted over the last 150 years. Schuell et al. (1964), Sarno (1981), Davis (1983), and Eisenson (1984) have reviewed comprehensively this vast body of information.

Changes of Affectual State: Neurological versus Psychological

Only relatively recently have researchers and therapists begun to ac-knowledge the significance of the psychodynamic factors associated with the individual who has incurred a cerebral vascular accident. Goldstein (1942) holds the view that many of the symptoms of brain damage are manifesta-tions of the patient's changed personality "and also an expression of the struggle of the changed personality to cope with the defect and with the demands it can no longer meet." He also believes that the brain-injured individual would have a "catastrophic reaction" or sudden and pronounced change in behavior when confronted with tasks he or she is unable to perform, resulting in "disordered behavior and anxiety" (1942, 1948). Goldstein, representing a holistic perspective, nonetheless believes that the patient's psychological instability is an essential aspect of neurobiological changes. We shall consider these latter factors first.

Neurological Changes

Lamendella (1977), in an extensive review of the role the limbic system plays in human communication behavior, also considers this system responsible for most nonpropositional speech and language as well. Evidence is presented that connects the communication and social function in primates to the limbic system. According to Lamendella, the dominant left hemisphere in some way inhibits affective function. He sees automatic speech to be relatively unaffected when there is damage to the left hemisphere with resultant disordered propositional language. A major reason is that automatic speech derives from areas within the limbic, thalamic, basal ganglia, or midbrain structure. He refers specifically to automatic speech of the scatalogical type, which he believes to originate in the limbic system.

Other investigators of brain injury have found a significant degree of functional brain asymmetry in the control of emotion, with the suggestion that definitive types of emotion are facilitated by each hemisphere. In a comprehensive review of the literature, Sackeim and Weber (1982), citing Gainotti (1972), Hecaen (1962) and Hommes (1965), declare that dysphoria is associated with left-side damage and an indifferent-euphoria reaction is associated with right-side damage. Patients with indifferent-euphoria reaction are characterized as carefree or placid, perhaps inappropriately humorous or socially disinhibited, whereas those with dysphoric reaction are anxious and/or depressed, self-reproaching, and socially withdrawn.

Summarizing the research of Rossi and Rosadini (1967), Terzian (1964), Milner (in Rossi and Rosadini 1967), and Tsunoda and Oka (1976), Sackeim and Weber report that barbituration of the left hemisphere is associated with a pronounced dysphoric response. Sedation of the right hemisphere is associated with euphoric behavior. With their own small group of patients, they too observed side-specific mood changes when administered barbiturates on one and then the other side of the brain.

Sackeim and Weber observe that mood changes associated with unilateral brain damage and unilateral barbituration share *common* features with classic psychiatric affective disorders but not *identical* ones. Geschwind (1975) found a high incidence of affective disorders among brain-injured populations. Continuing their review of case reports and clinical studies (Busch 1940; Hillbom 1960; Keschner, Bender, and Strauss 1936; Serafetinides and Falconer 1962), Sackeim and Weber found that primarily right-side damage was associated with inappropriate positive changes such as manic symptoms. Left-side damage was found to be associated with inappropriate negative emotional changes such as depression. Black (1975) and Gasparini et al. (1978) used the Minnesota Multiphasic Personality Inventory (MMPI) to contrast groups with right- and left-side lesions; they also found higher depression scores associated with left-side damage and increased tendencies toward extroversion associated with right-side damage.

Sackeim and Weber caution us in our interpretation of the research, suggesting that in many cases affective changes subsequent to brain damage may be secondary or psychological reactions to deficits in other areas. They state:

> It would not be surprising, for instance, to observe depression in a patient with left-side damage who is paralyzed and aphasic. Second, even if mood change in many of these cases is produced directly by changes in brain functioning, linking site of damage to type of mood change does not explicate the role of each side of the brain in subserving the altered emotional state. Unilateral destructive lesions may disinhibit emotional behavior subserved by the same or opposite side of the brain. (p. 185)

Sackeim et al. (1982), in a more recent study, examined these problems. Reporting on 119 cases in the first of three retrospective studies, they found pathological laughing associated with predominantly right-side damage and pathological crying associated with predominantly left-side lesions. In Wernicke's patients they found euphoric behavior, particularly in the acute phase. They further report that based on previous studies, the two sides of the brain differ in subserving contrasting emotional states. They suggest that mood changes are perhaps secondary reactions to associated sensorimotor and cognitive deficits rather than a direct result of brain mechanism disruption. In this same study they also found laughing and crying to be evident in sixteen of twenty-two patients with bilateral damage.

Among their conclusions are that indifferent-euphoric reactions and uncontrollable laughing are consequences of right-side damage. Dysphoric reactions and uncontrollable crying are consequences of left-side damage. They further conclude that emotional behavior is "subserved by integrated networks comprising cortical and subcortical regions." They finally conclude with the possibility that the expression of positive and negative emotions may reflect asymmetries in the content of, or responses to, particular neurotransmitters in the two sides of the brain. Davis et al. (1983) also discuss the possibility of a tentative relationship between altered neurotransmission and depression in the aged but admit to insufficient hard evidence to substantiate that relationship.

Psychological Changes

In discussing the psychological changes that manifest themselves following a cerebral vascular accident, we need to bear in mind the difficulty of isolating such changes from neurobiological alterations. Goldstein (1942, 1952, 1959) recognized the complexity of such a relationship by associating the loss of abstract attitude or cognitive processing with personality deviations. Eisenson (1984) reinforces Goldstein's earlier findings that personality changes accompany impairment of abstract attitude and states that "our clinical impression is strong that many aphasics who become predominantly concrete and ego-oriented in their behavior were premorbidly so inclined" (p. 90).

Consistent with the psychobiological reactions discussed above, several writers have examined the emotional lability factor. Emotional lability may be defined as the uncontrolled expression of the emotions, characterized chiefly by inappropriate crying or laughing. Although emotional lability has often been characterized as lacking true emotional significance Jenkins et al. (1975) believe that it does occur in an environmental context and that it relates directly "to something the patient has deep feelings or acute anxiety about" (p. 278). As Eisenson (1984) notes:

> The persistence of catastrophic emotional lability is a negative indicator for recovery. In the early, post-onset stages, however, such behavior is a response to disability and frequently a manifestation of the patient's awareness of his or her linguistic-communicative impotence. In the early post-onset period the expression of emotion—the reactions—should be accepted by the therapist and by the family as behavior that is quite in order and to be expected. It is far better for the patient to feel that he or she has the right to cry than to be discouraged from crying by any suggestion that crying is for children and not for an adult. (p. 94)

In comparing catastrophic reactions with emotional lability, we prefer to describe the former as an extreme response and the latter as a moderate or subdued one. Whether the concept of emotional lability can be considered a secondary reaction to associated sensorimotor and cognitive deficits or a direct result of brain mechanism disruption, therapists have observed the quality and intensity of the behavior to diminish in time. Moreover, it would be naive indeed for any investigator to suggest that the patient doesn't experience some direct psychological reaction to the physical, physiological, and social consequences of the brain insult. Let us, therefore, examine several representative studies.

Horenstein (1970), in his summary of the effects of cerebrovascular disease on the emotional behavior and personality changes of the patient, equates depression with a grief reaction. Horenstein describes its quality and severity in terms of the extent of the neural involvement, premorbid adaptability, intellectual level, and level of awareness. Horenstein, among others (Baretz and Stephenson 1976; Ullman 1962; Weinstein and Kahn 1955), discusses the patient's denial of illness in terms of psychodynamic reaction related to the premorbid personality. Adler (1980) developed a six-stage model based on the psychoperceptual disorientation of stroke patients during the acute postonset period. Citing stage 4 (psychoperceptual disorientation) as the most significant, he suggests that most disturbing to patients and family members are the schizoid symptoms reported. In light of the neuro-logical evidence discussed earlier, however, any definitive statement about a purely psychological reaction will have to await further experimental study.

PERSONALITY AND BEHAVIOR CHANGES

The research concerning the psychodynamic factors associated with cere-bral vascular insult has not clearly differentiated the neurological from the psychological in terms of primary or secondary determinants. Thus we need to consider the specific personality and behavioral changes that occur as patients react to their trauma.

Many investigators and therapists have written about or observed these profound emotional responses. Ullman (1962), in his three-year systematic study, found that among his 300 stroke subjects, feelings of depression, hopelessness, and futility were directly related to the duration and severity of the physical disability. He observed that although depression was associ-ated with the premorbid personality, it could also be attributed to the reality of the physical trauma. Friedman (1961) studied a group of aphasic patients in a Veterans Administration hospital and found all of them suffering diminished self-concept, loneliness, and feelings of isolation. Projecting feelings of rejection on others, they tended to exaggerate their own deficits and withdrew even in the group therapy setting. Perhaps most revealing was the sense of loss of their biological and psychological integrity, contributing to their alienation from other aphasics as well as nonaphasics.

Horenstein (1970) also describes the effects of stroke on the personal-ity by specifying depression as a manifestation of grief. He discusses the degree and quality of the depression relative to the patient's self-awareness and self-worth, type and severity of the neural deficits, intellectual level, and premorbid adaptive ability. Horenstein alludes to the profound sense of loss felt by the patient, particularly in regard to the personal and family situation. Probably the most extensive discussion of loss and grief in aphasia, ex-plained in terms of mourning theory, is provided by Tanner (1980). He reviews the states in the grieving process as variously outlined by Bowlby (1970), Engel (1964), Moustakas (1972), and Kübler-Ross (1969, 1975). With respect to the loss of self-respect, Tanner writes:

> The loss of some aspect of the self can involve changes in the individual's health, body function, sense of worth, self-concept, attractiveness and family loss. Loss of self is a broad dimension and includes functions which the individual can lose or perceive as lost. Automobile accidents, disease, stroke, congenital disorders, and amputation cause loss of some aspect of the self.
> Loss of some aspect of the self can have both an extra-dimensional and an intra-dimensional spreading of effect. Extra-dimensional spreading of effect can occur when the individual is placed in a nursing home or institution; as a result, loss is experienced in other dimensions such as security, loved ones

(symbolic), and loss of external objects. Intra-dimensional spreading of effect experienced as a result of paralysis could involve loss of a feeling of self worth, role, libido, and general reduction in self concept.

Aphasia is perhaps the most significant disorder seen by the clinician which results in loss in this dimension. In aphasia, loss is not limited to verbal expression; aphasics often have difficulty in reasoning, memory and comprehension. General reductions in ego, swallowing deficits, hemiplegia, and visual deficits are also common. In addition, many aphasics are institutionalized; grief can be expected not only relative to loss of speech but also as a result of the concomitant disorders and subsequent placement. (p. 92)

Coping and Defense Mechanisms

In describing the coping and defense mechanisms used by the patient, Davis (1983) believes these methods to be "a way of shielding the self from the disorder and from the difficult responsibilities of adapting to it" (p. 239). Among some typical responses are withdrawal and overconcern for the patient's spouse. Eisenson (1984) suggests that the patient may adopt either a negative or positive strategy if he or she feels inadequate when coping with life situations. Roskies and Lazarus (1979) describe coping as a dynamic process whereby the individual is actively involved in responding to what *has* happened but also helps determine what *will* happen when reacting to an event. Meichenbaum and Turk (1982), in referring to Lazarus and Launier (1978), recognize that sometimes improving a situation or escaping from one that is intolerable may be sufficient. They further note that rationalizing, being detached, or avoiding thinking about things, under some conditions, may be effective ways of coping.

Although Lazarus and Launier do not refer specifically to the defense and coping strategies of aphasic patients, the denial, withdrawal behavior, rationalizations, and overprotectiveness often seen in such patients may indeed be a very timely if not appropriate response to a seemingly intolerable situation. Eisenson (1984), in fact, believes that although a patient's euphoria may be inconsistent with truth or reality, it could be viewed as a means of self-defense. Eisenson (1984) and Sarno (1981) present self-accounts of patients who were able to describe the emotional impact of their experience with aphasia. Among the coping strategies described were euphoria, attention to only optimistic things, and denial of the disability. What was most revealing is how the premorbid personality often determined the method of coping.

It would appear that the reactive strategy or strategies used are unique to the individual and therefore should be considered when intervening therapeutically. It could certainly be argued that the defense and coping strategies employed by the patient are essentially psychobiological in nature. Although unique to the individual, they may reflect the structural and chemical changes in the brain. One, in fact, might support the notion of a psychological homeostatic reorganization, discussed earlier in this chapter.

Nonetheless, the therapist is still faced with the patient's own perceptual reality and all of its implications and needs to be prepared to intervene therapeutically according to the patient's emotional and linguistic needs.

Depression

It was noted earlier that the neurochemical changes induced by brain injury result in profound emotional changes manifested by depression (Sackeim and Weber 1982; Robinson and Benson 1981). Althought it may be difficult to differentiate depression in terms of secondary reaction or as a direct result of brain mechanism disruption, the literature is replete with reports of depression among the elderly in general. Salzman and Shader (1978) estimate that of the 20 million individuals over sixty-five years of age, at least 1 million suffer from depressive illness. Because of the stresses, defenses, and adaptations related to age, depression manifests itself differently in older than in younger age groups. They also note that because society often isolates the aged and places them in dependency roles, their feelings of inadequacy, exacerbated by physical and psychological decline, are reinforced. Thus symptoms of depression are further perpetuated by the loss of self-esteem and self-worth.

Breslau and Haug (1983) provide the most comprehensive account of depression among the aged, by the contributions of seventeen of the foremost authorities. Again, they indicate that individuals sixty-five years and older are more likely to suffer depression. They predict that with the increase of the elderly population, the incidence and prevalence of such depression could attain epidemic proportions. We would, therefore, not be remiss in assuming depression to be a direct psychological consequence to cerebral infarction and aphasia. Buck (1968) views depression as probably the most devastating response to the trauma, psychologically incapacitating the patient beyond even the physical effects. Baretz and Stephenson (1976) have noted the relationship of denial by the patient to the evolving depression. The reports of personal experiences of those who have suffered stroke and aphasia include depression as a grief reaction.

Anxiety, Guilt, and Anger

Discussion of the psychological forces operating in the patient would be incomplete without mentioning the varying degrees of anxiety, guilt, and anger experienced during the course of the mourning process. But, as Davis (1983) has noted, "The aphasic person is not always depressed and angry, or anxious. Though there may be some common phases of reaction to the condition and to interacting situations, people with aphasia are as different as people in general are different" (p. 294).

EFFECTS ON THE FAMILY

Webster and Newhoff (1981), in their excellent review of how families and family members are affected by the communication impairment of one family member, refer to a family systems model in explaining how the family balance is at first disrupted and how the family attempts to stabilize itself. Rollin (1984) developed a framework for understanding "aphasic families" within the context of a family systems approach and summarizes the literature describing the loss and devastation felt by the patient and the family.

Family reactions

Shontz (1965) formulated four stages that family members experience in reaction to the sudden impairment in communication of one member— shock, realization, retreat, and acknowledgment. We discussed earlier this grieving or mourning process with respect to the patient. In either case, we should bear in mind that whatever grief theory we may support, the varying stages are not necessarily discrete. Some patients or family members may get stuck anywhere along the continuum or even skip stages. Moreover, the time line during each stage may also vary from family to family and within the same family. In the preface to a description of their scale of Psychosocial Adjustment, Code and Muller (1983) also review the literature discussing the emotional effects the aphasic patient may have on the family and close friends.

We believe it would be of interest to list several notable authorities and summarize what they have written on the emotional effects on families and note the consistency among them.

Buck (1968): anxiety, guilt, psychasthenia, depression
Malone (1969): irritability, guilt, health problems, rejection, oversolicitousness
Lezak (1979): depression, unrealistic expectations
Kinsella (1978) and Kinsella and Duffy (1979): feelings of isolation, anxiety, overprotection, worry, disordered interpersonal relationships, sadness, irritability
Helmick, Watamori, and Palmer (1976): unrealistic expectations
Artes and Hoops (1976): hopelessness, nervousness, irritability
Mulhall (1978): frustration, sympathy, anger, depression
Shontz (1965): shock, anxiety, disorientation

Special note should be made of the work of Kinsella and Duffy (1979), who found psychiatric disorders in wives of aphasic patients. They found that spouses had increased difficulty in their relationships with their children, exacerbated by the tremendous demands put upon them and struggling to cope with increased guilt and resentment.

Shifting of family roles

Consistent with the family's initial disruption and attempts at reorganization or attainment of homeostasis, Lubinski (1981) stresses the importance of each individual within the immediate family to develop mechanisms to deal with the persistent emotional drain associated with the redefinition of the family after the onset of stroke in one of its members. After the immediate physical danger to the patient is resolved, the family faces the problem of integrating an unsuccessful communicator into the group. Unintentionally, the aphasia patient becomes the family member around whom all changes and accommodations are being made. Others assume new roles in the face of the decrease in responsibility of the patient's role. This is especially significant for the spouse, who must now assume the role of caregiver while also coping with a possible role reversal and the added responsibility of maintaining home, family, and finances.

The family of the aphasia patient is involved in a rehabilitation process made more demanding by the patient's sometimes antisocial behavior. Lubinski sees this as related to the aphasic's attempt to shun the "handicapped" role he or she is expected to fulfill. Such a role includes giving up responsibility, becoming dependent, and looking forward to rehabilitation therapy. If the patient does not wish to comply with these expectations, he or she may be "stigmatized as uncooperative, unmanageable, or hostile," compounding the problems the family must handle. Malone (1969) found among twenty-five families interviewed that role changes were particularly traumatic when the male patient was the chief means of financial support. When the wife assumed his role, she did so with either resentment or with enjoyment. The latter is not so surprising when we consider how, until recently, married women have not always been able to maximize their life potentials.

Porter and Dabul (1977) used a Transactional Analysis model to conceptualize the role changes that may take place in both patient and spouse. Using examples, they describe how the three ego states of Adult, Parent, and Child shift in the patient–spouse interaction. No longer able to maintain the responsibilities as "head of household" and as the "Adult," the male patient regresses to the "Child" state, feeling increasingly dependent and helpless. The female spouse, in turn, her own "Parent" state triggered, may respond by dispensing with her "Adult" state and take on a mother role. Obviously, the shifts in roles vary, depending on the premorbid family history, and become more complex when children are in the home.

Viewed in terms of family systems theory, the family's homeostasis as described by Satir (1967) has been disrupted. Satir believes that although typically each family member's role may be defined and perceived in terms of an unspoken, assumed consensus by other family members, it is possible for one member to be perceived differently by another. In an "aphasic family" behaviors may be seen as disturbing by one or more family members. This distress is then translated to identify the family member who is viewed as creating the problem and who becomes the "identified patient" or "identified symptom"—in this case the aphasic patient. (See Satir [1967] for her discussion of the identified patient and the dysfunctional family.)

Not only has the family reality changed, but so has the perceptual reality of each of the family members. There may no longer be the consensus originally established, and thus family members must struggle to satisfy a different perceptual reality, the latter being wrought with varying feelings of loss, helplessless, anger, rage, guilt, depression, and frustration. As Webster and Newhoff (1981) describe it in referring to the studies of Haspiel, Clement, and Haspiel (1972) and of Taylor (1976):

> This identified patient or scapegoat gives others a place to project family stress and/or blame for many of the family's failures. When the role of scapegoat or identified patient is essential to a unit's homeostasis, it may be impossible for other family members to participate in helping the imparied person to improve. (p. 230)

We would agree with Webster and Newhoff, however, that the aphasic patient may not necessarily be scapegoated, as long as the premorbid family system was functional or relatively stable and the family continued to be governed by previously established rules. Nonetheless, because the trauma is experienced by all, we would expect a necessary, if not dramatic, shift in roles to occur in order to satisfy the drive toward homeostasis. The key factor is that a crisis has occurred and the family may be desperately searching for a means of survival.

Each family member may develop different roles or ways of dealing with the new reality. For the preadolescent and adolescent whose world may also have been shattered, their needs and expectations can no longer be fulfilled in the style to which they had been accustomed. Not only must they readjust to the impaired parent but to the unimpaired parent as well. The family alignment now begins to shift dramatically, each member, including the patient, struggling to discover his or her own means to cope. Naturally, we do not assume that all families are as devastated as has been described. Healthy families have their own intrinsic mechanisms for coping despite the suffering they might endure.

We are also alert to the fact that the effects of a stroke on the family may not emerge immediately. Only the competence and sensitivity of and careful scrutiny by those therapists assisting in the recovery process may bring to light the underlying struggles, through counseling intervention. It is to this subject that we now turn.

COUNSELING INTERVENTION

Because the entire family has been affected by the stroke, we would immediately want to intervene so as to assuage some of the powerful feelings now surfacing, as well as to manage the continued adjustment difficulties the patient and family members may have throughout the recovery and rehabilitation periods. In doing so, we also focus attention on the spouse, as he or she has likely been the most significant person in the patient's life and will now be the probable caregiver.

Initial Considerations

Malone (1969) submits that family members cannot function effectively as part of the rehabilitation team until they have been advised of the many problems associated with aphasia and the various strategies for dealing with these problems. Conversely, in order to work meaningfully with affected families, the speech-language pathologist must be knowledgeable regarding the pervasive effects of aphasia on the family constellation. Armed with this information, the therapist is better able to assist family members in appropriately avoiding certain situations, changing situations that have the potential for changing, and accepting the unchangeable. In so doing, we would prefer to view the family dynamically rather than attempting to assign it a label of normal, neurotic, or psychotic. Family therapists generally consider this to be more realistic in terms of a continuum of dysfunctionality rather than hold to traditional absolute labels.

Importance of providing information   Skelly (1975), Linebaugh and Young-Charles (1978), Manuel (1979), and Goldberg (1980) concur that the most difficult problem for the family is their ignorance of the cause and effect of the stroke on the patient. Baretz and Stephenson (1976), in their description of practical management guidelines, highlight the importance of providing information about the disorder "to patient and family to allay fear, banish misconceptions, stress positive aspects, and provide the basis for a slowly developing recognition of the realities of the situation and a renewable adjustment" (p. 56). Interviewing fifty aphasic patients who had attained a functional level of speech, Skelly (1975) found that many believed they would have experienced less fear and anguish had they been given reassurance and a basic explanation of what had happened to them. In his study of twenty hospital inpatients, Goldberg (1980) found that none of those patients nor their families had received any explanation from the attending physician of the language problem before they met with the speech-language pathologist. He also found that interactions with family and staff reinforced patients' assumptions that they had "gone crazy." Such findings lend greater support for the necessity of providing families with information, as well as intensifying in-service programs for staff personnel.

We recognize the importance and value of providing information to both patient and members of the family. It is equally important to recognize that any one of them may not be able, during the initial stages of the posttrauma shock, to hear or understand all that is being communicated to them by the professional. The patient's cognitive-linguistic impairment or psychological state may prevent processing of information. Similarly, family members may be too numb, confused, or depressed to comprehend clearly what has occurred and what may be expected to occur in the future. Webster and Newhoff (1981) and Haspiel, Clement, and Haspiel (1972) have commented on this.

It appears to us that in these initial stages what is most important is not the information per se that is provided, but that the family senses caring, support, and understanding from the therapist. Testimony to this need comes from the wife of a patient with whom the author consulted: "If only they gave our family some information when he had the stroke, we wouldn't have felt so lost and frightened. We probably still wouldn't have understood what was going on, but at least we'd have some comfort in knowing that somebody cared, just by talking to us."

We agree with Sarno (1981) and Baretz and Stephenson (1976) that a rehabilitation team would be most desirable in dealing with the multitude of problems the patient and family must face. Considering the problems of health care cost, a more practical solution needs to be found. We address this issue later in the chapter.

Separating premorbid from postmorbid issues   It has been noted that because the spouse will probably have the greatest interaction with the patient, any counseling strategy employed should include a distinction between premorbid and postmorbid issues. This is all the more important for the speech-language pathologist who has had little training in psychopathology and yet most often becomes the essential agent in rehabilitation efforts. The therapist will need to keep a clear perspective on only those issues that refer specifically to the stroke, whether they include the wife's anxiety about her husband's withdrawal behavior, her feelings of resentment and guilt about her assumed burdens, or her feelings of sexual deprivation. For the therapist to delve into elements involving the premorbid marital relationship, such as money matters, lack of intimacy, and conflicts over the children, may not only be irrelevant but counterproductive and destructive. It is important to understand that, but for the stroke, the couple would most likely not have sought psychological assistance in the first place. The therapist must therefore honor the spouse's possible need to conceal earlier conflicts, while remaining attuned to the nuances, expressed or unexpressed, of premorbid marital struggles.

Although it is conceivable for the spouse now to ventilate pent-up feelings that refer back many marital years, given a willing and caring ear, the therapist will need to steer such discussions gently in the direction of what is happening in the present. This is not to suggest that the therapist should invalidate these powerful feelings, but first to acknowledge understanding of them and then deal in positive terms with ways of coping now. Ironically, in some cases the current crisis may actually serve to diminish, neutralize, or nullify elements of previous family conflicts. Some families that have been in constant turmoil may now put aside egocentric needs and unite to assist the afflicted member in any way possible.

Family involvement in rehabilitation efforts   The question now arises of how the family should be involved in rehabilitation efforts. We have already seen that in a very real sense the family must undergo its own rehabilitation regardless of the special needs of the patient. The extent to which the family should be involved directly in the rehabilitation process for the patient, however, depends on the following factors:

1. *Comprehensive analysis of the patient's linguistic abilities and communicative competence.* The therapist's definition and determination of the short- and long-range goals for the patient consistent with the nature and quality of the deficits revealed.

2. *Psychosocial analysis of the patient and family.* Through formal counseling and/or testing, the therapist's determination of the interpersonal perceptions of the spouse, therapist, and if possible, the patient (see the Code-Muller Scale of Psychosocial Adjustment [Code and Muller 1983]). Based on the analysis, the therapist may derive a clearer understanding of the attitudes that could hinder or facilitate the rehabilitation process and determine in specific ways how family members may participate. The therapist must also be alert to changing family circumstances and attitudes that positively or adversely affect the process.

3. *Communication environment analysis.* The therapist's determination of the patient's opportunities for communication and hindrances to communication in his or her environment as outlined in Lubinski's "Profile of the Communication Environment of the Adult Aphasic" (1981). We would include in this analysis a premorbid psychosocial linguistic history with particular emphasis on the patient's prior communicative style, for example, colloquial and slang usage, vocabulary, stereotyped expressions, and environmentally determined linguistic variations.

4. *Developing a rehabilitation plan.* The therapist's formulation of a short- and long-term therapy plan consistent with the patient's abilities, deficits, and ever-changing needs and his or her flexibility to change goals when deemed necessary. Input from family members is desirable insofar as it may positively contribute to the total rehabilitation process.

Once the level and degree of family involvement have been determined, the environmental goals for the entire rehabilitation program can be stated accordingly (see Lubinski 1981, p. 230).

Spousal and Family Counseling

Thus far we have discussed the importance and ramifications of giving information to the patient and the family. We have also noted the delicate relationship of pre- and postmorbid issues and guidelines for the therapist to initiate with the patient and the family in the recovery process. We are led now to consider the rationale and indications for continued spousal and family counseling.

The success of any rehabilitation program depends on the active cooperation of the professionals and the family. We concur with Lubinski (1981) that family counseling should be considered a reeducation process. Lubinski provides eighteen definitive communication strategies that both family and hospital personnel may use to enhance communication with the patient. Naturally, any successful efforts necessitate full cooperation by the family. Implied is a willingness by the family to adjust previous assumptions and behaviors and attitudes and to accept the necessity of defining different roles for themselves within the family constellation.

The presence of any hidden psychopathological elements could also undermine rehabilitative efforts. Kinsella and Duffy (1979) report the incidence of minor psychiatric disorders in wives of aphasic patients (but apparently not in husbands of aphasics). They indicate that the spouse must not only cope with the profound crisis of the stroke but that the spouse also loses "the protective function of an intimate relationship or a supportive social network. . . ," (p. 129) thereby increasing the likelihood of psychiatric illness. With children living in the home, spouses felt even more overwhelmed, becoming impotent in dealing with the children's own "reactive behavior problems," while coping with the patient's variable and oftentimes erratic emotional state. Caution should be taken in generalizing from these data because of the limited population used, but it should be considered an important indicator for counseling intervention nonetheless. In their study of sixty-five spouses of cerebral vascular patients, Artes and Hoops (1976) emphasize that the communication problems of the patient are not always the major concern of the spouse; that most wives were equally or more concerned about problems involving intrapersonal behavior and overall health care.

It is apparent from our discussion that family counseling in aphasia has two central goals: a reeducation process in which the family assists the patient and participates in those activities that will enhance the total rehabilitation efforts and an opportunity for the family to cope with their own emotional responses to the trauma, modifying previous behaviors and establishing a different mode of living. Implicit are the assumptions that family counseling can satisfy both goals simultaneously and that the speech-language pathologist can typically fill this counselor role.

As far as contributing to the family reeducation process, we acknowledge the role that the American Heart Association has played in sponsoring and establishing Stroke Clubs in communities throughout the United States. The club's major purpose has been to foster recreational and social activities for stroke families through group interrelationships and assist members in continuing to value themselves and to contribute to society. Other nonprofit support groups have begun to emerge, like the Family Survival Project, a San Francisco–based organization established to aid families of brain-injured adults in coping with various forms of brain disease through dissemination of information and initiation of self-support systems. A further goal of this public- and state-funded organization is to educate the public about brain injury and encourage the growth of other such groups throughout the United States.

Family Therapy

Thus far we have discussed the efficacy of traditional family counseling, which should not be confused with family therapy, a more systematic and interactional approach to the treatment of families that was introduced earlier. In this latter context we have recognized the importance and significance of determining the family's premorbid communicative interaction in order to facilitate the rehabilitation efforts. We propose that a family systems approach would be most appropriate to satisfy that end.

Rationale and value   Traditional family counseling typically excludes the direct participation of the aphasic in the actual process, thus perhaps isolating and alienating the patient further from the immediate family and thereby impeding the total rehabilitation procedure. We are not suggesting that family counseling is detrimental in any way; the literature has clearly demonstrated its value in helping the patient to recover and the family to readjust. What is suggested, however, is that family counseling per se may be omitting the very element that needs greatest attention—namely, the facilitation of language usage by the patient with the rest of the family.

It also appears obvious to us that it is far better to involve the patient in whatever changes are deemed necessary by the family and professionals alike. This would validate the person's role, albeit a different one, as an active member of the family. As the patient and other family members are provided the opportunity to explore areas of concern and conflict in an atmosphere of acceptance and safety, the patient may no longer feel singled out as the only problem or represented as being chiefly responsible for the family crisis. The patient's concern may now focus on his wife's struggle to "make ends meet," adding to his own feelings of guilt and inadequacy. But these feelings can be dealt with as a family issue, with the potential for each member to assist the other in reestablishing family equilibrium. Although the patient will need to take responsibility for the personal reality of the disability, he will know also that it is a family problem.

Family therapy motivates other family members, if only the spouse, to include the patient in all communicative transactions. They are aided in learning how to focus on the significant nuances and elements of the patient's communicative efforts, become more skilled in understanding aphasic messages, and adapt their own communicative efforts suitable to the patient. The patient, in turn, feeling related to the family and encouraged by them, is likely to feel more positive about him- or herself. Any small gains in communicative competence are positively reinforced by the family, strengthening the person's available assets and reducing the liabilities, thus giving the patient a sense of real progress. Those patients who cannot tolerate error in their linguistic attempts, but having family support, are more likely to take the risk and experience communicative reward.

Finally, family therapy provides not only a linguistic environment for reacquiring communicative competence but also serves as a rich source for the carryover of communicative skills gained through conventional speech therapy. It should be emphasized, however, that family therapy is not a panacea for all the difficulties the patient and the family may be having. Its appropriateness and value will be determined by the application of several criteria.

Criteria for family therapy Ideally, the patient and/or other members of the family should request help when they are unable to cope with the problems they are experiencing. Therapists have observed that many families do not require extensive counseling but merely an exchange of information. These families apparently have their own healthy internal mechanisms for coping with crisis and adapt easily to the rehabilitation program prescribed by the professional staff. With other families it may be only the spouse who requires counseling assistance.

The author counseled the sixty-year-old wife of a sixty-two-year-old severely impaired aphasic patient who described their sexual relationship prior to the stroke as virtually nonexistent for the last twenty years of their marriage. Frustrated and resentful over his pronounced dependency needs, she sought permission from the author to ease her burden and have transient sexual relationships with other men. Recognizing also her profound feelings of guilt, she needed to struggle with her conflict and arrive at some accommodation with which she could continue to be an effective caregiver to her husband and to herself. At her instigation, family therapy was also initiated to help her husband become more self-sufficient at home and to provide time off for herself. It was felt inappropriate and counterproductive to raise the sexual issue during family therapy, as, in reality, this was the wife's problem and her husband could not be expected to cope with that issue as well. Unsurprisingly, her need for sexual adventures diminished when she found that she could adapt and help provide a more positive home environment.

There may be times when the therapist will perceive elements that are interfering with speech therapy. The patient and/or spouse may or may not be aware of them. A therapist who has sufficient rapport with the family may delicately suggest that they seek further assistance to identify and resolve the problem in order to enhance speech therapy efforts. The author was treating a patient who had made significant and rapid progress in achieving limited communication but, after six months of speech therapy, had suddenly plateaued. Through gentle probing of the patient it was learned that he and his wife had been distressed about their son, who had dropped out of high school during his senior year. They were eager to participate in family therapy, particularly once the son agreed, though grudgingly at first, to do so.

The decision to initiate family therapy will depend on the degree of cognitive, receptive, or evaluative function of the aphasic patient. This may be very difficult for the therapist to ascertain because formal testing is of little value in determining the degree of communicative competence. Holland (1977) has been critical of language tests that do not measure communicative competence. She suggests that spouses may be more sensitive to the patient's verbal and nonverbal communicative attempts, particularly in a natural environment. We would concur and trust the occasion of the initial family session to decide continuation of the family therapy process. It may be argued that a severe Wernicke's or global aphasic patient would be totally confused, bewildered, distracted, and distant from the communicative process in family therapy. We would counter that the patient may be receiving valuable but unmeasurable input from other family members and perhaps is deriving some pleasure from the experience of being included in the family discussions.

Family therapy should not be considered a substitute for other speech therapy strategies. No research has yet documented the superiority of one approach over the other. It would appear, though, that family therapy can in fact enhance traditional speech therapy by revealing communicative competencies and personal attitudes heretofore undetected or undetermined.

During the course of family therapy sessions with a severe apraxic patient and his wife, the author learned of the patient's displeasure with the method his wife was using with him during home practice. The author had originally been consulted by the patient's speech-language pathologist, who reported that the patient had been vocally abusive to his wife. What had not been evidenced in formal speech therapy was now revealed so that steps could be taken to educate the wife to a different approach and, it was discovered, to a more positive attitude in helping. Family therapy had provided the milieu in which both the patient and his wife were able to verbalize their discontent and assuage their frustration after weeks of marital discord and inappropriate home therapy.

Guidelines for the therapist   Once the determination to intervene with family therapy has been made, the therapist (either a speech-language pathologist trained in family therapy or a psychotherapist with knowledge of aphasia) can follow a series of guidelines that best meet the needs of the patient and family. Rollin (1984) has developed such guidelines, which are outlined here:

1. The therapist must determine how much information the patient and/or family needs to be given about specific issues to be dealt with during therapy.

2. It must be recognized that the aphasic patient is not necessarily the only identified patient and that shifts to other family members may occur in order for underlying dysfunctional elements to be expressed.

3. Other family members must be aided in permitting the patient to function as a separate person during family therapy, communicating *with* the patient rather than *about* the patient.

4. The therapist must be prepared to verbalize thoughts and feelings the patient cannot readily express.

5. The therapist must be sensitive to what is being expressed nonverbally by all family members.

6. The therapist must gently facilitate the expression of feelings by all in order to uncover hidden angers, resentments, frustrations, or anguish.

7. The patient and other members of the family must be helped to confront self-destructive and self-defeating behaviors and to focus their energy on positive goals and the needs of other family members as well.

8. The therapist must help the patient and other family members to discover new roles for themselves consistent with the reality of the changed family circumstances.

9. The therapist, too, must struggle with his or her own role, avoiding the role of rescuer for either the patient or for other family members.

10. Finally, the therapist should have resolved or continue to work on his or her own personal inner conflicts, doubts about therapeutic competence, misjudged perceptions of the family, and other personal insecurities and uncertainties.

Counseling the Patient

As noted, family therapy should not be considered a panacea for all the problems and difficulties confronting the patient or, for that matter, the family. Oftentimes, direct or indirect counseling with the patient alone may be effective or beneficial in promoting real progress, particularly during the first several months following the trauma.

Initial considerations   Tanner (1980) has applied rules facilitating the grieving process with patients who have suffered a cerebral vascular accident. Suggestions are presented that the counseling therapist avoid certain behaviors that interrupt the grieving process and encourage behaviors that facilitate the process:

1. *Positive reinforcement of denial* should be avoided and the reality of current and possibly future circumstances discussed. Although a realistic prognosis may not always be determined, the patient must be given some degree of hope for recovery.

2. Recognizing and accepting rather than *punishing anger* will help to reduce and neutralize it. The patient must be helped to understand that what is felt is a natural consequence to what has been experienced.

3. *Bargaining with the patient* can be counterproductive in that it may present false hopes to the patient while assuaging the therapist's own uncertainty and insecurity.

4. Care should be taken to avoid *providing secondary gains* to the patient that may reinforce or interrupt the grieving process. The therapist must be alert to the fostering of unrealistic dependency by the patient on the therapist, and foster instead patient responsibility for decision making and ultimate progress.

5. The therapist should help the patient avoid *early distractions*, such as untimely suggestions that the patient get "his mind off things" or get immersed in other activities for which the patient may not be prepared.

6. The therapist must avoid *displaying anxiety about the patient's depression* and accept it as a natural consequence and a stage to be experienced before the patient can develop more constructive attitudes.

7. The therapist can *permit patient control* by encouraging specific decision making and responsibility taking in the therapy process.

8. The therapist must *provide the patient with perspective* so that a more realistic and rational understanding about reactions and attitudes that are quite normal for aphasia can be developed. Learning that what is being experienced is not unique will help remove the fright induced by personal reactions to the disabilities.

9. To *acknowledge the reality of the loss* of functions and to encourage the free expression of concerns the patient may have personally about the condition will strengthen the speech therapy program and further acceptance of the personal reality.

10. Therapists must *listen to the patient without defending or explaining their concerns* and not feel that they must have all the answers to the patient's problems. Unconditional positive regard and empathy without judgment are of the utmost importance.

Indicators and rationale for continued counseling   We now consider how counseling therapists can best respond to the ongoing emotional and language problems associated with aphasia, using appropriate counseling strategies while respecting their limitations.

1. *Dealing with continuing denial.* Patient denial manifests itself in several ways but may not be readily evident to the therapist. One such example is the patient's inability to accept the disability and the belief that full recovery is imminent. It is debatable whether or not this is similar to the "sleeping beauty syndrome" referred to elsewhere in this text, but it may be indicative of the patient's refusal to have speech-language therapy. A similar example is the patient who perceives himself or herself to have less of a speech-language disability than is objectively verified by formal and/or informal testing. Although this, like the previous example, represents self-protective or defensive behaviors and is perhaps highly resistant to change, the therapist can at least acknowledge verbally what the patient believes, even if the belief is not expressed verbally by the patient. This could instigate the patient to confront the contradiction between what is the reality and what is not, but it is the patient who must make the choice either to acknowledge the reality or continue to reject it.

As long as the patient is willing to continue in therapy, the greater the likelihood that a changed attitude will occur. The therapist will certainly have to exercise considerable patience and understanding so as to enable the patient time to consider all the facts and to ultimately make a personal decision either to continue or terminate therapy. Although the therapist may be tempted to enlist the aid of the spouse, we believe that may be counterproductive and could alienate the patient from therapy, the spouse, and the therapist. The therapist might, however, share with the patient his or her professional judgment and ask for permission to speak to the spouse about the issue. As long as the patient is conscious of and alert to the immediate environment, no interpersonal transactions between the therapist and the spouse should be secretive.

2. *Dealing with emotional lability.* Therapists frequently have difficulty in coping with their emotionally labile patients who weep persistently at what seems the slightest provocation. The response may be prompted by such apparently innocuous comments as, "Your husband tells me you have eight grandchildren" or "I understand you had a slight cold last week." Unlike the expected emotional response to depression or anxiety, it is best to neutralize it by either turning to another subject or, if the therapeutic task has instigated the response, by changing the task. The author also has found it helpful to acknowledge to the patient that "What you're experiencing now is natural for what you've been through" or "Because of your stroke it's hard to control things all the time," or "As you get better physically you'll also have better control of these things like crying when you don't want to." Most important is that the therapist help remove the affectual response to the weeping. If the labile response is only a momentary lapse of control, it is probably best ignored and continue on the planned therapeutic track.

We realize that emotional lability may sometimes be fused with the overall emotional status of the patient. In such a case it is important to verbalize for the patient as intuitively as possible, if necessary, that which is being experienced or felt.

3. *Dealing with guilt.* We are sometimes confronted with patients whose guilt in having gotten sick is so pervasive as to inferere with the overall therapeutic process. They are individuals who apparently are bearing the full burden of their illness as well as the burdens of the spouse or family. Although depression may be an obvious expressed emotion, the underlying feelings are of remorse, self-pity, self-denigration, and resentment. They feel as if they should not have survived their stroke and, feeling unworthy, will frequently resist therapeutic assistance or even spousal support.

Guilt can be traced back to premorbid unresolved interpersonal relationships, but it is likely that the therapist would encounter either patient or spousal resistance to discussion of these issues. Thus the therapist will need to focus attention on alleviating or modifying the patient's current attitude by providing the maximum in encouragement, support, and empathic understanding. The patient is helped to realize that none of us is responsible for all of the unfortunate events that befall us in our lives and were such an event as a stroke to strike another person in the family instead, we would certainly do all in our power to help.

By encouraging the patient to allow the spouse, in particular, to take on his or her own burden or responsibility is to show respect and love for that person. The therapist helps the patient understand that there is indeed enough burden for all to bear. In effect, the therapist attempts to neutralize the unrealistic or irrational concerns of the patient by directing him or her to take on positive and major responsibilities, such as trying to get better and helping others to cope.

4. *Modifying concrete responses.* Patients who are impaired in the "abstract attitude" manifest linguistic and emotional material concretely. Though the therapist may find it difficult to help the patient generalize more effectively because of the combined organic and emotional bases of the problem, some adjustments are possible. The patient who believes his spouse does not remain in the waiting room while he is having therapy because she does not care about him is perhaps an extraordinary example of a concrete attitude tinged with premorbid attitudes of paranoia. For a situation such as this the therapist can design a linguistic task that includes many of the possibilities for the spouse's absence. The patient is encouraged to contribute his own examples of reasons for her not remaining in the waiting room. Together the patient and therapist can identify other situations, particularly at home, in which she has helped him to improve. It will likely take many therapeutic sessions to strengthen a more abstract appreciation of reality, and much will depend on the extent of premorbid attitudes as well as on the degree of organic involvement.

Care should be taken to avoid judging the patient's attitude as foolish or malicious, but rather to acknowledge to the patient that such reactions are not unusual. If the patient's evaluative capabilities are impaired, the therapist's task will be considerably more difficult. In such a case, efforts will have to be directed at improving evaluative functioning first.

5. *Enhancing adjustment in the extended care facility or nursing home.* Speech-language pathologists are seeing more and more aphasic individuals in settings that have become permanent "homes" for them. Either because these persons can no longer care for themselves at home or because they have no families to which they can turn, they must rely on the often impersonal assistance of nursing personnel. Those facilities with social workers on their staff certainly help provide a richer support system for these patients, who feel lonely, depressed, and withdrawn. Although the speech-language pathologist's major objective is to help the aphasic patient gain the communicative competence necessary for functioning at least adequately in the facility, the daily emotional struggles cannot be ignored. Merely to work on language tasks that have little relevance to the patient's real environment, in order to satisfy Part B Medicare regulations, cannot be justified. We believe it is possible, however, to integrate meaningful language activities along with counseling support and yet fulfill the patient's needs and Medicare requirements as well.

One illustration of this approach can be drawn from the author's own experiences with aphasic patients in convalescent hospitals. A nursing aide is frustrated by her inability to determine what her patient is attempting to communicate. The patient in turn is also frustrated because she cannot get through to the aide. Rather than dwell only on the airing of the patient's frustration, we bring them both together and reenact the verbal interchange that had been attempted previously. This serves not only to satisfy the practical and emotional needs of both parties but also as an impetus for both to practice such interchanges throughout their daily contact. It is not difficult to establish appropriate baseline responses and demonstrate behavioral changes objectively.

The patient who is sad because he cannot go home may need to be assisted in sharing his concerns because his emotional state could interfere with further therapeutic intervention. This does not mean bombarding him with judgmental reassurances or unrealistic pronouncements but rather helping him to focus on improving the daily difficulties that prevent his going home. These may consist of being able to use the telephone for emergency purposes or to shop for himself. Ideally, a team approach, involving physical, occupational, and recreational therapy, would be most effective.

Some patients resign themselves to the reality of their hospital existence and to the realization that they will never go home. They present a considerable challenge to all caregivers who want to intervene in the patient's best interest. But do we really know what that best interest is? Several months ago the author evaluated a patient who showed considerable promise for becoming a limited communicator. After one month of traditional speech-language therapy, along with some client-centered counseling, it became clear that she did not wish to continue therapy. She appeared quite relieved, in fact, when told that therapy would be terminated.

Recently, the facility's social worker informed the author that shortly after termination the patient had been hospitalized with pneumonia but had since returned to the convalescent facility. What had been a depressed, noncommunicative patient was now one who attempted to communicate with others and who was delighted when asked if she would like to have speech-language therapy. Unfortunately, in this case, her physician refused to write orders because as he put it: "She doesn't know what she wants."

This anecdote, although perhaps somewhat disturbing to most readers, raises serious moral, ethical, and professional issues that cannot be readily dismissed. Whereas we do not believe that most physicians hold such an attitude, we nevertheless are challenged to determine objectively the efficacy of therapy when patient disengagement is a significant factor. Perhaps by providing the patient a therapeutic milieu in which she or he can air a particular desire consistently, and by periodically reviewing with the patient any change in attitude, an appropriate decision can be made. In the case discussed, this therapist need not have been so definitive in his original termination of therapy report.

6. *Dealing with sudden stress in the midst of speech-language therapy.* The therapist should feel free to suspend symptomatic therapy when the patient is observed to be distracted, depressed, anxious, or uncooperative. Therapist sensitivity to subtle verbal or nonverbal clues is most desirable so that the patient will not have to endure continuation of the session as planned. The therapist should share his or her perception that "something seems to be bothering you" and give the patient an opportunity to ventilate whatever is of concern. In some instances the patient may be hesitant in doing so, for fear of offending the therapist, who has a well-planned lesson. Or else the patient, unaccustomed to the expression of feelings, may feel uncomfortable in sharing personal feelings.

Insensitive coaxing or cajoling could alienate the relationship and thereby interfere further with the speech-language therapy process. In such instances the patient must be given the responsibility to make an independent choice as to how best to proceed, with the therapist accepting whatever choice the patient makes. If that means early termination of the session, so be it; the patient may be capable of working out the difficulty prior to the subsequent session or be more open to discuss his or her problem the next time. If the patient, on the other hand, welcomes the opportunity to talk about that which is disturbing, the therapist should listen and attempt to understand what the patient is experiencing. Providing instant solutions or professional value judgments will not only be counterproductive, because they could be wrong, but they may also inhibit the patient from revealing further information.

7. *Dealing with premorbid psychological problems.* It may be difficult for the therapist to identify premorbid deep-rooted psychological problems when they have been exacerbated by the cerebral vascular trauma. The situation becomes more complex when these problems are interwoven with problems resulting directly from the trauma. Even if the therapist has been able to sort them out, based on information gathered from the case history or from spousal and/or family therapy, focus can nonetheless be directed to the patient's immediate affectual state. The mere opportunity for the patient to express deep feelings to a trusting and accepting confidant may be sufficient to reduce the stress associated with the problem, regardless of solutions, if any, for it.

Frantic referrals to psychiatrists or clinical psychologists may not only be resisted by the patient and/or family but may also be interpreted by them to mean rejection by the therapist or raise doubts as to the therapist's competency. We do not suggest that the therapist attempt to bear the burden of the patient's deep-rooted conflicts and anxiety or assume the role of the professional psychotherapist. But neither do we suggest that the therapist unwittingly apply Band-Aids to pacify the patient and in all likelihood submerge the problem further. The therapist who is willing to listen and to understand first what the patient is experiencing is in a better position to suggest gradually and gently further psychotherapeutic consultation.

8. *Counseling the depressed or frustrated nonverbal patient.* On occasion, we have heard psychiatrists, clinical social workers, and psychiatrists refusing to see depressed nonverbal patients, with the apology that "I couldn't possibly help him because he doesn't speak, and anyway I don't really know anything about aphasia." Such an admission obviously places the speech-language pathologist in the position of assuming full responsibility for coping with that patient's depression. The therapist need not feel the burden of that imposition as long as the basic guidelines for counseling are followed and the therapist trusts his or her own skills for facilitating language. One of the most effective ways to do this is to verbalize for the patient in complete sentences whatever minimal verbal and nonverbal messages the patient is sending. If, for example, the patient tilts her head downward and appears sad when asked, "How are you feeling this morning?," the therapist might say, "It looks as if you're feeling down today." If the patient nods in agreement, the therapist could assist by having the patient say in unison, "I'm not feeling very well today," and then encourage her to say so independently or with some assistance.

Such an acknowledgment by the therapist of the patient's mood can then lead to further questions and responses that would not only help relieve the patient of several personal concerns but also contribute to functional language usage. Naturally, we may not always be that disconcerning in recognizing what the patient is feeling and may in fact miss the point entirely. Although perhaps momentarily frustrating for both the patient and the therapist, it need not deter us from continuing the process until the patient's feelings are discovered. Surely the aphasic patient recognizes that we too are human, that we are not always entirely accurate and can make mistakes. Even if the therapist cannot reach the heart of the matter by the end of the session, the patient might find some solace in the therapist's frustration so as to assuage the patient's own. It might indeed be appropriate for therapists to share their frustration in trying to understand the patient, commenting on their own limitations.

One further strategy the therapist might use to uncover hidden feelings is to share information surrounding an incident about which the patient may be concerned, thereby maintaining a constant flow of verbalization. In doing so the therapist should be alert to the patient's confirmation of that information and modify whatever is necessary to gain agreement. Such an approach can also serve to shift the emphasis to other therapy matters.

9. *Dealing with the patient's response to linguistic errors.* One of the most typical behaviors therapists encounter during speech-language therapy for the aphasic adult is the patient's emotional response to errors made while attempting linguistic tasks. These responses may be characterized by evocations of self-deprecation, frustration, anger, or the desire to cease the task. The quality and intensity of the affect will, of course, vary from patient to

patient, depending on a combination of such other factors as premorbid personality, postmorbid psychological attitudes, and the degree of overall deficits. Therapists often observe that such responses may mentally block the patient, thereby triggering further inaccurate linguistic responses. For example, it is not uncommon for perseverative behavior to increase at such times.

It is appropriate, then, for the therapist to "take time out" to comfort the patient by acknowledging the difficulty and frustration being experienced and encourage further responses regardless of accuracy. We are all familiar with our own need to respond accurately in a problem-solving situation and are well aware of the blocks that arise when we try too hard. We find that by being willing to risk error, we are more apt to arrive at the appropriate response. Similarly, for the aphasic patient, it is better to risk committing the error than to inhibit the attempt at all. Merely suggesting that the patient relax could contribute to further tension and subsequent blocks. We suggest that it is more productive to offer the person the thought that it is very natural and normal to want to be right and that if the correct response is not forthcoming then, it will perhaps be so later on or during further sessions. What is most important is not just the correct response but the development of a more positive attitude toward self and the tasks confronted. These considerations, we believe, will be most effective in reducing the patient's level of stress and enhancing continued retrieval of language competency.

10. *Dealing with patient attitudes toward therapy and options for behavioral changes.* The expectations of therapists are not always consistent with the expectations of their patients. Regardless of a particular issue, it is important for the therapist to open up discussion or provide the patient opportunity to do so. Those who restrict themselves to a particular therapeutic technique when patient progress is at a standstill may not be aware that it could be the patient's negative attitude about the technique that is inhibiting progress. What may be appropriate in the mind of the skilled professional may not necessarily be appropriate for the patient who knows "what works for me." The understanding, nonthreatened, creative therapist can take advantage of this opportunity to explore with the patient what isn't working, why it isn't working, and what could work. What may now lead to the use of a more fruitful technique can also provide greater patient responsibility for personal recovery.

Frequently, it is the patient who adheres to an unbending attitude, which may be counterproductive. Self-effacement, expressions of futility, resistance to home practice (no matter the techniques used)—all must be noted and brought out into the open. Here, again, the therapist can listen, understand, and clarify for the patient that these are normal attitudes to have, considering what the patient has been through. But at the same time the patient should be helped to realize that these attitudes can be self-defeating, delaying further progress. Counseling here demands great patience by the therapist, who must now guide the patient with persistence yet not sacrifice the rapport already established.

It is conceivable, however, that a patient's desire to terminate therapy may arise, thereby confronting the therapist with a difficult decision. Though not a life or death issue, it nevertheless presents the therapist with the choice either to acknowledge and accept the patient's resignation or to encourage the patient to continue therapy. This ethical issue is one to which we have no answer, given the communicative difficulty the patient may have in expressing the wish. Nonetheless, it is incumbent on us to respect the patient's feelings and to be sensitive to his or her persistence in the desire to terminate therapy. Whatever the obstacles facing the therapeutic relationship, the spouse or family members may be brought in to discuss the issue with the mutual consent of the patient and therapist.

Group Therapy

The efficacy of group therapy with aphasic patients has received some attention in the literature, and there are many positive reports of the emergence of such groups in hospitals, community agencies, clinics, and colleges throughout the United States.

Hurvitz (1970) studied groups that were organized around various self-destructive behaviors, such as drug abuse, alcoholism, and obesity, and found the effectiveness of group therapy to be related to the peer relationship itself, fellowship, explicit goals, and inspirational methods, among others. It appears appropriate to describe the objectives of group programs that have evolved over the last twenty years and how they might best serve the patient.

Purpose of group therapy   One of the chief objectives of group therapy for aphasic patients, it would seem, is to provide psychological support from participation in a group. A second objective would be to provide opportunities for patients to practice communicating with each other with the expectation that such experiences will enhance whatever the patient is trying to accomplish in individual therapy and/or at home. Because this chapter is not intended to deal with speech-language therapy per se, we focus our attention more on the psychosocial needs that may be satisfied through group treatment. We need to be cognizant of the fact, however, that even work on functional communication or on a specific language program may contribute to more productive psychosocial functioning.

Value of group therapy   On first glance, it would appear that although there has been a rapid growth of group therapy for aphasic patients, there has been only limited objective research to document its value in fostering language recovery. Davis (1983) and Eisenson (1984), in their reviews of the literature, cite the studies of Wertz et al. (1981), Redinger et al. (1971), and

Aten, Caligiuri, and Holland (1982), which did reveal limited value at least in contributing to enhanced use of language, particularly in conjunction with individual therapy.

Research supporting group therapy as a means for improving psychosocial behavior has been less definitive and also problematic. Albert et al. (1981) report the ineffectiveness of traditional group therapy techniques for aphasic patients but cite some psychosocial benefits to be derived. Jenkins et al. (1975), in discussing the effects of group therapy in Veterans Administration hospitals, view its greatest value to be in helping the patient feel less isolated and encouraged by the progress other patients are making. We might note that one disquieting feature might be the depression that could result in patients who are *not* progressing, particularly when they observe other patients who *are*. Eisenson (1984, pp. 236–238) cogently summarizes the value of group therapy for achieving the following social values:

1. *Group training provides an opportunity for socialization* which would include the singing of popular and well-known songs, and the practicing of "social gesture" speech. Participation by all should be the objective but it could be encouraged gently.
2. *Group training provides an opportunity for "motivation from peers" rather than from the unimpaired therapist.* Patients are more likely to be motivated to attempt verbalizations when encouraged by other patients rather than by the linguistically proficient therapist.
3. *The group approach provides a situation where awareness of certain aphasic speech "habits" such as telegraphic and agrammatical language structure, becomes apparent.* Patients would be able to better their self-monitoring skills through the corrective input of other patients as well as identifying with the incorrect "habits" of others.
4. *Group training provides an aphasic patient with an opportunity to observe the techniques of other aphasics for evoking speech and for getting speakers to make themselves understood.* The patient can learn either actively or vicariously without risking failures or detriment to his or her ego.
5. *. . .provides the aphasic with an opportunity in a learning situation to respond to more than one manner of speech and language usage.*
6. *. . .The group approach . . . provides for "ventilation of feelings" and "airing of grievances."* By identifying with the feelings of others in the group the patient is less likely to feel isolated and make a better adaptation to living with other members of his family.

Eisenson adds to his discussion of group therapy the following admonitions:

1. *Withdrawn patients may find it difficult to attempt expression as members of a group.*
2. *Group pressure may provoke some patients into talking about personal problems before they are entirely ready for such revelations.*
3. *The rate of a group is usually slower than the best member can manage and somewhat faster than the weakest member can progress.*

Eisenson concludes, as have other aphasiologists, by emphasizing that group therapy should be used only to complement individual therapy. We would concur, with the added suggestion that group therapy may not be appropriate for all patients and that the decision to institute it must depend on the therapist's awareness of the patient's emotional state and need. We should also bear in mind that group therapy can be a realistic, even if not an ideal, substitute for families who can ill afford the expense of individual therapy.

RESEARCH CONSIDERATIONS

This chapter has raised many issues regarding psychosocial correlates of aphasia and its resultant complications. Many inferences have been made based on the literature investigated as well as on clinical experiences. Consequently, we may wish to consider the directions research needs to take in order to validate several of the assumptions that have been made and collateraly discuss the design problems.

Personality Type

One interesting line of investigation might be the study of personality type as a precipitating factor in the onset of cerebral vascular attack. The value of such research could lead to definitive preventive measures, but also raises crucial questions regarding experimental design, among which are heterogeneity of population variance, difficulties with retrospective studies, and single-subject versus multisubject designs. Rollin (1972) has identified the heterogeneity factor as a confounding element in any aphasia research using control and experimental populations. Rabkin (1982) refers to the difficulties incurred by use of retrospective designs in terms of errors of recall by subjects, retrospective falsification to justify illness, and the differences between the evidence gathered by case study and results from prospective research. The problem she indicates is not so much the method as it is the misinterpretation of the results. Multisubject designs demand strict homogeneity and process delineation of personality patterns (whatever they are), psychosocial factors, and the complex interweaving of the two. Single-subject designs may be more precise, allowing for intensive clinical studies, but they hinder us in the generalization of the results to other subjects. Probably the most sophisticated, but unfortunately most costly as well, approach would be the longitudinal study in which a randomly selected and tested population is followed over a period of time, as in the Framingham studies.

Family Communication Scale

The development of a family functional communication scale for the measurement of pragmatic language competence in the aphasic adult would be another challenge to pursue. We have already alluded to the exciting work of Holland and Lubinski and their environmentally based testing and treatment strategies. We propose using the family therapy process as the model for determining how the family uses language in relationship to the patient's disordered use. We would attempt to measure the patient's functional usage over time, from onset, using a modification of the microanalysis method developed by Labov and Fanshel (1977). Such an approach would certainly not be free of obstacles. The complexity and uniqueness of "family communication" could defy standardization and predictability. As a measure of the way an individual's disrupted language system may recover, over a period of time, however, it presents us with challenging opportunities for constructive family participation in recovery and a method for complementing traditional speech-language treatment strategies.

REFERENCES

ADLER, R. Intrinsic psychoperceptual disorientation during the acute stage post-stroke and brain trauma. Unpublished doctoral dissertation. Walden University, Naples, Florida (1980).

ALBERT, M. A., GOODCLASS, H., HELM, N. A., RUBENS, A. B., and ALEXANDER, M. P. *Clinical Aspects of Dysphasia.* New York: Springer-Verlag, 1981.

ARTES, R., and HOOPS, R. Problems of aphasia and non-aphasia stroke patients as identified and evaluated by patients' wives. In Y. Lebrun and R. Hoops (Eds.), *Neurolinguistics, Vol. 4: Recovery in Aphasics.* Amsterdam: Swets and Zeitlinger, 1976.

ATEN, J. L., CALIGIURI, M. P., and HOLLAND, A. L. The efficacy of functional communication therapy for chronic aphasia patients. *Journal of Speech and Hearing Disorders,* 47 (1982), 93–96.

BARETZ, R. M., and STEPHENSON, G. R. Unrealistic patient. *New York State Journal of Medicine,* 76 (1976), 54–57.

BLACK, F. W. Unilateral brain lesions and MMPI performance: A preliminary study. *Perceptual and Motor Skills,* 40 (1975), 87–93.

BOWLBY, J. *Separation and Loss.* Englewood Cliffs, N.J.: Basic Books, 1970.

BRESLAU, L. D., and HAUG, M. R., (Eds.), *Depression and Aging: Causes, Care and Consequences.* New York: Springer-Verlag, 1983.

BUCK, M. *Dysphasia: Professional Guidance for Family and Patient.* Englewood Cliffs, N.J.: Prentice-Hall, 1968.

BUSCH, E. Physical symptoms in neurosurgical disease. *Acta Psychiatrica et Neurologica Scandinavica,* 15 (1940), 257–290.

CODE, C., and MULLER, D. J. Interpersonal perceptions of psychosocial adjustment to aphasia. In D.J. Muller and C. Code (Eds.), *Apahsia Therapy.* London: Edward Arnold, 1983.

DAVIS, G. A. *A Survey of Adult Aphasia.* Englewood Cliffs, N.J.: Prentice-Hall, 1983.

DAVIS, J. M., SEGAL, N. L., and SPRING, G. K. "Biological and Genetic Aspects of Depression in the Elderly." In L. D. Breslau and M. R. Haug (Eds.) Depression and Aging, Causes, Care & Consequences. New York: Springer, 1983.

DOHRENWEND, B. S., ASKENASY, A. R., FRASNOFF, L., and DOHRENWEND, B. P. The psychiatric epidemiology research interview life events scale. In L. Goldberger and S. Breznitz (Eds.), *Handbook of Stress: Theoretical and Clinical Aspects.* New York: Macmillan, 1982.

EISENSON, J. *Adult Aphasia,* 2nd ed. Englewood Cliffs, N.J.: Prentice-Hall, 1984.

ENGELS, G. L. Grief and grieving. *American Journal of Nursing,* 64 (1964), 93.

ENGELS, G. L. A unified concept of health and disease. In T. Millon (Ed.), *Medical Behavior Science.* Philadelphia: Saunders, 1975.

EVANS, J. G. Hypertension and stroke in an elderly population. *Acta Medica Scandinavica Supplementum No. 676* (1983), 23–32.

FRIEDMAN, M. H. On the nature of regression in aphasia. *Archives of General Psychiatry,* 5 (1961), 60–64.

GAINOTTI, G. Emotional behavior and hemisphere side of the lesion. *Cortex*, 8 (1972), 41–55.

GASPARINI, W., SATZ, P., HEILMAN, K. M., and COOLIDGE, F. L. Hemispheric asymmetries of affective processing as determined by the Minnesota Multiphasic Personality Inventory. *Journal of Neurology, Neurosurgery, and Psychiatry*, 41 (1978), 470–473.

GESCHWIND, N. The borderland of neurology and psychiatry: Some common misconceptions. In D. E. Benson and D. Blumer (Eds.), *Psychiatric Aspects of Neurologic Disease*. New York: Grune & Stratton, 1975.

GOLDBERG, S. A. The aphasic's need to understand his linguistic disability. Paper presented to the annual convention of California Speech-Language-Hearing Association, Los Angeles, 1980.

GOLDSTEIN, K. Functional disturbances in brain damage. In S. Arieti (Ed.), *American Handbook of Psychiatry*. New York: Basic Books. 1959.

———.The effect of brain damage on the personality. *Psychiatry*, 15 (1952), 245–260.

———.*Language and Language Disturbances*. New York: Grune & Stratton, 1948.

———.*Aftereffects of Brain Injuries in War*. New York: Grune & Stratton, 1942.

HASPIEL, M., CLEMENT, J. R., and HASPIEL, G. S. Aural rehabilitation for hard of hearing adults. San Francisco Veterans Administration Hospital, unpublished manuscript prepared for distribution, 1972.

HECAEN, H. Clinical symptomatology in right and left hemispheric lesions. In V. B. Mountcastle (Ed.), *Interhemispheric Relations and Cerebral Dominance*. Baltimore: John Hopkins University Press, 1962.

HELMICK, J. W., WATAMORI, T. S., and PALMER, J. M. Spouses' understanding of the communication disabilities of aphasic patients. *Journal of Speech and Hearing Disorders*, 41, (1976), 238–243.

HILLBOM, E. After-effects of brain injuries. *Acta Psychiatrica et Neurologica Scandinavica, Supplementum No. 142* (1960), 35.

HOLLAND, A. L. Comment on "Spouses' understanding of the communication abilities of aphasic patients." *Journal of Speech and Hearing Disorders*, 42, (1977), 307–310.

HOLT, R. R. Occupational stress. In L. Goldberger and S. Breznitz (Eds.), *Handbook of Stress: Theoretical and Clinical Aspects*, New York: Macmillan, 1982.

HOMMES, D. R. Stemmingsanomalien als neurologisch symptoom. *Nederlands Tijdschrift voor Geneeskunde*, 109 (1965), 588–589.

HORENSTEIN, S. Effects of cerebrovascular disease in personality and emotionality. In A. L. Benton (Ed.), *Behavioral Change in Cerebrovascular Disease*. New York: Harper & Row, 1970.

HURVITZ, N. Peer self-help psychotherapy groups and their implications for psychotherapy. *Psychotherapy: Theory and Research*, 7 (1970), 4–49.

JENKINS, C. D. Recent evidence supporting psychologic and social risk factors for coronary disease. *New England Journal of Medicine*, 294 (1976), Part I, 987–994; Part II, 1033–1038.

JENKINS, C. D., ROSENMAN, R. H., and FRIEDMAN, M. Replicability of rating the coronary-prone behavior pattern. *British Journal of Preventive and Social Medicine*, 22 (1968), 16–22.

JENKINS, J. J., JIMENEZ-PABON, E., SHAW, R. E., and DEFER, J. W. *Schuell's Aphasia in Adults*, 2nd ed. New York: Harper & Row, 1975.

KANNEL, W.B., and GORDON, T. (Eds.) *The Framingham Study*. DHEW Publication (NIH). Washington, D.C.: U.S. Government Printing Office, 1974.

KESCHNER, M., BENDER, M. B., and STRAUSS, I. Mental symptoms in cases of tumor of the temporal lobe. *Archives of Neurology and Psychiatry*, 35 (1936), 572–596.

KINSELLA, G. The spouse of the aphasic patient. In Y. Lebrun and R. Hoops (Eds.), *The Management of Aphasia*. Amsterdam: Swets and Zeitlinger, 1978.

KINSELLA, G., and DUFFY, F. Psychosocial readjustment in the spouses of aphasic patients. *Scandinavian Journal of Rehabilitation Medicine*, 11 (1979), 129–132.

KÜBLER-ROSS, E. *Death: the Final Stage of Growth*. Englewood Cliffs, N.J.: Prentice-Hall, 1975.

———.*On Death and Dying*. New York: Macmillan, 1969.

LABOV, W., and FANSHEL, D. *Therapeutic Discourse: Psychotherapy as Conversation*. New York: Academic Press, 1977.

LAMENDELLA, J. T. The limbic system in human communication. In H. Whitaker and H. A. Whitaker (Eds.), *Studies in Neurolinguistics*, Vol. 3, New York: Academic Press, 1977.

LAZARUS, R., and LAUNIER, R. Stress-related transactions between person and environment. In L. Pervin and M. Lewis (Eds.), *Perspectives in Interactional Psychology*. New York: Plenum, 1978.

LEZAK, M. D. Living with characteristically altered brain injured patients. *Journal of Clinical Psychiatry,* 39 (1979), 592−598.

LINEBAUGH, C. W., and YOUNG-CHARLES, H.Y. The counseling needs of the families of aphasic patients. In R. K. Brookshire (Ed.), *Clinical Aphasiology Conference Proceedings.* Minneapolis, Minn.: BRK Publishers, 1978.

LUBINSKI, R. Environmental language stimulation. In R. Chapey (Ed.), *Language Intervention and Strategies in Adult Aphasia.* Baltimore: Williams & Wilkins, 1981.

MALONE, R. L. Expressed attitudes of families of aphasics. *Journal of Speech and Hearing Disorders,* 34 (1969), 146−151.

MANUEL, M. Doing it the family way. *The Nursing Mirror,* 149 (1979), 28−34.

MEICHENBAUM, D., and TURK, D. Stress, coping and disease: A cognitive-behavioral perspective. In W. J. Neufell (Ed.), *Psychological Stress and Psychopathology.* New York: McGraw-Hill, 1982.

MOUSTAKAS, C. E. *Loneliness and Love.* Englewood Cliffs, N.J.: Prentice-Hall, 1972.

MULHALL, D. Dysphasic stroke patients and the influence of their relatives. *British Journal of Disorders of Communication,* 13 (1978), 127−134.

PORTER, J. L., and DABUL, B. The application of transactional analysis to therapy with wives of adult aphasic patients. *Asha* 19 (1977), 244−248.

RABKIN, J. G. Stress and psychiatric disorders. In L. Goldberger and S. Breznitz (Eds.), *Handbook of Stress: Theoretical and Clinical Aspects.* New York: Macmillan, 1982.

REDINGER, R. A., FORSTER, S., DOLPHIN, M. K., GOODDUHN, J., and WEISINGER, J. Group therapy in the rehabilitation of the severely aphasic and hemiplegic in the late stages. *Scandinavian Journal of Rehabilitation Medicine,* 3 (1971), 89−91.

ROBINSON, R. G., and BENSON, D. F. Depression in aphasic patients: Frequency, severity, and clinical-pathological correlations. *Brain and Language,* 14 (1981), 282−291.

ROLLIN, W. J. Family therapy and the aphasic adult. In J. Eisenson, *Adult Aphasia,* 2nd ed. Englewood Cliffs, N.J.: Prentice-Hall, 1984.

——.Oral responses of aphasics under different syntactical conditions. In M. T. Sarno (Ed.), *Aphasia: Selected Readings,* New York: Appleton-Century-Crofts, 1972.

ROSKIES, E., and LAZARUS, R. Coping theory and the teaching of coping skils. In P. Davidson (Ed.), *Behavioral Medicine: Changing Health Lifestyles.* New York: Brunner/Mazel, 1979.

ROSSI, G. F., and ROSADINI, G. Experimental analysis of cerebral dominance in men. In C. H. Millikan and F. L. Darley (Eds.), *Brain Mechanisms Underlying Speech and Language.* New York: Grune & Stratton, 1967.

SACKEIM, H. A., GREENBERG, M. S., WEIMAN, A. L., GUR, R. C., HUNGERBAHLER, J. P., and GESCHWIND, N. Hemispheric asymmetry in the expression of positive and negative emotions: Neurological evidence. *Archives of Neurology,* 39 (1982), 210−218.

SACIKEIM, H. A., and WEBER, S. L. Functional brain asymmetry in the regulation of emotion: Implications for bodily manifestations of stress. In L. Goldberger and S. Breznitz (Eds.), *Handbook of Stress.* New York: Macmillan, 1982.

SAHS, A. L., HARTMAN, E. C., and ARONSON, S. M. (Eds.). *Guidelines for Stroke Care.* DHEW Publication No. (HRA) 76-14017. Washington, D.C.: U.S. Government Printing Office, 1976.

SALZMAN, C., and SHADER, R. I. Depression in the elderly, Part I. Relationship between depression, psychologic defense mechanism and physical illness. *Journal of the American Geriatric Society,* 26, (1978), 210−253.

SARNO, J. Emotional aspects of aphasia. In M. T. Sarno (Ed.), *Acquired Aphasia.* New York: Academic Press, 1981.

SATIR, V. *Conjoint Family Therapy.* Palo Alto, Calif.: Science and Behavior Books, 1967.

SCHUELL, H., JENKINS, J. J., and JIMENEZ-PABON. *Aphasia in Adults.* New York: Harper & Row, 1964.

SELYE, H. *The Stress of Life.* New York: McGraw-Hill, 1966.

SERAFETINIDES, E. A., and FALCONER, M. A. The effect of temporal lobectomy in epileptic patients with psychosis. *Journal of Mental Science,* 109 (1962), 584−593.

SHONTZ, F. Reactions to crisis. *Volta Review,* 65 (1965), 364−370.

SKELLY, M. Aphasic patients talk back. *American Journal of Hearing,* 7 (1975), 1140−1142.

TANNER, D. C. Loss and grief: Implications for the speech-language pathologist and audiologist. *Asha* 22 (November 1980), 916−928.

TAYLOR, F. C. Project cope. In E. J. Webster (Ed.), *Professional Approaches with Parents of Handicapped Children.* Springfield, Ill.: Chas. C Thomas, 1976.

TERZIAN, H. Behavioral and EEG effects of intracarotid sodium amytal injection. *Acta Neuro-chirurgica*, 12 (1964), 230–239.

TSUNODA, T., and OKA, M. Lateralization for emotion in the human brain and auditory cerebral dominance. *Proceedings of the Japan Academy*, 52 (1976), 528–531.

ULLMAN, M. *Behavioral Changes in Patients Following Strokes*. Springfield, Ill.: Chas. C Thomas, 1962.

U.S. DEPARTMENT OF HEALTH, EDUCATION, AND WELFARE. National Center for Health Statistics. *Prevalence of Cerebral Vascular Disease*. Personal communication, 1984.

———.Public Health Service. *Prevalence of Published Chronic Conditions, Rates by Sex and Age. United States, 1981.* Unpublished data from the National Health Interview Survey, National Center for Health Statistics, Rockville, Md., 1983.

———.Public Health Service. *Prevalence of Chronic Circulatory Conditions. United States, 1972.* DHEW Publication No. (HRA) 75-1521, National Center for Health Statistics, Rockville, Md., 1974.

WEBSTER, E.J., and NEWHOFF, M. Intervention with families of communicatively impaired adults. In D. S. Beasley and G. A. Davis (Eds.), *Aging: Communication Processes and Disorders*. New York: Grune & Stratton, 1981.

WEINSTEIN, E., and KAHN, R. *Denial of Illness*. Springfield, Ill.: Chas. C Thomas, 1955.

WERTZ, R. T., COLLINS, M. J., WEISS, D., KURTZKE, J. F., FRIDEN, T., BROOKSHIRE, R. H., PIERCE, J., HOLZAPPLE, P., HUBBARD, D. J., PORCH, B. E., WEST, J. A., DAVIS, L., MATOVITCH, V., MORLEY, G. K., and RESURRECICION, E. Veterans Administration cooperative study on aphasia: A comparison of individual and group treatment. *Journal of Speech and Hearing Research*, 24 (1981), 580–594.

ZEGANS, L. S. Stress and the development of somatic disorders. In L. Goldberger and S. Breznitz (Eds.), *Handbook of Stress: Theoretical and Clinical Aspects*. New York: Macmillan, 1982.

3

PSYCHOLOGICAL CONSIDERATIONS OF THE TRAUMATICALLY HEAD INJURED AND THEIR FAMILIES

TRAUMATIC HEAD INJURY—THE NATURE OF THE INJURY

To understand the magnitude of traumatic head injury, we would define it as a cognitive, intellectual, emotional, and physical impairment resulting from multiple and/or diffuse lesions in the brain due to sudden injury from an external source. Griffith (1983), adapting from Rosenthal (1979), has created an extensive list of the postraumatic psychological sequelae of severe traumatic brain-injured patients (see Table 1).

Although precise figures are unavailable, the two major types of head injury are closed head or nonmissile injury, due to vehicular accidents and other blunt traumas to the head, and missile injury, such as gunshot wounds. As Levin, Benton, and Grossman (1982) state in the preface of their book on closed head injury:

> The personal, social, and economic consequences of head injuries, particularly those resulting from automobile accidents, assaults, and athletic mishaps, can scarcely be overestimated. Thanks to the remarkable life-saving capabilities of modern neurosurgical management of acute severe head injuries, the number of patients surviving such injuries mount steadily. . . . Hence in recent years,

TABLE 1. Psychologic Disabilities

A. Cognitive-intellectual
   1. Disorders of consciousness
   2. Disorientation
   3. Memory deficits
   4. Decreased abstraction
   5. Decreased learning abilities
   6. Language-communication deficits
   7. General intellectual deficits
   8. Deficits in processing-sequencing information
   9. Illogical thoughts
   10. Poor judgment
   11. Poor quality control
   12. Inability to make decisions
   13. Poor initiative
   14. Verbal, motor perserveration
   15. Confabulation
   16. Difficulty in generalization
   17. Short attention span
   18. Distractability
   19. Fatigability
   20. Perplexity
   21. Dyscalculia
B. Perceptual-perceptual motor
   1. Reduced motor speed
   2. Reduced eye hand coordination
   3. Poor depth perception
   4. Spatial disorientation
   5. Poor figure-ground perception
   6. Auditory perceptual deficits
   7. Anosognosia
   8. Autotopagnosia
   9. Tactile, auditory, visual neglect
   10. Apraxias
C. Emotional
   1. Apathy
   2. Impulsivity
   3. Irritability
   4. Aggressiveness
   5. Anxiety
   6. Depression
   7. Emotional lability
   8. Silliness
D. Behavioral-personality
   1. Lack of goal-directed behavior
   2. Lack of initiation
   3. Poor self-image, reduced self-worth
   4. Denial of disability or its consequences
   5. Aggressive behavior
   6. Childlike behavior
   7. Bizarre, psychotic ideation and behavior
   8. Loss of sensitivity and concern for others: selfishness
   9. Dependency, passivity

TABLE 1. *(continued)*

10. Indecision
11. Indifference
12. Slovenliness
13. Sexual disturbances
14. Drug, alcohol abuse

Adapted from: Rosenthal, M: *Psychological Deficits in the Brain-Injured Adult and Family.* Presented at Conference on Rehabilitation of the Traumatic Brain-Injured Adult, Williamsburg, Va, June 1979. (Griffith, 1983).

the focus of interest has shifted to a considerable degree from the fact of survival to the question of the *quality* of survival of the posttraumatic patient.

The effects of traumatic head injury are also experienced by the injured individual's family, resulting in often profound psychological and social changes in family members.

Comparison to Aphasia

In contrast to aphasia (discussed in Chapter 2), traumatic head injury presents a very different picture. Except for penetrating missile wounds, traumatic head injury generally results in diffuse lesions of the cerebral cortex rather than the characteristic focal ones in aphasia. In traumatic head injury, cognitive deficits in conjunction with emotional and behavioral changes are more pronounced. Although these persons may also be aphasic, as in the case of those who suffer a penetration wound, their prognosis for recovery appears more favorable than that of aphasia victims (Levin 1981).

A further distinguishing characteristic is that aphasia, which results from cerebral vascular disease, is related to the overall aging process, whereas traumatic head injury generally occurs in a much younger population. And, as we explain later, the psychosocial ramifications are much different. Finally, there is a greater likelihood of direct subcortical lesions and severance of the hemispheres at the corpus callosum in traumatically head-injured patients. These may have significantly greater neuropsychological consequences than in aphasia associated with cerebral vascular disease.

Incidence and Prevalence—Statistical Data

From the results of a major project conducted by the Santa Clara Valley Medical Center (SCVMC), a major regional head injury rehabilitation center in San Jose, California, it has been estimated that nearly 500,000 cases of head injury occur in the United States annually (1982). It has also been determined that between 1970 and 1974 more than 900,000 head-injured people were still suffering from the effects of their injuries. Thus, at any one time in the United States, one out of approximately 220 individuals is suffering the effects of head injury and requires medical, restorative, maintenance, or rehabilitative care. The figures cited do not, however, include those with permanent disabilities who are not using the health care services stated above. It is important to note that the data collected in the SCVMC study also do not include those individuals who, because of minor head injuries, were not admitted for hospital care despite significant cognitive impairment from transient loss of consciousness or severe concussion.

In fact, head injuries have been characterized by many specialists as the "silent epidemic," a term suggesting that the actual number of head injuries is much higher because physicians often fail to recognize head injuries when other injuries are more apparent. Recovery is impeded, and the head injured often do not receive needed treatment because of the absence of easily observable symptoms. These are people who generally look well and act appropriately, but who indeed may be suffering emotionally.

Fortunately, more and more physicians are recognizing the real damage that may be brought about by supposedly minor head injuries. Because of the development and refinement of new diagnostic instruments—computerized axial tomography scanners (CAT), positron emitted tomography (PET), nuclear magnetic resonance (NMR), brain electrical activity mapping (BEAM), regional cerebral blood flow (rCBF), and the magneto-encephalogram (MEG)—brain damage that escaped detection earlier is now revealed. Our increased knowledge of cranial physiology has further contributed to our understanding.

Profile of the Patient

According to Jennett and Macmillan (1981), the incidence of head injuries is highest among males between the ages of fifteen and thirty-five. Similar findings have been verified by Kraus (1980). Research by Kerr, Kay, and Lassman (1971) has shown the ratio of male to female patients admitted to hospitals is approximately 4:1, with an incidence rate peaking in the fifteen to twenty-four age range.

Kerr, Kay, and Lassman (1971) were able to establish a relationship between hospital admissions for head injury and a lower socioeconomic class in their Newcastle, England, study of 386 patients. They also noted a tendency toward a relationship between assault as a cause of injury and the lowest socioeconomic class, whereas sports-related injuries were common to upper socioeconomic groups. Findings in England and America have been supported by those in Australia, where Selecki, Hoy, and Ness (1968) found head injury admissions to predominate for laborers and craftsmen, with incidence among business people, clerical workers, and housewives being significantly lower.

Jennett (1983) reports in a study in the United States that 72 percent of head-injured patients had had alcohol upon hospital admission and 52 percent were intoxicated by legal definition. Kerr, Kay, and Lassman (1971) had earlier found alcohol to be a predisposing cause for head injury, particularly in motor vehicle accidents and in domestic accidents and assaults. Levin, Benton, and Grossman (1982) indicate that, based on previous studies, one-fourth to one-half of all severe head injuries are among chronic alcoholics.

Although the literature establishing precise relationships between specific psychiatric disorders and incidence of traumatic head injury is inconclusive, psychological factors appear to be a contributing factor to the occurrence of head injury. An early study by Fahy, Irving, and Millac (1967) in England revealed that 46 percent of the patients with head injuries admitted to hospitals presented evidence of social maladjustment. And in their study, Kerr, Kay, and Lassman (1971) found the incidence of head injury among the divorced to be four times that expected in the general population. One inference from such a connection is that some persons who have not recovered psychologically from their divorce might be more prone to serious accidents.

There appears to be some evidence also that individuals who have sustained one head injury are three times more likely to be head injured a second time and eight times as likely to have subsequent injuries, according to Annegers et al. (1980). They indicate that alcohol abuse is the predominant behavioral pattern contributing to repeated head injury in adults. These results must be viewed cautiously, however, considering the profound characterological changes that may occur after the first injury.

Although the research thus far has only begun to explain epidemiological aspects related to the incidence of traumatic head injury, it is apparent that socioeconomic and psychosocial factors play a major contributing role. It is with these factors that we must be concerned if we are to cope successfully with the posttraumatic patient. Also, less is known about the premorbid personality characteristics of the head-injured person, but it would be presumptuous for us to assume that there is a pre-accident—prone personality type, particularly when we consider the incidence of head injury among innocent victims. Nonetheless, we cannot ignore the cited evidence that suggests a prevalence of self-destructive individuals who have sustained traumatic head injury and who are being treated in hospitals and rehabilitation centers.

We view with considerable interest that falls are another major cause of injury, with two groupings: under age fifteen and over age seventy (Rimel and Jane 1983). Cartlidge and Shaw (1981) found that more than one-third of the over-seventy group of patients had recently taken alcohol and that the group is also more vulnerable to such hazards as unlit stairs, uneven pavement, and icy patches on the road, as well as confusion and unsteadiness.

The younger group is prone to injuries from falling for different reasons. In fact, Oddy (1984) stated that accidents in the home are the most common cause of head injury in children under three years of age, with "baby-battering" responsible for an unknown proportion. Falls occur so frequently that they are often used to cover up child abuse. Even sadder is the fact that child abuse is common enough that medical personnel have found skull fractures with particular features to be indicative of child abuse (Hobbs 1984). Hobbs acknowledges, however, "that more 'gently battered babies' might be indistinguishable from those having minor falls" (p. 251). Some authorities have advised consideration of head injury wherever abuse is suspected. The battered have recently been given the more socially accepted label of "nonaccidently injured" (Cartlidge and Shaw 1981).

It is worth noting, unfortunately, that injury caused by abuse is not necessarily unique to the younger population; the media have also brought to the public's attention in recent years that increased numbers of the elderly are physically abused by their adult children. Mention of this was not found in the related behavioral literature reviewed, however.

Rehabilitative Needs

During the last twenty years we have seen not only a dramatic increase of those individuals who have suffered traumatic head injury but also, as we noted earlier, the advent of almost miraculous medical procedures that have saved their lives. The modern efficiency of paramedic emergency teams and hospital trauma centers has played a part, along with the medical knowledge gained in battleground surgical theaters of the Vietnam War. Consequently, the need for acute and long-term care and rehabilitation has been accompanied by a demand for new procedures and techniques to cope with the personal, social, and economic needs of the patient.

The nature and extent of the injury   Throughout the United States and abroad, rehabilitation programs, often part of major medical centers, have been established to assist survivors of traumatic head injury and their families. Because these programs vary in magnitude, breadth, and kind, the patient may not always receive the individualized attention necessary for multidimensional recovery.

Levin, Benton, and Grossman (1982), citing reports by Najenson et al. (1974, 1978) and Rosenbaum et al. (1978), describe one of the foremost rehabilitation programs established. Responding to the casualities suffered by Israel in the Israeli-Arabic conflicts, the Lowenstein Rehabilitation Hospital in Raanana, Israel, was established to provide the most comprehensive treatment facility for the brain injured.

Active management begins with physical therapy for comatose patients, and during the transition from coma to normal orientation, the patient is encouraged to cooperate more actively. With wakefulness also emerges behavioral disturbances, which to an extreme may consist of transient psychoses. The patient's family is always included and encouraged to participate in providing a supportive and calm environment in order to facilitate a sense of security and reorientation for the patient. The recovery program also includes a comprehensive cognitive, intellectual, and communication assessment based on formal testing, family interviews, and informal behavioral observation.

Among the goals of treatment are helping the patient to develop skills that are indirectly and/or directly related to holding a job, to acquire adaptive behavior to deal with personal problems, and to enhance cognitive skills. The psychotherapist is primarily responsible for the patient's total rehabilitation program, and the therapist–patient relationship is considered the key to encouraging the widest range of skills and activities.

A team approach   We believe that the elements that should characterize the best of rehabilitation centers is a team approach. Because of the wide range of problems encountered with traumatic head injury, and because of the different types of injuries that vary along differing stages, many disciplines need to be involved in patient care. Among these we would include medical-surgical, nursing, neuropsychology, speech-language pathology, audiology, learning disability, physical, occupational, and vocational therapy, and social work. Although each of these areas has its own distinctive goals to pursue with the patient, no one of them can be totally effective without interfacing with the others.

It appears to us that the convergence of all of these disciplines must occur at the loci of the cognitive-emotional-behavioral changes. For the purposes of this chapter, we prefer to emphasize the psychosocial components, recognizing the difficulty in separating these from purely cognitive elements.

PSYCHOSOCIAL FACTORS SUBSEQUENT TO INJURY

The enormity of the psychosocial consequences of traumatic head injury has been described by many investigators. Lishman (1973), among them, presents considerable evidence "that the *long-continued* [sic] 'posttraumatic syndrome' rests principally on psychogenic mechanisms" (p. 316), and the degree to which the symptoms are prolonged is not dependent on the extent of severity of the brain damage. Levin, Benton, and Grossman (1982) not only believe that residual psychosocial behavioral disturbance persists even with partial recovery of cerebral dysfunction but that pretraumatic personality and extrinsic factors like litigation and family reactions can prolong and intensify many of the symptoms. Rosenthal et al. (1983), with chapter contributions from leading authorities, provide further evidence that the psychological problems of the head injured are more common and last longer than the physical ones.

In one of the most recent books on the subject, Brooks (1984) presents a comprehensive data base and conceptual framework for understanding the psychological, social, and family consequences of closed head injury.

With contributions from experts in the field, the most recent evidence is discussed relative to the psychiatry of closed head injury, attentional deficits, the psychological implications of head injury during childhood, and the psychological management of behavior disorders following severe head injury, among other related topics.

Changes in Affectual State

The quality and the degree of changes in the affectual state following head injury may vary from acute psychosis through neuroticisms to maladjustments.

Levin et al. (1982) describe the psychiatric consequences in terms of four states:

1. *Acute posttraumatic psychosis* in which the patient may manifest such behaviors as depressive psychosis, manic depressive psychosis, paranoid psychosis, or reactive psychosis. These may be observed in patients who are not comatose but who are confused and stuporous.
2. *Acute confusional state*, which includes acute agitation, traumatic delirium, disorientation, increased psychomotor activity, incoherent talkativeness, and indiscriminate movements, with perhaps transient periods of coma. "Agitation in these patients was manifested by thrashing of extremities, truncal rocking, dislodging intravenous tubes and catheters, yelling, combativeness, and attempts to get out of bed" (p. 175).
3. *Affective psychosis* in the subacute phase of recovery may include euphoria, depression, and prolonged disinhibitory behavior.
4. *Postconcussional syndrome*, which includes combined psychological and somatic symptoms characterized by "headache, anxiety, insomnia, hypochondriacal concern, hypersensitivity to noise, and photophobia."

Levin et al. note, however, that differentiation between neurological and psychological changes is not clear, as is reflected in the literature on the subject.

Neuropsychological Changes

Gronwall and Wrightson (1975, 1980) support the view that even after minor head injury, there is pathological evidence of microscopic lesions and that concussion is related to both a breakdown in information processing and characteristic behavioral symptoms. Bukay and Glasauer (1980) view postconcussion syndrome in minor head injury as a constellation of headache, irritability-restlessness, depression, insomnia, defective memory, fatigue, impaired concentration, dizziness-vertigo, and alcohol intolerance.

Blumer and Benson (1975) report on the now famous case of Phineas Gage who was head injured as a result of an explosion that sent a crowbar through his frontal lobe, penetrating his corpus collosum. Though he was thought to be a premorbidly psychologically healthy person, the injury was responsible for profound personality changes and regression intellectually.

His behavior was characterized by fitful moods of mania with associated childlike tantrums, inability to respond to advice from his friends, and marked impatience. He lived for twelve more years, never returning to his premorbid state, and meandered directionless until his death. In Chapter 2 we discussed the direct and indirect changes that occur in cerebral vascular accidents and that would be applicable in head injury.

Rosenthal (1983) considers the behavioral effects of closed head injury to the frontal lobes. Among the behavioral consequences discussed are "decreased drive, lack of goal-directed behavior, apathy, lethargy, social disinhibition, childish behavior, poor judgment, inappropriate sexual and aggressive behavior, and dull or flat affect" (p. 198). Because the frontal lobes apparently fulfill an "executive" function, it is understandable why frontal lobe–injured persons are unable to regulate and integrate their behavior and characteristically wander aimlessly with little sense of identity and lack of self-esteem. Rosenthal cites Harlow (1868), who originally documented the Phineas Gage case, and Blumer and Benson (1975), who considered the destruction of the prefrontal convexity, basal ganglia, and thalamus to result in antisocial, childish, and euphoric behavioral patterns somewhat akin to a "pseudopsychopathic" personality.

Although Lishman (1973) reports that the persistence of behavioral symptoms two or three months after a mild injury may reflect a constellation of premorbid neurotic symptoms, he also notes the occurrence of a disinhibition of aggression with temporal lobe lesions (Lishman 1968). Rosenthal (1983), citing Sweet, Ervin, and Mark (1968), discusses the disinhibition process associated with temporal lobe damage, characterized by violent verbal and physical outbursts in head-injured persons who experience minor environmental stresses. Although the aggressive behaviors appear to resemble behavioral changes associated with temporal lobe seizures, Rosenthal states that the incidence of posttraumatic epilepsy in head injury is minimal statistically (5 percent), and may not necessarily conform to classic temporal lobe seizures.

Most crucial to our understanding of the relationship of focal neurological evidence of destructive lesions with the presence of behavioral dysfunction is Rosenthal's (1983) admonition:

> Problems such as fluctuating depression, irritability, poor frustration tolerance, inability to deal with stress, and sexual dysfunction are often seen in head-injured persons, irrespective of the neuropathology of their injury. These behavioral changes may be attributable to the diffuse and widespread organic damage, the presence of pre-existing emotional and behavioral problems, or perhaps the response of the environment to the newly head-injured person. (p. 200)

It is the response of the environment, in conjunction with the secondary psychological manifestations, we shall now address.

Environment and Psychological Changes

Regardless of focal or diffuse head injury, the individual is thrust into a strange, frightening, and unfamiliar world, with the body and the brain struggling to regain a grip on reality. The perception of the actual reality by the patient is colored by the unique features that characterize that person's premorbid state and previous environment and certainly by the nature of the injury itself.

Bond (1983), citing the extensive review of the literature by Lezak (1978b), categorizes five major effects on personality and behavior:

1. *Capacity for social perceptiveness:* The patient loses the ability to be empathic with others, generally is self-centered, and does not appear capable of self-criticism.
2. *Capacity for self-control:* The patient is impatient, randomly restless, and impulsive.
3. *Learned social behavior:* The patient is impaired in the ability to organize, plan and make judgments with concomitant loss of initiative.
4. *Ability to learn:* Learning capacity is reduced, the patient demonstrating a slowing down and rigidity of mental processing abilities.
5. *Emotion:* The patient becomes labile, apathetic, often silly, and irritable, with reduced or increased sexual drive.

Indicating the obvious overlapping of these categories and the apparent connection between other cognitive-behavioral-social changes, Bond also cautions us that there is significant variation in the defects among the head injured. Furthermore, the pretraumatic personality characteristics certainly must be considered.

Recall our discussion of premorbid profiles of head-injured patients in which we noted that specific factors and certain personality characteristics appear to predispose many of them to injury. Thus such premorbid features as aggressiveness, anxiety, and anger are likely to be exacerbated. It is obvious, also, that depending on premorbid personality, patients will respond to their immediate hospital, rehabilitation center, and family environment in a particular manner. We need to bear in mind, however, that the nature of the physical injury itself may cause devastating psychological changes regardless of premorbid tendencies and postmorbid reactions.

There is no available evidence to suggest how neural reorganization occurs in individual patients and how these same patients establish their own organismic homeostasis. Perhaps many of the behavioral changes occur relative to the way in which each patient must adjust to the trauma experienced. What we have previously discussed as pathological behavior may in part be described as a quite normal reaction to an extraordinary shock to the brain, psyche, and body. Certainly even less is known about the overall recovery process after head injury in individual patients. Nevertheless, we are left with the task of understanding as much as possible about the personality and behavior changes in order to assist all head-injured patients toward recovery.

Specific Personality and Behavioral Changes

In discussing personality and behavioral changes, it is necessary that we consider them in the light of the various levels of change each patient undergoes. Further, because severity of injury determines in part the extent of the various disabling characteristics, we discuss personality and behavior changes regardless of injury type.

Impairment of judgment   Luria (1980) has described deficits in judgment in patients with damage to the prefrontal area. These patients may not be aware of all that is occurring in their immediate environment and often appear to act impulsively and hyperactively, without regard for others. They do not appear to process all the information that is available to them. Ben-Yishay and Diller (1983) describe impaired judgment in terms of loss of a cognitive function. These patients are unable to use good judgment in self-care activities such as dress, eating, and elimination needs. Verbal and nonverbal expressions or gestures are often inappropriate to the occasion, and such patients will often invade the privacy of others. They seem unable "to maintain 'friendliness' or 'chuminess' within proper bounds" (p. 175).

Denial   According to Rosenthal (1983), patients in a later stage of recovery (three to six months postmorbidly) tend to deny the extent of their disability, particularly when they have made substantial progress in ambulation and performance of daily activities. Disturbed by restrictions placed on their behavior, they become confused and upset.

It is not so much the physical disability that is being denied, but the cognitive and other mental concomitants to the brain insult. Although the patient may cooperate with members of the rehabilitation team in assessment and treatment procedures structured to deal with cognitive and other mental difficulties, he or she continues to deny overtly their existence and significance. The degree and quality of denial may range from an extreme euphoric "all is well" reaction to an opposite one of depression, that is, one of self-denigration and disavowal of intact abilities already present. As we shall discuss presently, the degree to which patients manifest denial may often be dependent on the family's own response to the patient and the injury.

Denial may be viewed also as an adaptive mechanism that may fend off a major emotional disorder. Further, it should not be confused with the patients' disordered thinking that interferes with their awareness of their actual deficits. Because patients are not reacting emotionally in a manner we think appropriate does not necessarily mean they are denying but, rather, that they are coping. Finally, we must be cautious in not equating real memory loss with denial, particularly when patients cannot recall unpleasant events.

Impaired capacity for control and self-regulation   Under this rubric, patients demonstrate impatience, impulsiveness, and random restlessness, according to Lezak (1978b). In the extreme state, patients are confused and agitated, detached from the present, and unable to process information. Less extreme is the tendency for patients to respond prematurely and/or inappropriately to requests or input from others. As Ben-Yishay and Diller (1983) describe it, patients demonstrate an inability to attend and concentrate. They are abnormally "stimulus bound" (distractible), disinhibited, and unable to modulate their responses.

Apathy and withdrawal   Under the heading of initiative, activity level, and emotional "tone," Ben-Yishay and Diller (1983) describe several subclasses: (1) the inability to initiate simple behaviors, verbal or nonverbal, without assistance from others; (2) the abnormal slowing down of responses, manifested by "laf" and waning rhythm; (3) the abnormal reduction in the way activities are carried out, which includes passivity and displays of "lack of stamina"; and (4) manifestations of an inability to relate emotionally to others as characterized by "flatness" of affect or "remoteness."

These patients also appear to be self-involved, that is, they are preoccupied with self or extraneous stimuli from their immediate environment. Their inability to remain tuned in may often give others the impression of severe intellectual impairment when it may actually represent a defense coping mechanism. Withdrawal from and apathy to activities structured by caregivers should not be interpreted as necessarily indicating stubbornness, rigidity of thought, or uncooperativeness, but may be the manifestation of complex primary and/or secondary effects.

Irritability, paranoia, and hostility   The degree to which head-injured patients demonstrate any one or combination of the above traits depends on the interrelationship of many factors, including the premorbid, neurological, and family elements. Caregivers can significantly help to extinguish such behaviors as long as they do not personalize them when bearing the brunt of attack from their patients. To do otherwise is to reinforce the patients' attitudes, thus causing greater frustration for all. Certainly it may be very difficult to determine what triggers irritable, paranoic, and hostile responses and how much is actually based on reality. Sometimes nothing more than uncaring handling by a rude aide may unleash a torrent of rage, out of proportion to the provocation.

Depression   The onset of depression may be viewed from either a primary deficit viewpoint or as a secondary manifestation. Levin et al. (1982), citing studies by Van Woerkom, Teelken, and Minderhoud (1977), Boismare, LePoncin, and LeFrancois (1977), and Grossman et al. (1975), report that neurotransmitter changes in the form of disturbance to brain catecholaminergic and cholinergic metabolism may bring about marked affective symptoms, including depression.

Viewing it as a secondary manifestation to brain injury, Rosenthal (1983) declares that patients experience a profound feeling of loss. Less able to function physically and feeling impotent and more dependent socially, they find safety in the depressed state. Rosenthal is quick to point out that in the rehabilitative phase of recovery such depression should be viewed positively "in that it signals the lessening of denial and usually reflects the patient's growing understanding and insight into the realization of the extent of the disability" (p. 204). He further notes that it may "be more related to the acknowledgment of the physical impairments caused by the injury, rather than the mental sequelae" (p. 204). Although the depression may not interfere profoundly with the patient's rehabilitation program as physical recovery continues, the prospect of new adjustments socially, vocationally, and educationally may bring on further depression. Once physical recovery plateaus, the likelihood of anxiety, frustration, sadness, and anger increases. In some cases suicide is contemplated.

In a very real sense the patient experiences a partial death, and, while not mourning in the way the family may (as we will discuss later), nevertheless passes through the stages of shock, denial, anger, and depression. The head-injured patient feels overwhelmed, finds the problem insurmountable, and realizes that life may never return to quite the way it was. The extent to which head-injured patients come to the latter realization cannot be determined, however, given the paucity of scientific investigations in this area.

Regression to childlike behavior and dependency   It is not unusual to see a regression to childlike behavior in head-injured adults. Their behavior is characterized by a desire to have needs satisfied immediately, to be unusually affectionate, and to demand constant attention. They will often defer from taking responsibility, relying on others to do things for them. They might also ignore the needs of others, and seem unconcerned with expressions of others' problems. Family members often feel as if they are talking to a stone wall. Interestingly, some young head-injured adults will acknowledge to family members or caregivers that they realize what they are doing, but add that they find it difficult to control their behavior. The degree to which primary or secondary effects of the brain injury are operating cannot be ascertained at the present time.

Other personality and behavioral changes   Varying degrees of anxiety, hypochondria, hypersensitivity, and poor self-esteem are also noted in some cases of head injury, but as with other behavioral changes, these may subside following the subacute stage. According to Levin, Benton, and Grossman (1982), cerebral dysfunction may be partly reversible, but in cases of psychoses, residual behavioral disturbance is more likely. Regardless of the degree and quality of the initial brain insult, the premorbid personality and psychosocial environment, along with postmorbid factors such as family reactions, personal problems, and poorly conceived rehabilitation attempts, may exacerbate and extend the symptom complex.

ADJUSTMENT PROBLEMS FOR THE FAMILY

The psychological and social upheaval to the family brought about by head injury to one of its members is well known. In terms of family systems theory (discussed in Chapter 2), the equilibrium of the family has been traumatically disrupted, creating not only profound changes in other members but also altering the interpersonal relationships of all members, including the patient. Regardless of the extent of the initial insult, the family shares with the victim the long and tedious process of recovery. Barry (1984) describes the early period of the medical crisis as a time when everyone's energy is geared toward surviving the initial crisis. As the patient proceeds through the recovery period, family members also experience varying stages of recovery. The way in which each family member copes with the recovery process and the reality of the life situation affects all family members, including the patient and the family as an entity. Because family members differ from each other, no one member will respond similarly, so the adjustment process and its time line vary for each.

The Grieving Process

Not unlike the grieving process experienced by family members in response to the physical death of another family member is the response to brain injury when actual death does not occur. Grief is both a natural response to loss and an important aspect of the recovery process. As described by Kübler-Ross (1969), the family goes through various stages to reach a point where the loss can finally be accepted. Because the "death" is within the personal system and not complete, it has been characterized by Muir (1978) as "mobile mourning." Unlike definitive death, there appears to be a more diffuse process involving the various stages through which the family passes. Nonetheless, these stages can be determined.

The first stage is shock caused by what has happened and the denial of its occurrence. Denial may assume the form of optimism that the patient has survived a life-threatening injury and thus has taken on aspects of immortality (Lezak 1978a, b; Bond 1983). Unrealistic pressure may later be put on the patient in efforts to deny the reality of the condition, for example, the patient's limitations may be criticized as caused by "laziness."

Following this is anxiety or panic where the family feels helpless in coping with the disruption in their lives. According to Bond (1983, 1984), the family transforms the anxiety or panic into anger and may express this to members of the hospital staff when the staff refuse to confirm the family's false hopes and to the victim himself when he becomes irritable and egocentric or when spontaneous recovery begins to plateau. The anger toward others transforms into anger at self, resulting in feelings of guilt, particularly when family members contrast their good health with the precarious health of the patient (Lezak 1978; Barry 1984).

Bargaining, according to Lezak (1978b), is evidenced as the family exhausts itself in providing excess care in hopes and expectations for a rapid recovery. This may have a negative effect on the patient, who may now make unrealistic demands on the family, when in fact she or he should be initiating self-care.

Eventually, depression becomes part of the grieving process. Overwhelmed by all that has happened, the reality of loss—that life for the patient may never be the same—is finally realized. Finally, the bewildered family gradually accepts what has happened, attaining a realistic understanding of the patient's assets and liabilities. The patient is accepted and dealt with in his or her present reality. According to Barry (1984), the family recognizes the actual limits dictated by the disability.

In a study of thirteen head trauma patients over a four-year period, Romano (1974) found negligible movements through the grief stages as described above. She found denial to be the predominant stage, evidenced in the common fantasy (the "sleeping beauty" syndrome) that the injured patient would awaken from the coma in the premorbid state. Families also fantasized improvement when, in fact, none had occurred. Once the patient emerged from the coma, denial would persist that the patient had altered in any way. Romano maintains that anger—at the hospital staff, doctor, and patient—was still a denial of the patient's condition. Denial was further manifested in isolation from social activities as the family defensively protected the patient's "normalcy." As the injured victim began the recovery process, the family would deny to the patient personal limitations and thus would do the patient (and themselves) irreparable harm. Romano suggests that persistence of this denial stage indicated rejection of the mourning process because, though the body was still alive, the family could not accept that the person known premorbidly was essentially dead.

The author's own experience with families of head-injured patients over twenty-five years, as well as reports from fellow workers, confirm the extent of the denial process. We would remind the reader, however, that it may be important for the family to deny, to an extent, in order to re-establish family equilibrium. Virtually no published data indicate how long a family can remain stuck in the denial stage without it being characterized as abnormal. Perhaps, as with the other stages of grief, each family responds uniquely with its own internal adjustment process, so that any absolute norm may be impossible to establish.

Though little significant data have been published indicating the value of the family to the patient's recovery, according to Diehl (1983) there is little doubt that family support is critical to satisfactory progress. Fahy, Irving, and Millac (1967) surveyed twenty-six families six years posttrauma and concluded that where family support was lacking, patients became socially withdrawn. Romano (1974) also appears to support these findings, suggesting that social deprivation may lead to depression in the patient.

Thomsen (1974) did a follow-up study of fifty young head-injured patients and reported that most patients continued to suffer from lack of family contact and nearly all relatives complained of the patients' change in personality and behavior. Thomsen stresses the need for long-term treatment and support of the patient as well as the family.

The Plight of the Spouse

In Chapter 2 we discussed the profound effects a stroke has on the family and in particular on the female spouse. We believe the effect is even greater for the spouse (usually the wife) of a head-injured patient because the patient is typically much younger than the stroke victim. Further, because the use of excessive alcohol shortly before injury is the most firmly established correlate as noted by Levin, Benton, and Grossman (1982), as well as a history of impulse-control and antisocial behavior problems, the significance of the premorbid marital relationship cannot be underestimated.

The premorbid relationship   Although there is virtually no research, prospective or retrospective, to isolate a characteristic dysfunctional premorbid marital relationship, environmental difficulties that may have long been present will have to be identified in order to enhance rehabilitation efforts more effectively. Just as premorbid traits of instability and inadequacy contribute to the form that postmorbid dysfunction takes (Lishman 1973), so must the nature of the premorbid marital relationship.

The postmorbid relationship   Romano (1974), Lezak (1978b), Bond (1983), and others report the spouse to be particularly victimized by the plight of the head-injured patient, as she agonizes over the loss of a partner for whom she cannot mourn in the typical sense. Her attempts to mourn are unsuccessful because the "body" (that is, the patient) is still functioning. The wife's despair is intensified by a society that neither acknowledges her grief nor provides support and comfort as would benefit a widow.

Rosenbaum and Najenson (1976) discuss how the wife's role changes abruptly from equal partner to mother surrogate or nurse. Emotions ranging from desolation to hostility are responses that accompany such role changes as she copes with the social isolation, after initial support by friends and extended family. Increased responsibility for household affairs, and childrearing, as well as having to deal with often critical and overprotective in-laws, may also result in a conflict between hostility toward the patient and guilt at having such feelings.

According to studies by Oddy, Humphrey, and Uttley (1978b), Thomsen (1974), and Painting and Merry (1972), the primary cause of depression in the spouse is related to the personality changes of the injured victim. Bond (1983) sees the wife enjoying little in her life now that she no longer has a husband as confidant. Because she receives little positive reinforcement from others in caring for her husband and children, she easily becomes vulnerable to depression. In the Rosenbaum and Najenson study (1976), the wives of brain-injured servicemen were considered to be more depressed and socially isolated than those of physically disabled servicemen, because the former had lost their intellectual capabilities, which more profoundly limited their function in society.

Further stress is brought to bear on the spouse when the patient becomes emotionally dependent and demands constant attention. As described by Rosenthal (1984), the spouse may reinforce this behavior to avoid further distress in the patient, herself, and/or the family. Often this encourages a negative situation, as "pampering will foster dependency, resentment and behavioral stagnation" (Lezak 1978b, p. 594). Other significant causes of stress to the wife might be the patient's poorly controlled behavior, such as pathological laughter and/or emotional lability, fear of epilepsy, dealing with associated physical disabilities, concern for the patient's prognosis, and fear of another accident (Oddy, Humphrey, and Uttley 1978b).

The incidence and prevalence of sexual dysfunction have been reported in several studies. Lezak (1978b) describes how the spouse's sexual and affectional needs are frustrated by the injured husband's inability to empathize and be sensitive to those needs. Childlike and dependent, the patient may be self-involved, unintentionally inconsiderate, or demanding for purely physical sexual relief. In research by Rosenbaum and Najenson (1976) concerning wives of brain-injured survivors one year after the Yom Kippur War, there was a drastic reduction in sexual relations. Although Oddy, Humphrey, and Uttley (1978a), claim that sexual dysfunction was not indicated in their six-month posttrauma study, a decrease as well as an increase in intercourse was evidenced. We would question, however, what is meant by their use of the term *dysfunction*.

Mauss-Clum and Ryan (1981), citing their own research and that of others, indicate that approximately 47 percent of the spouses reported either sexual disinterest or preoccupation in their brain-injured husbands. Either, we believe, could be considered "dysfunctional." It must be recognized, however, that because of the very personal nature of sexual activity, any definitive findings would be contaminated by subjectivity and/or misrepresented reports.

Prospects for the future relationship   Many factors will determine the outcome of the marital relationship, among which are (1) degree of personality and behavioral change in the victim; (2) premorbid marital relationship; (3) the spouse's attitude and level of support; (4) level of support for both victim and spouse from members of the extended family; and (5) the degree and quality of formal rehabilitation efforts, with particular emphasis on family counseling and/or therapy.

Oddy and Humphrey (1980) found in their study of fifty-four patients who had suffered closed head injury that, after one year, of the seven patients who were married, three spouses were rated as feeling less affectionate toward their partners. After two years one spouse and two patients reported their marital relationship to be worse than before the trauma. Thomsen (1974), in her follow-up study of fifty patients, found that the relationship between single patients and their mothers was essentially better than between married patients and their spouses. In six families where car accidents were involved, persistent feelings of spousal guilt continued to affect the relationships.

Bond (1983), summarizing earlier studies, concludes that the mental problems persist longer than the physical ones and have a more profound effect on the marital relationship. In time, as the reality of the new circumstance is acknowledged, the recovery plateaus, and as the marital couple no longer receives the support given earlier by outside sources, a new family equilibrium is established. Although Painting and Merry (1972) report a divorce rate of 40 percent, there is no definitive evidence that describes how the head-injured and their spouses relate to each other within the context of their changed lives. Perhaps many of these relationships will be characterized more by toleration than by mutual understanding and acceptance. Certainly, those couples who premorbidly were functioning well would be more likely to resume their lives, albeit differently.

In general, patients with less severe injuries will in time be more likely to settle into acceptable relationships with their spouses. Those with more severe injuries, who are likely to be more dependent, may have less satisfactory relationships, unless adequate counseling and support have been given to the spouse and family to help them with the adjustment. People with unsatisfactory premorbid relationships are likely to find such adjustment very difficult to cope with, and these may be families where separation and divorce are inevitable.

It would seem from Oddy and Humphrey's findings that the period when the family, and the spouse in particular, need the most support is usually when services are being withdrawn and the patient is returning home to face the future. This needs to be recognized by the rehabilitation team, and provision made for counseling services to be available even when the patient is no longer receiving direct services.

Specific Effects on the Family

Having discussed the possible effects of head injury on the spouse, it is important to consider what effects there may be on other members of the family as well. Although to a degree some similarities exist, the intrinsic nature of the patient and family member relationship will determine a different outcome. Of considerable interest are the effects on the children and parents of head-injured persons.

The children   When the father has been injured, it is not unusual for the children to suffer silently as attention is drawn to the victim and the plight of the spouse. The unbalancing of the family system may bring about temporary or permanent changes in family interrelationships, depending on the nature of the family system, the various premorbid roles of each member, and how each copes with the distress caused by the trauma.

Unfortunately, there have been few systematic studies of the effects of head injury on children in the family other than in those families when the parent has died for other reasons. Bowlby (1975), in his formidable essay, tracks the child who progresses through the stages of denial, euphoric hope, despair, and resignation.

Lezak (1978a, 1978b), one of the few writers who discusses the plight of children, describes them as being confused, fearful, and desperate. The young child tends to rely more on the mother for stability and comfort, thus increasing her burdens still further. The wife finds herself caught in a web of conflicting loyalties that she may resolve by either abandoning her mate or passively abandoning her child. The situation is further aggravated by the head-injured patient, who may deliberately tease or upset the child by immaturely competing for the wife's attention. The patient is likely to have an abnormal reaction to noise stimuli, making house play impossible. Large family gatherings during the holidays may have to be discontinued as the patient becomes withdrawn and/or irritable. Pathological laughter and outbreaks of verbal abuse and/or crying may make the home and home life intolerable.

Often the child's personal agony is reflected in truancy, delinquency, failure at school, or psychosomatic illness. Oddy, Humphrey, and Uttley (1978b) indicate that 25 percent of the relatives of brain-injured patients reported an illness at intervals of six months and twelve months postmorbidly. Older children may attempt to cope with their own feelings or the family's feelings by leaving home prematurely.

Rosenthal and Muir (1983) found that the social isolation of the family is felt most keenly by the adolescent and young adult, because they tend to lose peer contacts that are so vital to them. They also found that the child who sustains head trauma has a marked effect on siblings. Poor performance in school accompanied by guilt is not unusual, particularly when there have been unresolved premorbid sibling issues. There may also be a role reversal for the children whereby the big brother becomes the youngest child.

Rosenthal (1984) also found guilt in the siblings of head trauma patients. In addition, he found that the patient who played a significant positive role in his or her sib's life, but now who "can no longer be relied on for emotional support and assistance," will have profound effects on the uninjured siblings.

The parents Lezak (1978b) found that the families of brain-injured patients often have unrealistically high expectations regarding how much the patient will recover. The inability to understand and appreciate fully the profound changes that have occurred is related to the "family's natural optimism," which is "abetted by its conceptions of the disease." Bond (1983) has noted that families may develop overly high expectations for two reasons. First, in the beginning, patients do recover rapidly; second, the hospital staff may be reluctant to be specific about the long-term outcome. In this case, the family may push the patient too hard. For many people, particularly parents, the concept of irreversible disease is alien to their past experiences. After all, children, when they do get sick, usually get well. Lezak also believes that overly low expectations may be related to the family's need to protect the patient. However, this can lead to the patient's dependency, resentment, and behavioral stagnation.

Regardless of the reasons, parents of brain-injured patients often do have unrealistic expectations. Whether too high or too low, such expectations can interfere with the patient's recovery.

Intertwined with the unrealistic expectations of the parents is their denial of the severity or long-range effects of the injury. Romano (1974) found that in families of brain-injured patients, denial did not give way to anger, bargaining, and grief, as is usually the case in loss. Instead, it persisted for months, even years. She found that denial manifested itself in many ways—first, in fantasies: families would actually state that "He is only sleeping"; and second, in verbal refusals: "He always did have a temper." Often the family can recognize and even accept the physical, but not the mental, limitations of the patient. Third, family members responded inappropriately by overprotecting the patient.

Denial, as we have seen, may be a normal reaction of the head-injured person's family. However, if it lasts too long, as is frequently the case, it can produce an unstabling psychological condition that prevents the patient from accepting the disability and resuming a productive role in society.

A Case Study

The twenty-year-old son of a family personally known to me suffered severe head injury as a result of speeding on his motorcycle on a narrow curved street and hitting a tree. Rendered unconscious, Kevin spent one month in a coma close to death. Neurological findings revealed severe diffuse lesions involving the right frontal parietal cortex. Within one year of the accident, after intensive rehabilitation efforts, Kevin was ambulating independently, but with marked left-sided spasticity and with slowed dysarthric and dysarthrophonic speech and voice. He continued to demonstrate impaired judgment, memory, and attentional difficulties. Most evident was his decreased initiative and flat affectional state.

Having known this young man, albeit casually, premorbidly, I found him in marked contrast to the young man who had been gregarious and friendly, but in constant difficulty with the law for drug and alcohol abuse. I had also been aware of constant bickering with his parents, Joe and Ella, but a close relationship with a thirty-five-year-old sister, Diane. Somewhat from afar, I had viewed this family as one in which all members would characteristically "do their own thing" and one where the parents were essentially passive toward the activities of their children. Even the arrests were met with parental rationalizations and attempts to manipulate the legal authorities.

Although I had not been directly involved in Kevin's rehabilitation, Joe and Ella sought me out for assistance, knowing my professional position. The two counseling therapy sessions I had with the entire family eight months postmorbidly were characterized by extreme denial of the physical and mental changes that had occurred in Kevin and the belief that somehow everything would return to normal, in time. Joe, always jovial, friendly, and good-natured, could not acknowledge that anything had really changed. Ella, always aloof, distant, and superficially pleasant, could not allow the traumatic events of the past year to interfere with her active social life. Though Kevin still lived with them by necessity, they were not ready to discuss his future, nor could he.

A junior college dropout before his injury, Kevin appeared to accede passively to the rationalizations presented and did not share his own concerns. The second session ended with Joe and Ella expressing no further need to meet with me again. My suggestion of referral to another family therapist was met with: "We'll work things out."

This case study is an example of a perhaps not uncommon situation in which the premorbid family system is a major contributing element to the postmorbid outcome of one of its head-injured members. Unfortunately, my limited professional contact with them prevented me from concluding a definitive family assessment, but enough data were revealed to explain, in part, the nature of their family process. It should be noted, as a closing note, that although a supportive and nonjudgmental therapeutic approach was used, it is doubtful that a more challenging and confrontive approach would have been of any greater value.

The Abused Child as Head-Injured Patient

Earlier we documented the extensive epidemiological evidence suggesting the high incidence of head injury in children, with physical abuse as a major determining factor. The implication of such evidence will significantly influence the child's recovery, particularly if the child is to live with the abusing parent(s) once again. Although not addressing the needs of the abused head-injured child per se, Levin, Benton, and Grossman (1982) report that the postmorbid behavioral disturbances found are related to an unclear combination of primary brain injury, premorbid characteristics, and the postmorbid family milieu.

Unfortunately, because of the legal-medical complications and ramifications surrounding child abuse in general, the difficulties in providing a safe, healthy, and encouraging environment conducive to recovery are obvious. Only with the close-working congruent relationship of the caregiving team and legal authorities can the child have at least the chance for a positive outcome.

COUNSELING INTERVENTION

The need to intervene psychotherapeutically with head-injured children and adults and their families is justified not only by the marked behavioral and personality changes that occur but also by the neuropsychological changes. Although our attention will be directed mainly to procedures focusing on emotional adjustment, we cannot ignore the influence of cognitive deficiencies on such an adaptation. The rehabilitation effort, as we see it, is both educational and therapeutic in that each contains elements of the other. For this reason, we do not believe any one caregiver can lay claim to any one strategy. It does imply, however, that all caregivers have at least some knowledge of all the procedures that constitute the rehabilitation process.

Educating the Family and the Patient

We have already inferred from our earlier discussion that the family must play a significant role in the overall and specific aspects of the rehabilitation program. Diehl (1983) believes that the program should be flexible and varied enough to adapt to the specific needs of the patient and the family, with input from all members of the rehabilitation team. Of utmost importance is the establishment of "careful environmental control" in both the home and treatment facility, as both the victim and the family will have their own distinctive time line for adjustment and adaptation to the injury.

Providing information   In Chapter 2 we discussed the value and importance of providing information about stroke to aphasic patients and their families. Although we believe it is as valuable to provide information about head injury to these victims and their families, qualitative differences between the two types of brain insult dictate a somewhat different approach. To begin with, denial of the head injury and its concomitant sequelae appears to be more intense and of longer duration. It is doubtful that the patient or the family could process and assimilate any substantial amount of information during the initial stages of grief. Yet it is certainly important to provide basic data concerning the initial impact of the injury on all members of the family.

Also, because the course of recovery in head-injured patients is much less predictable than in cases of aphasia, prognostic indications by the information provider must by necessity be deferred or be given with great caution. The profound behavioral and personality changes that often occur in head injury, either immediately postonset or later, are unlikely to be understood by either the patient or the family, even when discussed by the most sensitive and expert caregiver. Furthermore, the younger age of the head-injured patient would oblige us to direct our attention to the far-reaching implications on both the patient and the family and cautions us to withhold our opinions until such time as when some stabilization has occurred.

Of utmost importance during the early and later periods postonset is that opportunities for continued communication between caregivers (or their designated spokesperson) must be maintained. Nothing is more frustrating and insulting than for family members to be kept ignorant of all that is occurring during the rehabilitation program, of changes in their own feelings and attitudes, and particularly what is in store when the patient comes home.

Probably the greatest challenge to the information provider, however, is the often unstated ambiguities and the incongruent messages family members give regarding their desire for information. We must understand that such behaviors are not necessarily psychopathological but rather natural defenses related to coping with the tragedy. It entails great patience in attempting to understand exactly how much information and what kind family members may indeed wish. It has been this author's experience to have worked with some head-injured families who two years postonset had not yet reconciled themselves to exactly what they wanted to know. In some cases, the head-injured victim himself has also been uncertain.

We will discuss presently how this problem and others can be dealt with during the counseling process.

Major areas of information   In addressing the needs of the family, Millard (1983), the parent of a twenty-four-year-old head-injured man, provides us with several guidelines that we believe are particularly useful:

1. Encourage the family to make use of their own knowledge of the patient to ascertain even minimal return of awareness.
2. Inform the family of the function of the acute care and rehabilitation facilities and particularly the extended care facility (ECF) if that will be an interim requirement.
3. Prepare the family for the necessary financial requirements so that the transfer process between facilities will be facilitated and the family given enough time to make whatever arrangements are necessary.
4. Help the family understand that they are dealing with an adult (if such is the case) and an intelligent person regardless of the current behavior and to treat the patient appropriately.
5. Inform them that the uniqueness of individuals, different types of injuries, and different recovery factors will determine the possible outcome, and all of what they observe now may not necessarily be permanent.

6. Explain exactly what constitutes the various therapies to be employed and what values they serve. We would add, explain how the family may assist in the various therapeutic processes.

7. Encourage limited home visits by the patient, when appropriate, with the understanding that such visits would not necessarily be under the best circumstances. These visits will give the family a better understanding of what may be in store for them, but they should also be made aware that the permanent reality will be experienced only after the patient is discharged.

8. Discharge planning must include continuous open communication with the family. We would add that families must have access to advice, long after discharge.

Specific areas of information   Lezak (1978b) has consolidated definitive problem areas we need to cover with the family:

> (1) Anger, frustration and sorrow are natural emotions for close relatives of brain injured patients; (2) Caretaking persons must take care of themselves first if they are going to be able to continue giving the patient good care; (3) The caretaker must ultimately rely on his own conscience and judgment in conflicts with the patient or other family members; (4) The role changes that inevitably take place when an adult becomes dependent or irresponsible can be emotionally distressing for all concerned; (5) The family members can probably do little to change the patient and thus need not feel guilty or wanting when the care does not result in improvement; (6) When it appears that the welfare of dependent children may be at stake, families must explore the issue of divided loyalties and weigh their responsibilities. (pp. 595−596)

It has already been noted that many head-injured families in the beginning have difficulty in assimilating all the information provided. Nevertheless, it is important to give information on some topics that the family could process. Among those are several that the author has found significant for families to know:

1. A basic description of the physical trauma with reference to which part of the injured brain may affect which behavior.

2. An explanation of incontinence and how the patient may be responding to it. Emphasis must be placed on the fact that such physiological behavior is likely to correct itself in time.

3. An explanation of any one or combination of typical behaviors, such as patient self-centeredness, depression, paranoia, hostility, and inability to respond to family members as they would wish. Here we would also include patient apathy, withdrawal, confusion, agitation, disorientation, and clinging to family members.

4. A clarification of the nature of the patient's memory problems and how these interfere with personal day-to-day functioning.

5. An explanation of the cognitive-linguistic changes and how these influence, or are influenced by, other behaviors.

We will presently see how providing information about head injury to the family becomes a vital aspect of the entire counseling process for the entire family as well as for the patient.

A Framework for Psychotherapeutic Counseling

As we discussed in Chapter 1, the rationale and justification for intervening psychotherapeutically when a brain insult has occurred are quite different from those for typical intervention procedures. In the case of traumatic head injury we feel that its effects on the patient and the family system generally to be more profound than in the cases of cerebral vascular insult. Rosenthal and Muir (1983) believe that the patient's "emotional regression," "inappropriate social behaviors," and, in the case of frontal lobe syndrome, maladaptive behaviors such as lethargy, reduced drive, flat affect, irritability, lack of spontaneity, and inappropriate goal-directed behavior are the most devastating to the family system.

The spouse, family, and traumatically head-injured person can be seen to react to the initial event and ensuing circumstances in a discernible pattern. Recognition of the effects on the individual, the family, and their lifestyle by the rehabilitation team is vital for the patient's progress. It would appear that the team's support of the family and the patient, and the adjustments they make, are important factors in successful rehabilitation. It is also clear that information and support for the head-injured person and the family need to continue well after the patient has completed a rehabilitation program and returned home. The need for individual counseling and for family education and family counseling/therapy is clear; by this means the family and the head-injured person will receive emotional support and will be assisted in understanding and accepting the disability and its potential long-term consequences. Most important will be the establishment of a reorganized but functional family system.

Guidelines for Intervention

1. The degree and quality of counseling intervention will depend on the way in which the family is mourning. The therapist must be sensitive to the need of some families to cope independently and to the needs of others who want help but have difficulty in asking for it.

2. Counseling must be conducted within the context of understanding the pretraumatic family system and the behavioral and personality characteristics of individual family members and the patient in particular. As Rosenthal and Muir (1983) note: "The 'diagnosis' of the family and 'prescription' for treatment will aid in preventing secondary disability produced by maladaptive interactions between patient and family" (p. 410). (We would add particularly when such maladaptive patterns were there previously.)

3. The quantity and complexity of information to be provided the patient and the family depend not only on their need to know but also on how necessary it is for them to have the information in order to assist in the rehabilitation process. For example, the spouse who gets upset with her head-injured husband over his childish behavior should be informed of its

meaning so that she can not only assist in perhaps modifying that behavior but can at least be assisted in understanding it.

4. Determining the degree to which the patient should be counseled, or be involved with the family in the counseling process, will be based in part on the feedback from members of the rehabilitation team and from family members. Many speech-language pathologists find that counseling is an intrinsic aspect of cognitive retraining, and occupational therapists find counseling to be helpful in encouraging self-help skills. It is important that counseling, no matter to what degree utilized, be coordinated by one professional sufficiently trained in counseling psychotherapy and in the subject of head injury.

5. The choice of family intervention techniques, which include patient–family education, family counseling, and family therapy, is based on the appraisal of the particular head-injured family by the various rehabilitation personnel. As Rosenthal and Muir (1983) and Rosenthal (1984) have indicated, patient–family education would be of considerable benefit to most families, particularly in the early stages postmorbidly. The decision to use family counseling should be based on the need of the family to cope with their mourning and to understand the consequences of head injury, according to Rosenthal and Muir. We believe that family therapy should be the method of choice, but only if the patient can be included. Criteria for use of aphasia family therapy that can apply to head injury family therapy have been outlined by Rollin (1984).

6. The role of nonprofessional support groups for families of head-injured persons should not be underestimated because they are beginning to play a major role in providing the emotional support and practical assistance such families need. For the head-injured family it is probably the least threatening method psychologically and, practically speaking, the least expensive. We hesitate to imply that it should replace other counseling intervention strategies, but suggest that it complement professional approaches.

Family Counseling

Initially, family counseling should be convened to provide whatever information is deemed necessary for the family to have and/or whatever information it requests immediately after the head injury. We would not expect the process to be particularly dynamic at that time because the family may be resistant to counseling intervention. Nonetheless, as long as the family is aware that such services are available, and if they are aided in the understanding that such therapy will be of value to their injured member, they are more likely to be willing participants in the process.

Mauss-Clum and Ryan (1981), based on their experiences with families of the brain injured in the brain injury rehabilitation unit at a Veterans Administration hospital in California, found that families unanimously "ranked their need for a clear and kind explanation of the patient's condition as first priority" (p. 166). Most important, however is the need to include families in the planning of acute and long-term care of their injured member. We believe this to be fundamental to family counseling in that it can help reduce the guilt-ridden, self-pitying, and defeatist attitudes aroused in the grieving process by reinforcing all of the positive possibilities. Excluding families from the rehabilitation process will not only induce negative consequences for the patient but will also distance family members from the patient, thereby alienating them from each other.

Caution must be exercised, however, in the manner in which and the degree to which the therapist involves the family. Consideration of the unique and complex dynamics that constitute a particular family must be a determining factor.

Family Therapy

Family therapy is a far more dynamic and complex process than family counseling in which the focus is away from individual family members and towards the entire family system. Unlike in family counseling, the head-injured person must be included so that all members may interact in order to grow and develop together. The rationale, justification, and guidelines for family therapy in the case of the aphasic family as discussed in Chapter 2, as well as in the work by Rollin (1984) and Webster and Newhoff (1981), also apply to the head-injured family, except for certain modifications.

Because the evidence identifies clearly defined premorbid psychosocial patterns that may be present—social maladjustment, alcoholism, marital/family instability, and so on—the therapist would have to give careful consideration to these factors in the quest for family harmony. Long established individual and family patterns are not readily modified regardless of the postmorbid reality and in fact may become more firmly entrenched. Of course, it is also possible that the trauma may produce such a dramatic shift in the realignment of family members that some positive changes may ensue. In the case of Kevin and his family described earlier, there certainly was no longer the problem of alcohol, drug abuse, or run-ins with the law, but whether or not such self-destructive behaviors were now being channeled either positively or negatively is still questionable.

A second major consideration in regard to family therapy is the younger age incidence of the trauma. Unlike the aphasic patient, the head-injured patient is likely to have many more years of life ahead and thus educational, vocational, and social factors become more crucial to the overall family therapy process. In the case of older or elderly parents of the victim, the issue of future independent living must be recognized and acknowledged by all and dealt with in a constructive manner. Younger marital relationships in head trauma cases further dictate considerations of sexual and role adjustments, as well as realistic vocational possibilities.

A third and perhaps even more important consideration is the quality and degree of the cognitive-emotional-communicative deficit. Edelstein and Couture (1984) provide a comprehensive rehabilitation approach in their text. The often profound changes in behaviors will certainly challenge the family therapist to establish and maintain interpersonal family communication conducive to family homeostasis. Although the temptation might be to exclude a patient who evidences inappropriate language, affect, and behavior from the family therapy process, we believe it is unwise to do so because all will need somehow to cope with the reality of living together. Unless participation by the victim in the family therapy so interferes with the process, we would advise that the therapist be steadfast in the commitment to the procedure and purpose, particularly if family therapy is to be used to enhance the communicative ability of the patient.

A final consideration is the recognition that certain high-risk families may not be amenable to any form of counseling intervention. Although Rosenthal and Muir (1983) do not preclude such families from counseling assistance, we believe that the severe "maladaptive behavior patterns," "prolonged use of denial," and "severe chronic physical and/or mental deficits" that they describe would resist well-intentioned psychotherapeutic efforts.

As a concluding note, we agree with Rosenthal and Muir that regardless of postmorbid problems, not all families require extensive counseling intervention and would add that we must trust such families to determine their own livable reality apart from our presumably objective and professional judgments.

Family Caregiver Support Groups

Because of the mutual frustration, dissatisfaction, helplessness, and financial strain often experienced by families in their search for appropriate facilities and support in returning head-injured family members to their realistic potential, several family survival programs have sprung up across the United States. Among the goals of the National Head Injury Foundation, a nonprofit corporation formed to advocate for head-injured persons and their families, has been the development of a support group network to assist families in organizing local support groups in all states.

Levy (1979) describes the function of a support group in which a trained facilitator is used. He defines such groups as

> . . . composed of members who share a common status or predicament that entails some degree of stress, and the aim of these groups is generally the amelioration of this stress through mutual support and the sharing of coping strategies and advice. There is no attempt to change their members' status; that is taken as more or less fixed, and the problem for members of these groups is how to carry on in spite of this. (p. 242)

Employing a health model, the support group focuses on current problem situations, not on the dynamics that created the situation or on the interpersonal relationship among members. The approach is essentially nonconfrontational, supportive, and nonjudgmental, in which the members take responsibility for their own actions. Networking and socializing among members are encouraged in order for them to learn how to cope from each other, particularly when grief is still being experienced.

The role of the facilitator is to[1]

1. *Foster cognitive and emotional communication* by encouraging members to talk to each other and focus on feelings about specific situations. These feelings are verified by one another.

2. *Encourage mutual support among group members* by modifying and emphasizing special aspects of each situation in order to decrease competitiveness, advice giving, or rescuing.

3. *Encourage exploration of problems* through practical problem solving, alternative choices, brainstorming, and similar activities. All aspects of each individual member's problems are explored and interrelated in order to obtain a complete picture.

4. *Encourage the sharing and trying out of coping strategies and support efforts to change* by moving from exploring problems to making change, often very difficult. The facilitator uses as models those members who have made changes in their situation and asks how they accomplished it. The main focus is on flexibility and individual ways of achieving the desired goal.

5. *Focus on improvement* by giving respect and supporting efforts to change, to grow, to adapt, to fight the system if necessary, *to care for self*.

6. *Maintain the group duties* by encouraging members to define and maintain ground rules. There is also the *structuring process*—helping members develop appropriate norms, goals, roles, and values by providing structure and allowing structure to emerge.

7. *Gatekeep or maintain balanced participation of members* by keeping group discussion on topics pertinent to the focused group concerns.

8. *Mediate* (also done by members) when an inappropriate level of friction is observed.

9. *Coordinate* by handling arrangements, overseeing the newsletter, arranging the room, and so on.

How members of the group are helped to deal with the emotional difficulties of caregiving includes

1. *Coping with depression by decreasing the feeling of helplessness and hopelessness* through taking action to control parts of the situation when that is possible.

2. Reducing feelings of being overwhelmed by having a place to ventilate feelings with others can help put them into perspective and help *provide a structure for dealing with the problems.*

---

[1]The role of facilitator and how emotional difficulties of caregiving are handled have been adapted, in part, from M. L. Boreing and L. McKinney-Adler, "Facilitating Support Groups—An Instructional Guide, Copyrighted." NIMH Training Grant 15718, "Group Facilitation Skills for Health Professionals," made to Pacific Medical Center, 1981.

3. *Guilt* can be decreased by sharing common themes and seeing them as natural by-products of caregiving—"I want my husband to die," "How can I place my husband?" or taking time for *themselves.*

4. *Decreasing anger and frustration* by provision of a place to ventilate and get validation for the reality of many frustrating situations, such as dealing with bureaucracies—difficult for all of us and not our fault. It may not necessarily decrease the frustration but can help provide a better perspective on it, and it may decrease if a better understanding of how the system works is achieved.

5. *Anger and resentment* can be decreased through education gained in the group, for example, being angry at a spouse because he can't perform a certain task. The group member may learn this is a common symptom of the injury and by an increase in understanding will feel less angry and helpless.

6. Members have a place to express *grief* and work through it with others and view it as natural.

It is obvious that support groups cannot necessarily change the basic situation of caregiving, but members of different families can learn to cope more effectively by gaining increased control of their situation, a continuous process over time. We must also recognize that these groups are not a panacea and that individuals may require either individual psychotherpay or therapy within the context of family therapy. It should be noted further that some individuals may resist all forms of counseling intervention.

Individual Counseling

In treating the individual patient, it is apparent that psychological dimensions are involved in every aspect of the rehabilitation process and that the chief provider of services (very likely the speech-language pathologist) must take on the task of integrating the cognitive-emotional behaviors psychotherapeutically.

The Adult Head Trauma Team of Rancho Los Amigos Hospital (see Malkmus et al., 1980) in California, one of the foremost and earliest rehabilitation teams to work with the head injured on the West Coast, states the responsibilities precisely:

> All personnel, regardless of their specific disciplines, are psychotherapists in that they possess human qualities of warmth, understanding, empathy, genuineness, caring and respect and as such, set the therapeutic environment. It is most important to view the patient as a person, to understand and respect his confused and fractured state of identity and his struggle and frustration to regain his previous identity and place in life. One does not have to be a psychologist to be facilitative. Often because of failure to understand behavior, one becomes fearful and uncomfortable and the tendency is to refer such problems to a psychologist to diagnose and "cure." Psychotherapy, more often than not, is a lengthy process in that a person must be allowed time to progress and reassess ways of being in light of his consequences and life dynamics. The psychologist does not possess any magical power or potent words that will somehow transform a situation and miraculously cause the patient to perform and "behave". (p. 51)

We would concur and add that not only is it possible to combine cognitive treatment strategies with psychotherapeutic ones, but it is of the utmost necessity to do so. To act otherwise is to neglect the very needs presented by the patient. Of course, how much emphasis is to be given to cognitive retrieval and how much to psychological adjustment is not so simple to determine. The speech-language pathologist may choose to use traditional symptomatic procedures that can strengthen cognitive processes as well as emotional ones. Or it is possible to rely more on counseling procedures to do the same thing, if the therapist is trained in these methods. Unfortunately, we have no definitive answers to the best approach. Until we have, we will need to rely on those methods we know best and with utmost consideration for the unique needs of each patient.

We are well aware that the behavior problems presented by the patient, according to the Rancho Los Amigos team, are made more complex by the variables of premorbid psychosocial factors; the presence of postmorbid primary organic variables, including cognitive deficit; and the necessity for long-term psychotherapeutic treatment, often impossible to sustain if hospitalization is short term. The team believes the focus should be on using psychotherapy to prepare the patient for discharge and reentering his family and community and on helping him determine a redefinition of his life.

We believe that although many of the psychotherapeutic guidelines described in Chapter 2 for the apshasic patient, as well as the principles outlined in Chapter 1, are applicable here, there are some major differences. These differences are highlighted by the fact that emotional reactions in the head injured are often mediated by disordered thought processes, and that to assign "neurotic" explanations to aberrant behaviors can be misleading and counterproductive. There are, nevertheless, psychodynamic factors that can be dealt with and we present them as follows:

1. *Marked egocentricity and inappropriateness of behavior.* The patient is aided in becoming aware of exactly what constitutes such behavior. Although informed that these behaviors are natural consequences of the injury, they can be altered by recognizing that they occur; acknowledging their effects on others, and modifying them to produce more acceptable behaviors. Use of feedback through videocassettes has been found to be an effective means to achieve this end with many patients, and can readily be utilized during the course of cognitive retraining procedures.

2. *Concrete thinking and impaired judgment.* A similar approach to that above is used. Modeling by the therapist can help the patient more clearly recognize individual behavior and how it interferes with communication and interrelating with others. To be sure, the patient may not always have the ability to modify the behavior accordingly, but any positive change must be rewarded and reinforced.

3. *Confusion, disorientation, and restlessness.* Work being done on orienting the patient to reality should be carried over during counseling. We refer

not only to the identification of such concepts as time, events, and places but also to the concentration on clarity of communication between the patient and the therapist. For the patient to be confused by the psychotherapeutic process will add to personal confusion surrounding other aspects of reality, particularly if feelings about being confused and disoriented are discussed.

4. *Anxiety and insecurity.* The therapist will need to distinguish between anxiety and insecurity that is based on actual reality from anxiety and insecurity that is a reflection of the personality pattern of the patient. For example, it is certainly understandable if the patient becomes anxious when not being informed of schedule changes of various therapies, and it is incumbent on the counseling therapist to help correct the situation. If, on the other hand, the patient is unable to risk expanding the individual range of experiences, say, to going home on weekends, then such fears should be carefully scrutinized and analyzed by the patient and the therapist.

Especially important is that the therapist also be aware of any developing transference and/or countertransference relationship. It is not unusual for head-injured patients to cling to the professional caregiver who is most "there" for them or appears to understand them best. Weaning the patient away from the dependency, yet still maintaining the therapeutic relationship, is a challenge to even the most experienced counselor.

5. *Denial and unrealistic expectations.* It is not uncommon for the head-injured patient, because of disordered thinking, to believe that a return to the premorbid state is imminent and that life will continue as it had left off. We need to be cautious not to assign such a belief to a maladjusted emotional state, because it could well be the organism's attempt to reestablish homeostasis. Similarly, when we believe that the patient is not reacting in an appropriate emotional way, we must be careful not to assume that the problems are being denied. The therapist must attempt to help the patient identify the disparity between thought and feeling with the understanding that their reconcilation can indeed be very difficult to achieve.

6. *Memory problems.* Long-or short-term memory difficulties can also hinder the psychotherapeutic relationship in that anything processed, understood, or learned in one therapy session may be readily forgotten in another. There is no simple solution to this problem, except to help the patient be aware that it is a natural consequence of the injury and that by maintaining a diary or log of learned insights and/or practicing new behaviors, some retention is possible. Maintenance of a stable environment and schedules will also be helpful to the patient.

7. *Depression.* It is important to reinforce any slight gain the patient makes in order to minimize the effects of primary and/or secondary depression. The therapist must sometimes cope with the patient who becomes depressed about being depressed. Such a state of mind is very complex, and the patient should be helped to understand that what is being experienced is a natural consequence of the injury and that it could be a positive sign of progress. To be oblivious to it may in fact be counterproductive.

8. *Disinhibition.* Because of the injury, the inhibitory function of the cerebrum is reduced. Violent outbursts and temper tantrums typically occur, and the therapist will have to be acutely sensitive in distinguishing these from secondary acting-out behaviors and behavioral manifestations of frustration and anger. As with depression, the patient must learn to reconcile the primary and secondary behaviors and, in doing so, gain some degree of control over them. Although many factors, such as resistance, avoidance, denial, or even euphoria, might mitigate against recognition, awareness, and control of disinhibitory behavior, the therapist will find confrontive cognitive-emotional techniques, used judiciously, helpful.

The neuropsychodynamic processes and psychotherapeutic strategies we have just described cannot be viewed discretely in every case, and therefore the therapist is urged to use the best professional judgment in intervening accordingly.

Furthermore, the therapist will have to determine judiciously how much the family must or should know of the patient's struggles. Counseling or family therapy is used to complement individual counseling. Regardless, the patient's individual rights should be honored and respected while directed toward independent living. With those cases where independent living and/or reentering family life is contraindicated because of the extent of the disability, the therapist as well as other caregivers will be challenged to help the patient adapt cognitively and emotionally to whatever living environment is deemed appropriate.

A Case Study

Brian K. was twenty-six years old when he ran off a remote country road into a culvert, after a long night of imbibing. Although the friend he was with was uninjured, Brian suffered brain concussion and scattered damage to the cortex. Comatose for several weeks, he emerged with spastic hemiparesis, severe cognitive dysfunction, childlike behavior, and impulsivity. After one year and a half of rehabilitation efforts, he rapidly progressed to the point where he was fully ambulatory, albeit with spastic movement of the right side. His cognitive-intellectual behavior was characterized by distractibility, poor judgment, and difficulty in processing and sequencing information. Emotionally, he often acted silly, inappropriately, and generally insensitively to others but was overly friendly and often ingratiating. His speech was mild to moderately dysarthric, and his voice breathy and aprosodic.

Prior to the injury, Brian lived at home with his father and stepmother, and had been employed as a cook in a local coffee shop. Postmorbidly, he was still living at home. Clinical reports indicated some family counseling during the course of rehabilitation but no individual counseling per se for Brian except for some tangential work connected to cognitive retraining. Brian was referred to me by a social worker who believed Brian needed more help in adjusting to his changed circumstances and in acknowledging his deficits. Apparently, the family, his father in particular, was still caught up in the so-called "sleeping beauty" syndrome whereby it was believed that soon all would be normal again. The family had refused further family counseling and family therapy, but agreed to individual counseling for Brian.

The following clinical protocol is intended as an example of the psychotherapeutic process that may be used in such cases as the one described above. It illustrates the complexity of dealing with the psychodynamics posed by some head-injury victims and represents an excerpt from Brian's and my fifth session together:

B: You know what my father told me yesterday?
T: What was that?
B: As soon as I'm able to drive again, he's getting me a new TransAm.
T: You sound very pleased about that.
B: You bet!
T: Do you remember last week when we talked about realistic expectations for yourself? Have you thought much about that?
B: And you know another thing, it's gonna have all the equipment on it.
T: What was it that I just asked you, Brian?
B: If I know what to expect.
T: Yes, if you thought about things you can realistically achieve with respect to your difficulties.
B: I know I'm getting better.
T: Up to now, you've come a long way and have worked very hard at getting better.
B: I know. And you want to know another thing, Walter?[2]
T: Yes?
B: I like you.
T: Oh?
B: Yeah. You're really gonna get me on my feet again.
T: Do you know what you're doing now, Brian?
B: Yeah, I'm getting off the subject.
T: Yes, it's really hard for you to stay on the subject, but it's important that you stay focused on what we need to talk about—like realistic expectations.
B: I get distracted.
T: Yes you do, but it's good that you recognize that as you do now. I know you work very hard at doing that. Keep it up.
B: Do you think I'm going to get better?
T: You've made a lot of progress already and I know you'll make more. How much, we don't know. You have to take one day at a time.
B: You bet! Like, I'd like to meet a nice girl.
T: You have strong feelings about that.
B: I keep thinking about it all the time.
T: And that's very natural for you to do.
B: Maybe when I get my TransAm.

[2]*Note:* Typically, in the initial counseling interview, I introduce myself with my full name, allowing the client to choose whatever form of salutation he or she finds comfortable. In Brian's case I felt his choice was characteristic of his need to be liked and to establish a "buddy" relationship with me.

T: What do you mean?

B: I'll be able to impress her (laughs boastingly).

T: A relationship with a girl means much more, Brian, and I think you know that.

B: I do, but I need something to get it going.

T: Like you feel that you personally won't attract her? That you need some kind of artificial object to begin the relationship?

B: I guess so. It's easier that way.

T: Is that how you want it?

B: I don't care which way.

T: I have trouble understanding that.

B: What do you mean?

T: Because I think you want to be accepted for who you are, in spite of your disability.

B: And I'm better off now than I used to be, aren't I?

This therapeutic transaction identifies several aspects of cognitive-intellectual-emotional behavior sometimes characteristic of head injury. To what degree such behaviors relate to the premorbid state is not readily determined. In Brian's case, he had graduated from high school and was generally an affable young man but prone to immature outbursts of anger. The latter behavior virtually disappeared following his injury, but other premorbid characteristics were evident.

Brian was counseled for eight months, during which time he gradually but slowly began to respond more appropriately to others and became more willing to look realistically toward his future. It should be noted that during the course of counseling, I had the persistent feeling that he was making a greater effort at pleasing me and acquiesing in fulfilling contract goals while not really modifying his inappropriate behavior. How much of this was due to my own counseling competence and/or the nature and persistence of primary and secondary neuropsychological factors cannot be fully ascertained.

Certainly we do not wish to infer that all such counseling interrelationships in the case of head injury will have such outcomes. The author, in fact, has had and seen many definitely successful results. We merely suggest that the reader be fully cognizant of the manipulative behaviors that often characterize the head-injured person's quest for survival in a differently perceived world.

CONCLUSION

It is clear that traumatic head injury presents the counseling therapist with the most formidable challenge to his or her expertise in dealing with the complex issues manifest in the patient and his family. It demands not only the highest degree of competence in individual and/or family psychodynamics but also a sound knowledge of all the related physical, cognitive, perceptual-motor, intellectual, and communication concomitants. The re-entry of the traumatically head-injured patient into family and social life, virtually nonexistent twenty-five years ago, invites us to devote our interdisciplinary efforts in designing and carrying out the research necessary to discover the most effective means to cope with a problem that has attained epidemic proportions.

REFERENCES

ANNEGERS, J. F., GRABOW, J. D., KURLAND, L. F., and LAWS, E. R. The incidence, causes, and secular trends of head trauma in Olmstead County, Minnesota. *Neurology,* (1980), 912–919.

BARRY, P. *Family Adjustment to Head Injury.* Framingham, Mass.: National Head Injury Foundation, 1984.

BEN-YISHAY, Y., and DILLER, L. Cognitive deficits. In M. Rosenthal, E. R. Griffith, M. R. Bond, and J. D. Millers (Eds.), *Rehabilitation of the Head Injured Adult.* Philadelphia: Davis, 1983.

BLUMER, D., and BENSON, D. F. Personality changes with frontal and temporal lobe lesions. In *Psychiatric Aspects of Neurologic Disease.* New York: Grune & Stratton, 1975.

BOISMARE, F., LEPONCIN, M., and LEFRANCOIS, J. Memorization et catecholamines centrales apres un traumatisme cranio-cervical experimental chez le rat: Influence d'une administration d'imipremine. *Psychopharmacology,* 55 (1977), 251–256.

BOND, M. R. The psychiatry of closed head injury. In N. Brooks (Ed.), *Closed Head Injury: Psychological, Social and Family Consequences.* Oxford: Oxford University Press, 1984.

———. Effects on the family system. In M. Rosenthal, E. R. Griffith, M.R. Bond, and J. M. Douglas (Eds.), *Rehabilitation of the Head Injured Adult.* Philadelphia: Davis, 1983.

BOWLBY, J. Attachment theory, separation, anxiety and mourning. In S. Arieti (Ed.), *American Handbook of Psychiatry,* Vol. 6. New York: Basic Books, 1975.

BROOKS, N. (Ed.). *Closed Head Injury: Psychological, Social and Family Consequences.* New York: Oxford University Press, 1984.

BUKAY, L., and GLASAUER, F. *Head Injury.* Boston, Little, Brown, 1980.

CARTLIDGE, N. E. F., and SHAW, D. A. *Major Problems in Neurology,* Vol. 10: *Head Injury.* London: W. B. Saunders, 1981.

COOPER, P. R. Epidemiology of head injury. In P. R. Cooper (Ed.), *Head Injury.* Baltimore: Williams & Wilkins, 1982.

DIEHL, L. N. Patient-family education. In M. Rosenthal, E. R. Griffith, M. R. Bond, and J. D. Miller (Eds.). *Rehabilitation of the Head Injured Adult.* Philadelphia: Davis, 1983.

EDELSTEIN, B. A., and COUTURE, E. T. *Behavioral Assessment and Rehabilitation of the Traumatically Brain-Damaged.* New York: Plenum. 1984.

FAHY, T. J., IRVING, M. H., and MILLAC, P. Severe head injuries: A six year follow-up. *Lancet,* 2 (1967), 475–479.

GRIFFITH, E. R. Types of disability. In M. Rosenthal, E. R. Griffith, M. R. Bond, and J. D. Miller (Eds.), *Rehabilitation of the Head Injured Adult.* Philadelphia: Davis, 1983.

GRONWALL, D., and WRIGHTSON, P. Duration of post-traumatic amnesia after mild head injury. *Journal of Clinical Neuropsychology,* 2 (1980), 51–60.

———.Cumulative effect of concussion. *Lancet,* 2 (1975), 995–997.

GROSSMAN, R., BEYER, C., KELLY, P., and HABER, B. Acetylcholine and related enzymes in human ventricular and subarachnoid fluids following brain injury. *Proceedings of the Fifth Annual Meeting of the Society for Neuroscience,* 76 (1975), 506.

HARLOW, J. M. Recovery from the passage of an iron bar through the head. Publications of the Massachusetts Medical Society, 2:329, 1868.

HOBBS, C. J. Skull fracture and the diagnosis of abuse. *Archives of Disease in Childhood,* 59 (1984), 246–252.

JENNETT, B. Scale and scope of the problem. In M. Rosenthal, E. R. Griffith, M. R. Bond, and J. D. Miller (Eds.). *Rehabilitation of the Head Injured Adult.* Philadelphia: Davis, 1983.

JENNETT, B., and MACMILLAN, R. Epidemiology of head injury. *British Medical Journal,* 282 (1981), 101.

KERR, T. A., KAY, D. W. K., and LASSMAN, L. P. Characteristics of patients, type of accident, and mortality in a consecutive series of head injured admitted to a neurosurgical unit. *British Journal of Preventive and Social Medicine,* 25 (1971) 179−185.

KRAUS, J. F. Injury to the head and spinal cord: The epidemiological relevance of the medical literature published from 1900 to 1978. *Journal of Neurosurgery* (suppl.), 53 (1980), 3−10.

KÜBLER-ROSS, E. *On Death and Dying.* New York: Macmillan, 1969.

LEVIN, H. Aphasia in closed head injury. In M. T. Sarno, *Acquired Aphasia.* New York: Academic Press, 1981.

LEVIN, H. S., BENTON, A. L., and GROSSMAN, R. G. *Neurobehavioral Consequences of Closed Head Injury.* New York: Oxford University Press, 1982.

LEVY, L. H. Processes and activities in groups. In M. A. Lieberman and L. D. Borman (Eds.), *Self-help Groups for Coping with Crisis.* San Francisco: Jossey-Bass, 1979.

LEZAK, M. D. Subtle sequelae of brain damage: Perplexity, distractibility and fatigue. *American Journal of Physical Medicine,* 57 (1978a), 9−15.

─────. Living with the characterologically altered brain injured patient. *Journal of Clinical Psychiatry,* 39 (1978b), 592−598.

LISHMAN, W. A. The psychiatric sequelae of head injury: A review. *Psychological Medicine,* 3 (1973), 304−318.

─────. Brain damage in relation to psychiatric disability after head injury. *British Journal of Psychology,* 114 (1968), 373.

LURIA, A. R. *Higher Cortical Functions in Man.* New York: Basic Books, 1980.

MAKMUS, D., BOOTH, B. J. and KADIMER, C. *Rehabilitation of the Head Injured Adult: Comprehensive Cognitive Management.* Downey, CA: The Professional Staff Association of Rancho Los Angeles, 1980.

MAUSS-CLUM, N., and RYAN, M. Brain injury and the family. *Journal of Neurological Nursing,* 13, (1981), 165−169.

MILLARD, A. The family and communication: A letter from the mother of a head trauma victim. *The Coordinator,* (June 1983), 6−11.

MUIR, C. A. Mobile mourning: Psychodynamics of family and patient in brain trauma. Paper presented at the Western Psychological Association, San Francisco, April 1978.

NAJENSON, T., MENDELSON L., SCHECHTER, I., DAVIV, C., MINTZ, N., and GROSSWASSER, Z. Rehabilitation after severe head injury. *Scandinavian Journal of Rehabilitative Medicine,* 6 (1974), 5−14.

NAJENSON, T., SAZBON, L., FISELZON, J., BECKER, E., and SCHECHTER, I. Recovery of communicative functions after prolonged traumatic coma. *Scandinavian Journal of Rehabilitative Medicine.* 10 (1978), 15−21.

ODDY, M. Head injury during childhood: The psychological implications. In N. Brooks (Ed.), *Closed Head Injury: Psychological, Social and Family Consequences.* Oxford: Oxford University Press, 1984.

ODDY, M., and HUMPHREY, M. Social recovery during the year following severe head injury. *Journal of Neurology, Neurosurgery and Psychiatry.* 43 (1980), 798−802.

ODDY, M., HUMPHREY, M., and UTTLEY, D. Subjective impairment and social recovery after closed head injury. *Journal of Neurology, Neurosurgery and Psychiatry,* 41 (1978a), 611−616.

─────. Stresses upon the relatives of head-injured patients. *British Journal of Psychiatry,* 133 (1978b), 507−513.

PAINTING, A., and MERRY, P. The long-term rehabilitation of severe head injuries with particular reference to the need for social and medical support for the patient's family. *Rehabilitation,* 38 (1972), 33−37.

RIMEL, R. W., and JANE, J. A. Characteristics of the head injured patient. In M. Rosenthal, E. R. Griffith, M. R. Bond, and J. D. Miller (Eds.), *Rehabilitation of the Head Injured Adult.* Philadelphia: Davis, 1983.

ROLLIN, W. J. Family therapy and the aphasic adult. In J. Eisenson, *Adult Aphasia.* Englewood Cliffs, N.J.: Prentice-Hall, 1984.

ROMANO, M. D. Family response to traumatic head injury. *Scandinavian Journal of Rehabilitative Medicine,* 6 (1974), 1−4.

ROSENBAUM, M., LIPSITZ, N., ABRAHAM, J., and NAJENSON, T. A description of an intensive treatment project for the rehabilitation of severely brain-injured soldiers. *Scandinavian Journal of Rehabilitative Medicine,* 10 (1978), 1–6.

ROSENBAUM, M., and NAJENSON, T. Changes in life patterns and symptoms of low mood as reported by wives of severely brain-injured soldiers. *Journal of Consulting and Clinical Psychology,* 44 (1976), 881–888.

ROSENTHAL, M. Strategies for intervention with families of brain-injured patients. In B. A. Edelstein and E. T. Couture (Eds.), *Behavioral Assessment and Rehabilitation of the Traumatically Brain Damaged.* New York: Plenum, 1984.

———. Behavioral Sequelae. In M. Rosenthal, E. R. Griffith, M. R. Bond, and J. D. Miller (Eds.) *Rehabilitation of the Head Injured Adult.* Philadelphia: Davis, 1983.

———. Psychological deficits in the brain-injured adult and family. Paper presented at Conference on Rehabilitation of the Traumatic Brain-Injured Adult. Williamsburg, Va., June 1979.

ROSENTHAL, M., and MUIR, C. A. Methods of family intervention. In M. Rosenthal, E. R. Griffith, M. R. Bond, and J. D. Miller, (Eds.). *Rehabilitation of the Head Injured Adult.* Philadelphia: Davis, 1983.

ROSENTHAL, M., GRIFFITH, E. R., BOND, M. R., and MILLER, J. D. (Eds.) Rehabilitation of the Head Injured Adult. Phila., PA.: F. A. Davis, 1983.

SANTA CLARA VALLEY MEDICAL CENTER. Head Injury Rehabilitation Project. Final Report. San Jose, Calif. 1982.

SELECKI, B. R., HOY, R. J., and NESS, P. Neurotraumatic admissions to a teaching hospital: A retrospective survey, Part 2. *Head Injuries Medical Journal of Australia,* 2 (1968), 113–117.

SWEET, W. H., ERVIN, F., and MARK, J. H. The relationship of violent behavior to focal cerebral disease. In S. Garuttini and E. B. Sigg (Eds.), *Aggressive Behavior. Proceedings of the International Symposium on the Biology of Aggressive Behavior.* Milan, May 1968.

THOMSEN, I. V. The patient with severe head injury and his family. *Scandinavian Journal of Rehabilitative Medicine,* 6 (1974), 180–183.

VAN WOERKOM, T. C. A. M., TEELKEN, A. W., and MINDERHOUD, J. M. Difference in neurotransmitter metabolism in frontotemporal-lobe confusion and diffuse cerebral contusion. *Lancet,* 1 (1977), 812–813.

WEBSTER, E. J., and NEWHOFF, M. Intervention with families of communicatively impaired adults. In D. S. Beasley and G. A. Davis (Eds.), *Aging: Communication Processes and Disorders.* New York: Grune & Stratton, 1981.

4

PSYCHOLOGICAL CONSIDERATIONS OF PEOPLE WHO STUTTER AND THEIR FAMILIES

INTRODUCTION

Over the last fifty years, at least, the quest by speech-language pathologists for answers to the mystery and dilemma of stuttering has not been unlike Jason's search for the Golden Fleece. The discussion in this present chapter is no exception to that adventure except that it will attempt to trace one further route to the source and explore some familiar and some unfamiliar paths toward discovery of the stuttering phenomenon.

One major hypothesis that will underscore our discussions is the assumption that people *are not stutterers* and that if we are to understand the stuttering process we must focus on what people *do*. To assume otherwise is to pigeonhole people categorically and in a real sense deny them the prerogative to represent something more than only their stuttering. To define people as "stutterers" not only defeats our own professional purposes but forever guarantees the perpetuation of their stuttering behavior.

We do not claim to have discovered the ultimate solution to the problem of stuttering. We merely suggest that we shift our thinking and give more attention to a different aspect of the process itself. We would not deny that the stuttering process has received considerable emphasis over the last several decades, except that the value of such research has been undermined by our persistence in labeling. We view, with great irony in fact, Wendell Johnson's own constant use of the term *stutterer* in his landmark work, *People in Quandries* (1946), yet elsewhere in his text he discusses *evaluative labeling* as follows:

> This term is designed to emphasize our common tendency to evaluate individuals and situations according to the names we apply to them. After all, this is a way of saying that the way in which we classify something determines in large measure the way in which we react to it. We classify largely by naming. Having named something, we tend to evaluate it and so react to it in terms of the name we have given it. We learn in our culture to evaluate names or labels, or words, quite independently of the actualities to which they might be applied. (p. 261)

We would agree with Johnson, who further suggests that by naming the individual who stutters, and who is evaluated by others in the environment as a stutterer, the problem becomes self-perpetuating. Later, influenced by one of his former students, Dean E. Williams (1957, 1971), Johnson extended his semantic orientation to therapy. He challenged the stuttering person's view of self as a *stutterer* and described how that view set the person apart from others merely on the basis of the stuttering behavior. Dare we consider the possibility that, as speech-language pathologists, we have contributed as well to the self-perpetuation of stuttering?

Morgan (1980) and others have written extensively on the iatrogenic factor that frequently occurs in doctor–patient relationships in the health care professions. Iatrogeny is the production or inducement of a harmful change in the somatic or psychological condition of a patient or client, by means of the words or actions of the doctor or therapist. Aronson (1985) has decribed how iatrogenic voice disorders may be caused as the result of injudicious medical advice regarding voice rest following laryngeal surgery. Conceivably, in our attempts to treat the stuttering person we may be focusing too much on all the negative things (dysfluencies) that these individuals do rather than on the positive elements (fluencies). Thus these individuals could be inclined to perceive themselves as more different than similar to those who do not stutter.

We prefer to leave the solution to this problem for consideration by individual practitioners and focus more positively on how speech-language pathologists may approach their clients from a cognitive-emotional counseling perspective. Before doing so, however, we will look briefly at several etiological perspectives to establish a rationale for treatment course to be followed.

ETIOLOGICAL CONSIDERATIONS

Several writers have devoted considerable energy to documenting the many theories of stuttering that have evolved over the centuries, and in particular during the latter half of the twentieth century (Hahn 1956; Eisenson 1975; Rieber et al. 1976; Van Riper 1971; Bloodstein 1981). Today most theorists would categorize the major trends as breakdown, repressed needs, anticipatory struggle, and learning theories. We will briefly review these, drawing together several components of each, and introduce family systems theory as a contributory explanation for the stuttering process.

The Breakdown Hypothesis

Modern-day investigators who support the breakdown hypothesis view stuttering as essentially constitutional in nature. That is, they believe stuttering individuals to have had a predisposition to its occurrence or to the breakdown of speech. Although these theorists differ with regard to the exact predisposing factor, they all agree that stuttering is an inner organic condition that may be precipitated by any one or a combination of environmental circumstances. Research has yet to confirm the breakdown hypothesis, however, and researchers continue to search for the definitive factor that would explain all stuttering behaviors.

Among the various explanations put forward in the twentieth century are lack of cerebral dominance (Orton 1927; Travis 1931), biochemical causes (West 1958; Kopp 1934), perseveration (Eisenson 1958), lateral auditory dominance (Tomatis 1963), and laryngeal dysfunction (Schwartz 1976). Representing an intriguing neurofunctional theory of stuttering, Blum (1984) postulates that stuttering individuals have an intermittently dysfunctional auditory monitoring system that interferes with the ballistic function of articulation, resulting in a breakdown of speech fluency. According to Blum, the integrity of the auditory feedback process is dependent on external environmental influences and stressors. That is, the stuttering individual's auditory monitoring does not function continuously but is invoked when going from silence and by his or her own perception of a change in the environment. The difficulty the stuttering individual has is in modulating personal speech to varying moments of silence and external stimuli, which in turn contributes to the disruption of the phonemic process.

Genetic Factors

We have chosen to identify genetic factors as necessary components toward a fuller appreciation of the stuttering phenomenon, but only in the context of other significant factors to be discussed later.

Ludlow and Cooper (1983), in the most recent survey of the genetic literature, contend that stuttering as a genetic disorder has gained in popularity. They caution that methodological problems prevent us from drawing significant conclusions about etiology. Nonetheless, they note that studies of familial incidence, spontaneous recovery, parental dysfluencies, and twinning suggest a connection between stuttering and a family history of stuttering. Ludlow and Cooper cite several studies that suggest the risk of stuttering is almost four times higher for individuals whose relatives stutter than those in nonstuttering families. They further note that if one parent stutters, the risk is even greater that one of the children will stutter. Confirmation of significant sex differences is cited in their review of the literature, with males four times more likely to stutter than females.

Based on a series of genetic studies, Kidd (1977) found that a genetic factor in stuttering represented by a "single major locus" is highly likely. Although his research and the research of others provide substantial support for the contention that genes play a part in stuttering, environmental factors were also found to be related. With this gene-environment interaction model, it has been possible to predict accurately the scope of stuttering among the various members of families. Further, Sheehan and Costley (1977) suggest that heredity might account for only about 25 percent of all those who stutter. Thus there is yet the open question of what role family environment, cultural factors, and learning processes play in stuttering behavior.

Individual adaptability to stress It is obvious that we have not reached that level of understanding that would allow us to determine which genetic precursors account for stuttering behavior. Having a genetic blueprint will not be enough, as we will need to determine how environment can activate or inhibit the blueprint in order to bring about specific behaviors. Farber (1982) cautions us in our use of the term *heritability*, which "refers to the proportion of variance in a group that can be associated with genetic variance." She notes that heritability is a population statistic and tells us nothing about individuals. Thus, even if we were able to determine that a certain percentage of those who stutter do so because of a genetic predisposition, it still would not mean that among that population environmental factors would not be as significant. She notes: . . . heritability statistics are based on a cross-sectional, nondevelopmental approach and frequently are interpreted as though the actions or genes (or environment) were static and indeed immutable from the moment of conception" (p. 124).

We are led, then, to consider how, given a genetic component, psychogenic and cognitive stress may play a part in activating the stuttering process. Hamilton (1982) defines *cognitive stressors* as "those cognitive events, processes, or operations that exceed a subjective and individualized level of average processing capacity" (p. 109). Using an information processing model, he suggests that we vary in our abilities to process the content to which we are exposed, as well as in the degree to which we utilize, extend, or overload our processing system. As an example, he explains how the ego-threatening content of the word *failure* may be received through the process of hearing and how the individual identifies the auditory features in order to understand the word. He further notes that short-term memory is the most vulnerable to overload.

Hamilton defines *psychogenic stressors* as "internal stimuli deriving from internal sources of information that is unpleasant, aversive, threatening, or dangerous for the person" (p. 112). He views psychogenic stressors as related to distinctive thought processes a person has about self in relation to the actions of others or to objects, situations, and events in the immediate life space of the person. Thus the person described is one who will be most sensitive to attacks to self-esteem, failing to achieve goals, or vulnerable "to situations in which performance may be adversely evaluated, or to any situations that are ambiguous with respect to meaning or personal implications that therefore signal unstable or uncertain events" (p. 113).

Hamilton reasons that psychogenic and cognitive stressors must be considered jointly because anxiety contributes to the information processing load of the cognitive processing system. Similarly, with stuttering behavior, we would infer from Hamilton's research and the research of other cognitive psychologists whom he cites that the child learning language makes interpretations and assigns meaning not only in terms of a developing lexicon but in relationship to the environment to which the child is exposed. Adaptability to whatever stressors are present depends on unique constitutional factors, be they biophysiological or a specific diathetic factor as originally put forth by West (1931).

Related to Hamilton's conceptualizations, Andrews et al. (1983), based on the research of Neilson, hypothesize that a central processing inadequacy is inherited. They believe that the development of stuttering depends on a special relationship between sensory-to-motor and motor-to-sensory transformations and on the capacity with which the individual copes with the speech act itself.

A considerable body of research by speech scientists has strongly hinted at a possible relationship between language acquisition and the development of dysfluency or stuttering in children (Murray and Reed 1977; Westby 1979; Stocker and Parker 1977; Andrews et al. 1983). Among the evidence found have been delay in language development, greater risk of articulation disorders, and poor performance on some tests of language. It is too early to draw any definitive conclusions regarding the nature of the relationship between the two except to suggest continued investigations. What is of interest, however, is that researchers from different disciplines appear to be drawing similar inferences about some type of relationship between cognitive development and stuttering. How individual adaptability to the stresses placed on the child in his or her early development certainly demands our attention and continued investigation.

Repressed Needs Models

Most repressed needs models suggest that neurotic behavior is at the basis of all stuttering behavior. If we define neurotic lexically, it generally means a functional disorder of the mind or emotions involving anxiety, phobia, or other abnormal behavior symptoms. Such a definition hardly provides us with any definitive explanation as to the differentiation of behaviors manifest at varying times in most of us, the stuttering individual notwithstanding. Moreover, we would have to define what we mean by abnormal behavior.

Probably the classic repressed needs model is most clearly represented in the psychoanalytic explanation of Glauber (1958), who sees stuttering as essentially a neurosis in which a basic conflict emerges between satisfaction of the ego and the superego. Stuttering is viewed as a symptom manifestation, represented by anxiety, in which the ego has become fixated in its early childhood state. Representing a neoanalytic viewpoint, Barbara (1954) believes that stuttering resides in the child's inability to resolve inadequate interpersonal relationships. Anxiety is produced by parental pressures and inconsistent rearing practices creating inappropriate means of coping. Stuttering is essentially a neurosis in which aberrant personality patterns develop as a means of reducing anxiety.

The research thus far has given us little reason to support the contention that stuttering per se is a neurosis, particularly when we reconsider the definition of neurosis noted earlier. We prefer to support the contention made by many learning and nonpsychoanalytic theorists that stuttering is a maladaptive behavior brought about, in part at least, by interactional elements occurring in the individual's early childhood. We would not, of course, rule out the possibility that stuttering for some is associated with unresolved deep emotional conflicts and that stuttering itself, again for others, may bring about severe emotional hardship, which in turn could exacerbate the stuttering behavior. We need to examine, therefore, other explanations for its occurrence and development.

Anticipatory Struggle Models

One of the most popular explanations for the onset of stuttering is the belief that individuals who stutter interrupt the manner in which they are attempting to speak because they believe they will have difficulty speaking. As a somewhat self-fulfilling prophecy, it is the anticipation of the stuttering that creates the stuttering.

This viewpoint is best illustrated by the diagnosogenic theory put forth by Johnson and elaborated upon by his associates (1959). According to his theory, stuttering is not brought about by what comes from the child's mouth but what is interpreted by the parents' ears. In essence, parents identify their child's normal dysfluencies as stuttering. Evaluated as such, the child tries to speak in a way to satisfy the parents' expectations for more fluent speech. The child perceives the parental criticisms and anxieties and begins to speak differently in order to be relieved of the pressures felt. Support for Johnson's theory has come from years of research, which tends to identify the parents of those who stutter as perfectionistic, demanding, and overanxious.

The major problem with such generalizations is that not all children of such parents develop stuttering. Moreover, self-reports by others who stutter have not always identified such parents, nor even such significant others, in their early environment.

Bloodstein (1981), in summarizing his own earlier research involving stuttering children, has expanded the anticipatory struggle hypothesis. He goes beyond mere labeling and believes stuttering to be brought about by the child's perception of communicative failure. He suggests that anticipatory struggle reactions develop regardless of either a diagnosis of stuttering or normal dysfluenices in the child's speech. He notes: ". . . what is first identified as stuttering usually begins as a response of tension and fragmentation in speech, not sharply different from certain types of normal dysfluency, and is brought about largely by the provocation of continued or severe communicative failure in the presence of communicative pressure" (p. 56).

Going beyond just communicative pressure, we would suggest that other stressors within the child's environment could well contribute to the onset of stuttering and/or other maladaptive behaviors. But these we will discuss later.

Learning Theory Models

Learning theory models cover a broad range of hypotheses that include formulations based on operant and classical conditioning and approach-avoidance conflict. Though these various theories give little attention to etiology per se, they do relate in part to other models discussed earlier. Because thorough descriptions of these models have already been given in depth by others, we will take only a cursory view of them here.

Sheehan's double approach-avoidance theory   Based on Miller's work with rats, in which approach-avoidance conflict was first demonstrated, Sheehan applied a similar paradigm to stuttering behavior (1953, 1975). In essence, during any specific moment the individual has a desire to speak and not to speak. But for each desire there are both negative and positive components that contribute to the conflict. The resulting vacillation is represented in the stuttering phenomenon. Although Sheehan's theory is essentially an attempt to describe the behavioral event of stuttering, it appears to fit the anticipatory struggle theory and repressed needs theory etiologies.

Sheehan viewed the conflict as occurring on various levels: *the word level*—sounds or words that have unpleasant meanings or are feared; *the situation level*—fear reactions to threatening speech situations; *the emotional level*—conflicts that include guilt, anger, and anxiety about speaking; *the interpersonal level*—involving anxiety with others, particularly with authority figures; and *the ego-protective level*—avoidance of competitive behaviors, which are viewed as threatening in terms of success or failure. We shall refer to these later in our discussion of therapeutic intervention.

Operant behavior theory Goldiamond (1965) applied Skinnerian behavioral conditioning principles in bringing stuttering and dysfluency under "operant control" through the use of negative and positive reinforcers. In operant conditioning, the voluntary or spontaneously emitted (operant) behavior such as stuttering is strengthened by positive reinforcement (reward) or is discouraged by negative reinforcement (punishment) or lack of reinforcement (failure to reward either positively or negatively). The conditioned behavior (stuttering) operates on the environment or is instrumental in obtaining the reinforcement or the reward. Shames and Sherrick (1963), although presenting no new etiology of their own, acknowledge the importance of psychosocial processes and suggest that stuttering behavior is maintained by complex schedules of positive and negative reinforcements, but do not believe there is any single contingency for stuttering. That is, there may be a variety of prior events and conditions under which the stuttering may occur and the consequences to follow.

Two-factor theory Brutten and Shoemaker (1967) represent a more classic conditioning viewpoint in stating that the disruption of speech is precipitated by stresses in particular situations in which the negative emotions aroused are linked to neutral stimuli. Thus generalization of word and situational fears occurs through a complex series of stimulus-response conditions. As the child is penalized for abnormal speech behaviors, the communicative act produces conditioned negative reactions. In time, the child learns to associate words and people with communication failure.

This theory is described as "two-factor" in nature because the means by which the child attempts to cope are instrumentally conditioned. That is, the child attempts to avoid or escape fluency failures and thereby secondary stuttering features are developed. Although these avoidance reactions may lessen the anxiety about speaking, they are also reinforced and therefore maintained. Such operant behaviors, when combined with classical conditioning behaviors, define the process through which stuttering develops and is perpetuated.

Though two-factor theory does not identify any one etiology, it seems to come close to a breakdown hypothesis. As Bloodstein (1981) notes: "The development of stuttering is ascribed, not to speech anxiety, but to stress in essentially any form, and constitutional predisposition, in the form of innate conditionability and autonomic reactivity, is considered to play a part" (p. 65).

A Family Systems Theory

The likelihood for stuttering to have a biochemical or genetic base in conjunction with familial incidence has already been noted. Nonetheless, the relationship becomes somewhat obscure when we consider the influence of family environment. That is, neither a nature nor a nurture hypothesis can stand alone, given the present evidence.

Bloodstein (1981), in surveying the literature through 1976, finds support for stuttering to be linked to environmental pressure for conformity and achievement. The exact nature of that relationship is not yet clear, particularly when we try to determine if we are dealing only with parental demands for verbal communication, or parental pressures for a standard of behavior beyond the capabilities of the child, or both.

Andrews et al. (1983), based on their research and the research of others, find little evidence to support a relationship between personality factors and neuroticisms in studies of unselected groups of those who stutter. We prefer not to debate this issue because not all the facts are yet available. We do maintain, however, that the major issue is not one of holding to preconceived labels of neuroticisms, whatever those are, but one of identifying behavioral factors that characterize family relationships where stuttering is present. What is important from our viewpoint is that we attempt to understand the complex processes that occur and that perhaps instigate and perpetuate stuttering behavior.

It seems appropriate, therefore, for us to consider the role of the family within the context of how families operate as a system, given the data we have already gathered. In doing so, we hold to the proposition stated by Van Riper (1971) that "the greater the stress, the more likely it is that the sequencing of speech will be disrupted at a more basic level of integration" (p. 424).

Family functioning: a review of major concepts   Although many theories of family functioning have been developed during the last thirty years, it is possible to identify the themes common to most of them. We summarize these here.

1. *The presence of symptoms to characterize family conflict.* Dysfunctional behavioral patterns may be manifest in one family member, an indication that the growth of family members in general is being thwarted. Whereas symptoms may be present in all, there is usually one member who becomes scapegoated. It implies a breakdown of the ability of the family to share feelings and work out solutions to family problems. Despite the overt distress caused, the symptoms serve to maintain the status quo or homeostasis of the family.

2. *Homeostasis as a process that maintains family equilibrium through interaction.* Dyadic or triadic interactions represent the various interpersonal and intrapersonal processes that characterize families. Each family has its own rules that imply how each member must function in order for the entire family to function and survive. This adaptational process, while covertly maintaining family equilibrium or stability, actually contributes to family dysfunction. Thus any therapeutic attempts to modify family interactions or symptomatic behaviors are frequently met with considerable resistance. Only functional families are likely to change their rules in order to satisfy changes and needs of various family members.

3. *Family strengths and weaknesses.* Every family has tendencies to reinforce either wellness or emotional sickness, depending on the unique characteristics of the family as a whole or of one or more family members. Also implied is the ability or inability for one or more members to tolerate and cope with the strengths and weaknesses of other family members. Thus in some families it may be difficult for one family member to be well unless another is sick.

4. *Family communication.* The way family members communicate with each other reflects the underlying system by which the family functions. In functional families, relationships and attitudes are characterized by congruence, clarity of communication, mutual respect, love and trust, support, and encouragement. In dysfunctional families, while some aspects of these traits may be present, family communication is characterized more frequently by incongruence, distortion of meaning, projection, and conflicts that get expressed through disagreements regarding oftentimes innocuous situational events.

5. *The marital relationship.* The nature and quality of the marital relationship are prime determinants of behavior of the children. Concealed or unresolved marital conflict not only influences the whole family system but may also get expressed by acting-out behavior of other family members. Such conflict also instigates projection by one or both marital partners on other family members as well. Conversely, a functional marital relationship is characterized by mutual caring and acceptance where marital conflict gets resolved through a dynamic give and take process that appropriately excludes the children. Parental decisions regarding the children are made as a team.

It is important to point out that no single concept stands apart from any other; the various structures and processes overlap. Family events are multi-determined, and the configuration of the various structures and processes will determine the degree to which family dysfunction may occur.

Stuttering as an identified symptom Our discussion of disturbed behavior and the dysfunctional family has referred to behaviors and/or internal events that are considered distressing by one or more other members of a family. Such distress may lead to the unwitting selection of one individual to become the disturbed "identified patient." This person, often the child, becomes a scapegoated victim who symbolizes the interfamily conflict. The child becomes part of a process in which attention is directed away from the underlying family conflict and/or from other family members. We are not suggesting that such a process is a conscious decision made by any family member, but it does imply the active involvement by all in which the child gets parental attention in any way possible. The child is merely representing a homeostatic means of coping with perhaps an intolerable or distressful series of family events.

We contend that stuttering in a child may be a behavioral manifestation produced by family tensions, particularly between parents, that have not been resolved through other means. This is not to imply that the child, or for that matter the parents, are necessarily neurotic; simply that on a continuum of emotional functioning, this particular family is functioning in the only way it thinks and knows possible, albeit dysfunctionally.

It could certainly be argued, as Andrews et al. (1983) have pointed out with regard to childhood stuttering, that "no differences in personality factors related to neuroticism have been demonstrated in controlled studies of unselected populations" (p. 229). Yet we would question Andrew's implied assumption that these studies meet his criteria for "Class A facts—findings replicated in two or more research centers, there being no negative reports" (p. 226). (The reader is referred to Wingate (1983) for an extensive and provocative discussion on the Andrews's et al. paper.) We do not consider the use of the various personality scales reported to be exact replications. We would further argue that the scales referred to may not necessarily measure the complex interfamilial dynamics to which we are presently referring.

We therefore hypothesize that stuttering in childhood is a complex developmental process involving a predetermined neurobiophysical factor or factors associated with interfamily distress that becomes identified in the child through the disruption of communicative behavior. Although a comprehensive search of the literature in family systems theory and therapy has failed to reveal any discussion or documentation of stuttering, we believe it is useful to explore the role that family environment may play in its development. In so doing we do not presume to have discovered the multicausal answer but are merely raising several dynamic issues that we believe are unavoidable.

Scapegoating and tolerance to pressure   We have already suggested that scapegoating of a child is effective in managing roots of family tension. It is also understood that this may lead to disturbing secondary complications.

Let us assume that in Family A, the three-year-old child is evidencing signs of dysfluent behavior, not unusual for most young children. Let us further assume that the parents do not appear to be particularly upset with such behavior, but they are enwrapped with personal tensions and perhaps minimal conflict in their relationship. (Thus far, we are describing a not untypical set of circumstances in our society of the 1980s.)

Broadening this scenario, the child, as part of the family system, begins to reflect the tension and/or conflict with an increase of dysfluency and possibly with other behaviors. The focus now turns to the child, who is overtly manifesting the unresolved and perhaps undiscussed parental tensions. As the parents' concern is now directed toward the child, their anxieties about themselves diminish (for the moment, anyway) but become symbolized in the child. The parents also bring into play projections emanating from their own past (whether or not there is a family history of stuttering).

As the child's dysfluency or other behavioral changes increase in sever-ity, the parents' attitudes change also in the form of overprotection and/or disapproval, and/or demands for fluency perfection, and/or "suffering in silence." What is particularly important for us to understand is that the parental attention may not necessarily be directed at the increased dys-fluency per se, but at the overall manifest changes in the child's behavior. Superficially at least, this parental reaction appears to conform to Johnson's diagnosogenic theory, but not really. In the family systems theory we are proposing, labeling is considered only one of several possibilities.

Regardless of the nature of the parental concern, the child's tolerance to the internal and/or external pressures now being experienced is depen-dent on his or her own combined innate and adventitiously developed capabilities. The child's coping behavior is thus seen as an individualized and complex set of dynamic factors that could explain the many multicausal and multimodal theories in the literature.

Theory notwithstanding, it is not difficult to comprehend how the hypothetical child's speech we have described may develop into the full dimension we recognize as stuttering. But we must be careful not to presume a simple cause and effect relationship either in terms of etiological theory or in the developing pattern of stuttering in the family. We hope we have made evident that it is the family interactional process that dominates and that changes of behavior are contiguous to all family members. Finally, we must acknowledge that even with our hypothetical family we must consider not only the influences of the extended family and family of origin but also the possible effects of other external environmental conditions.

DEVELOPING A STUTTERING PERSONALITY

Regardless of etiological theory, most workers in the field would agree that varying combinations of dynamic factors in the environment, as the stutter-ing child develops, will contribute generally to some difficulties in emotional adjustment. As Bloodstein (1981) has pointed out, however, after a compre-hensive search of the literature, there seems to be no definitive character structure or fundamental personality traits to characterize stuttering indi-viduals. Yet he further reports, based on studies carried out for several years at the University of Iowa, that parents of stuttering individuals tend to exhibit certain parental traits and attitudes that could contribute to the stuttering.

The Continuing Influence of the Family

We stated earlier that family relationships must be considered when attempting to understand how stuttering may be perpetuated in the young child. We also indicated that the contiguity of these dynamics can be under-stood without the assignment of neurotic labels to either the child or the parents. We do postulate, however, that stuttering families can be differenti-ated from nonstuttering families on the basis of unique family systems pro-cesses irrespective of psychopathology per se. That is, our stuttering families constitute a special and often unique combination of circumstances, re-actions, conditions, behaviors, and personalities from which stuttering itself has evolved. In some cases, stuttering occurs as a primary instigator for effecting changes in family dynamics, whereas in others, stuttering mani-fests itself as one possible response to family conflict.

It should be pointed out, however, that there are probably many families from which stuttering does not emerge even though all of the dynamics for its development are present. We can offer no explanation for this except that perhaps there are one or more undetermined extenuating factors that differentiate these families from those in which stuttering is generated. Nevertheless, it is possible to explore how the self-image of a stuttering or "identified" child can be molded and the stuttering pattern perpetuated.

The Molding of Self-Image and Perpetuation of the Stuttering Pattern

It is important that as we consider the molding of self-image in the stuttering individual we make clear that we refer not to a unique "stuttering personality," but to a special way in which that individual perceives the self.

Referring back to our hypothetical Family A, we found that the identi-fied child became more and more frustrated in the ability to communicate. The parents, in turn, responded to the best of their ability by "helping" the child. This does not mean that all of their concerns are directed at the child or even that other aspects of the child's development are ignored. Certainly, life continues to go on for the parents, including coping with their own relationships, and so does the child continue to go on in his or her own way. Definite, however, is the fact that child begins to develop secondary symp-toms typical of stuttering behavior that can readily be explained by the learning theory position of Brutten and Shoemaker (1967).

More significant, though, is that while the child is in the process of formulating a self-image as a person, the stuttering becomes an inherent aspect of that development. How much so depends on the nature, quality, and kind of family and social influences.

Although the experimental literature surveyed by Bloodstein (1981) cannot confirm a negative self-image that is distinctive to those who stutter, few therapists would deny that the stuttering individual in time develops feelings of frustration, rejection, and self-doubt while attempting to commu-nicate. That the reactions of others contribute to these feelings and attitudes is evident as well.

But we must remember that the child we describe in Family A is not necessarily condemned to a life of stuttering that precludes the positive development of other aspects of the personality and the self, despite the nature and quality of parental involvement. After all, most of us do survive to varying degrees the effects our parents' struggles have on us. It is no different for the child who stutters and who also typically grows to be a functioning human being. It is little wonder, therefore, that some find such profound meaning in their stuttering behavior to lead them toward a professional life dedicated to solving the stuttering riddle.

What cannot be ignored, however, are the negative features of the child's communicative behavior that shape the perception the individual has of self. Our clinical experiences with stuttering children and adults tell us of the domination stuttering has over all else in terms of how they see themselves and what they can or cannot accomplish in life.

Considering the child in Family A, it is important to recognize that although early and later stuttering behavior may serve to distract the parents from their own struggles, a homeostatic state of affairs is accomplished, at least temporarily. In time this too changes, and the child may soon cease to satisfy the family status quo. But even if the parents direct their attention to other matters, like the birth of another child, the stuttering process has nevertheless taken hold, and, depending on the child and/or the nature and quality of continued family involvement, the stuttering pattern is set and a distinctive self-image established.

It is not surprising that workers in our field find such wide variations among children and adults who stutter. We maintain, however, that the abrupt cessation of stuttering, or the presence of varying degrees of psychopathology, can be explained by the distinctive and dynamic system that characterizes the family in which stuttering occurs. Little wonder that the vast numbers of experimental studies have failed to establish many definitive commonalities among those who stutter or in stuttering families because the boundaries of homogeneous groupings are yet unclear.

A Cognitive Learning Theory Explanation

Thus far we have used family systems theory to explain partly the development and perpetuation of the stuttering pattern through childhood and how a stuttering self-image is shaped. We also offered several learning theory explanations that could account for the development of the phenomenon. That stuttering often continues through childhood and into adulthood could readily be explained by its self-reinforcement and by its reinforcement from external sources, including parental influence.

We have strongly hinted that stuttering behavior is not only an emotional process but a cognitive one as well, as supported in part at least by diagnosogenic theory interpretations. It is possible to pursue this line of reasoning through the work of Ellis and his rational-emotive theory.

In Chapter 1 we described Ellis's theory, which contends that personality is characterized by the development of constructs, beliefs, or attitudes that are included in childhood and maintained through adult life, "and that absolutistic, perfectionistic values tend to make you feel emotionally disturbed" (Ellis 1976, p. 22). These beliefs, which he describes as irrational, are learned through a cognitive mediating process not unlike that described by Johnson, who, like Ellis, expands on the original semantic concepts of Korzybski (1933). Though Ellis focuses mainly on therapeutic change rather than on etiological theory or early cognitive processing, we could readily apply his constructs to the development of stuttering behavior and a stuttering self-image within the context of family systems theory.

As the recipient and expression of parental conflicts and concerns, the dysfluent child soon begins to perceive the self as different. Because of all the negative connotations associated with disruptive communication, feeling and believing oneself as different takes on the meaning of being worse than others. Consequently, the child's developing self-image is defined in terms of "stutterer." All other aspects of the developing value system are perceived in the light of the stuttering self-image.

Should the child have the good fortune to be exposed to more positive, rational, or empirically based values, because of either changing and more positive perceptions by the parents or changes in their value system, there is greater likelihood for the cessation of the stuttering behavior and the enhancement of a more positive self-image. If, on the other hand, should the former circumstances continue into adolescence and adulthood, the earlier irrational value system and the stuttering behavior become fixed, with or without any continuing influence of the nuclear family. The adult then persistently perceives the self in terms of "being a stutterer" and acts in other ways that he or she has always associated with stuttering. Thus it becomes an irrational excuse for such problems as not meeting people, not being able to obtain a desired job, or feeling less worthy than those who do not stutter. Paradoxically, the individual nonetheless appears to others to be functioning adequately and in fact often does, except for the ongoing self-defeating perception that he or she is not. The reality is that the individual is preventing oneself from fulfilling the personal potential that actually exists.

A Case in Point

The author was referred a family in which the chief complaint by the parents was their "stuttering child." An initial, traditional evaluation of the five-year-old boy revealed marked dysfluencies with little indication of secondary struggle behavior, though the child was aware of his unacceptable speech. Articulation and language testing revealed normal linguistic functioning and through diagnostic play therapy portrayed a child who was fairly intelligent with no apparent psychopathological signs but who was somewhat reticent and withdrawn. As the diagnostic session progressed, the dysfluencies decreased, and the child participated more actively and with pleasure in the evaluative process.

Following the interview, the entire family was seen, which provided the opportunity for all members to share with the therapist what their expectations were in getting together and what they wished to accomplish. Both parents indicated that their chief concern was their child's inability to "speak clearly." The child did not express exactly what he wanted initially, but increased dysfluency was demonstrated in his attempt to respond.

After the therapist provided basic information about speech and language development with the concomitant appearance of normal dysfluencies, both parents expressed difficulty in accepting such an explanation. They thereby formed a coalition, albeit unwittingly, against the child and certainly the therapist. What emerged as well were distinct differences of opinion about referring to the child as a stutterer and how to cope with his communication behavior at home. The father was insistent that the child not be called a stutterer, while the mtoher was resolute in affirming that he was. The father's stance was revealed to be one of "suffering in silence," and the mother's was one of "trying to correct him."

What soon emerged was an argument between them about parenting styles that immediately developed into angry recriminations of how they, the husband and wife, treat each other. The revelation of the underlying conflict that had been submerged by "identifying" the child had now surfaced and, fortunately for all, received predominant attention. Their willingness to discuss their own conflict was a sign of their own basic emotional health and genuine concern for the needs of their child. That they both expressed an ardent desire to return the following week for further definition and discussion of the major issue, their own conflict, portended well for the child. The child, for the most part, expressed very little verbally during the session, but through his nonverbal behavior revealed tension and sadness.

The family entered the second session very differently than they had the previous one. To begin with, both mother and father reported a marked decrease in their child's dysfluent speech. This was obvious from the child's ebullient behavior and constant, fluent chattering. Apparently, the intervening week was a time for husband and wife to talk intimately about the things that had been bothering them, which in this case was their current respective relationships with their own parents.

The real issues that emerged in our second family session were difficulties both young parents were having in asserting their independence from their own families of origin. It was unnecessary for the therapist to describe how their child became the recipient of their own troubled relationships, as they were already apparently aware of the effects they had been having on him. They also were able to listen to and process more attentively further information about dysfluency in childhood. It was agreed by them, with the therapist concurring, that further meetings were unnecessary, except that the child desired to return again to "play." He appeared willing to accept being told that he could perhaps return at some later day.

It is important to note that although differences in parenting obviously still existed, the therapist did not consider that to be detrimental to the overall family functioning.

A follow-up meeting was scheduled three months hence. On the day prior to that meeting, the mother called to say that everything was going fairly well at home, and although the relationships with their own parents were still fragile at best, she and her husband were no longer "dumping" on each other. Also, the child's speech was "just fine." A follow-up phone call by the therapist one year later confirmed that "everything was well and even better."

The preceding scenario is representative of how childhood dysfluency can relate to relatively minimal family dysfunction without deep psychopathology being present. One might venture that, if left alone, the marital relationship would have deteriorated and the child's dysfluency increased, but we do not necessarily believe so. Many families have an inner health and although they may struggle toward equilibrium, the end result without therapeutic intervention can indeed be the same. In this case, brief family therapy was an answer—but not the only one.

THERAPEUTIC INTERVENTION

Most workers in the field would agree that as a result of the many experimental investigations and individual empirical case findings, no one therapeutic strategy has surfaced that could be identified as the answer to the elimination of stuttering behavior. In fact, it would appear that some investigations have more likely served to satisfy the individual bias of the investigator who hides behind statistical design manipulations to justify a presumably objective position and for whom a self-fulfilling prophecy is achieved. Certainly, we do not wish to imply that all scientific studies related to stuttering should be so attacked, but merely that all studies must be evaluated and analyzed with greater scrutiny, with cautious avoidance of conclusive overgeneralizations. Too often have so-called objective investigations been the subtle manifestations of deeply felt or unconscious subjective personal attitudes.

Review of Current Strategies

Although we will not discuss at length the various treatment strategies that have evolved over the last several decades, it is nonetheless useful to review the major ones before we consider the one most pertinent to the philosophical position taken in this chapter.

In their interesting study in which a meta-analysis of the effects of various stuttering strategies was used, Andrews, Guitar, and Howie (1980) designated prolonged speech, gentle onset, airflow, and attitude techniques as the four major prevailing strategies. We have difficulty in clearing differentiating among these because ancillary treatments were included among them and seem to contaminate the attempted distinctions. A further difficulty is that Andrews et al. (1983) in a later study refer to *five* major treatments designated in the earlier study, including precision fluency among them. Curiously, in the earlier study precision fluency shaping is not mentioned. Finally we are troubled by the term *attitude therapy*, which in the earlier study was used to designate 12 percent of the studies analyzed. In their 1983 study Andrews et al. continue to use the term, which Wingate (1983) criticizes for its vagueness.

Because of these apparent inconsistencies and lumping together of apples and oranges, we prefer to designate the major treatment modalities as symptom modification, fluency enhancement, and client-centered psychotherapy, for the purposes of discussion. It should be understood that in doing so we readily acknowledge the overlapping of the various strategies by individual practitioners.

Symptom modification By *symptom modification*, we mean the reduction, alteration, and/or elimination of the secondary characteristics commonly associated with secondary stuttering behaviors. Among the strategies used are chewing, pullouts, cancellation, gentle onset, bouncing, shadowing, prolongation, negative practice, relaxation, rhythmic speaking, drugs, hypnosis, easy stuttering, controlled airflow, and counseling.

An inherent feature of symptom modification programs is the notion that stuttering behavior can be controlled and that the individual is expected to live with the problem. Naturally, the degree to which the person is expected to eliminate all aspects of dysfluency depends on the personal orientation of the individual therapist.

Fluency enhancement We would define *fluency enhancement*, not so much as the reduction of stuttering behavior, but rather as the emphasis on achieving completely fluent speech. There is no attempt to manage dysfluent speech; rather, the effort is to encourage and develop the fluent speech of which the individual is capable. The various strategies used include delayed auditory feedback, fluency shaping, cognitive retraining, systematic desensitization, drugs, counseling, prolongation, token rewards and syllable-timed speech. An implied assumption of fluency enhancement therapy is that increased fluency also brings about a more positive self-image as a nonstuttering individual, which will further enhance the maintenance of fluency.

Client-centered psychotherapy *Client-centered psychotherapy*, as we would generically define it, is a process whereby a client–therapist relationship is established in which the client's inherent potentialities for change and growth are activated. The major assumption is that the client is responsible for his or her own destiny and has the right of choice in solving problems. Among the various strategies used are family therapy, nondirective counseling, cognitive emotional counseling, Transactional Analysis, psychoanalysis, systematic desensitization, and assertiveness training. Typically, client-centered psychotherapy may include the use of combined counseling strategies with or without symptom modification and fluency enhancement approaches.

Stuttering in Children

Consistent with our cognitive-emotional and family systems theories approach discussed earlier, with respect to etiology and the development of the dysfluent speech patterns, we propose a combined application with stuttering children in general. We are not convinced, however, that only a cognitive-emotional, family systems, or combined approach is applicable to all of these children. Unique family circumstances and/or special needs of the child would guide our choice of methods.

A family systems approach   The decision to employ a family systems approach would be determined by consideration of the following criteria: (1) evidence of continued family dysfunction; (2) mild to moderate degree of secondary stuttering characteristics; (3) evidence of parental pressure on the child; (4) motivation—the desire by all family members to participate in the family therapy process; and (5) no evidence of severe psychopathology in the child or other family members. Although the choice of family therapy method may be difficult to decide, because of the many approaches described in the literature, we have selected a general approach that would be most appropriate for the "stuttering family." We present it only as a guide that should be supplemented by further study of the subject.

Ackerman (1966), one of the early leaders in the development of family therapy, presents us with a useful model that is summarized with regard to the therapist's function.

1. The therapist formulates a new network among family members, including himself or herself, in which rapport, empathy, and communication play a major part.

2. Through rapport, the therapist clarifies and brings into sharp focus the major conflicts and coping behavior of family members. Through removing obstacles, disguised defenses, disagreements, and disorganized modes of thinking and behavior, the therapist makes the conflict clear. Family members learn, by stages, what has been misunderstood and what the real problem is.

3. Defensive attempts by the family to deny, rationalize, and displace conflict are thwarted by the therapist.

4. Hidden and inert interpersonal conflicts are transformed into open interactional communication.

5. Intrapersonal conflict is raised to the level of interpersonal communication.

6. Scapegoating, which strengthens one segment of the family while weakening another, is neutralized.

7. Playing, in part, the role of a real parent figure, the therapist provides elements that the family lacks but needs and provides the basis for emotional support.

8. Emphasizing confrontation, and to a lesser extent, interpretation, the therapist penetrates and sabotages resistances and lessens the intensity of anxieties, guilt, and conflict.
9. The therapist becomes the major figure on which the family tests reality.
10. The therapist serves as a teacher and exemplifies an ideal model reflecting healthy family functioning.

One "stuttering family" The author was referred a family in which the major complaint was the "stuttering of our twelve-year-old child." The family consisted of the father, Bill, a clinical psychologist; Diane, the mother, a clinical social worker; Andy, the stuttering child; and his ten-year-old brother, Dan, who had no apparent problems. Frustrated by several years of unsuccessful remediation efforts, the parental complaint was that "Andy's stuttering is getting worse."

The initial interview with Andy alone confirmed a clinical picture of secondary stuttering characterized by intermittent hesistations, repetitions, and blocks with associated eye blinking and body twitching. Although Andy's pattern was severe during the stuttering loci, he tended to be fluent approximately 80 percent of the time during the course of our interview. His own chief complaint was the stuttering and his inability to get along with his brother. He otherwise appeared to be a bright, congenial, and sensitive young person.

In a meeting of the entire family, it was immediately evident that the focus of attention was on Andy and "his problem." Bill monopolized much of the early part of the session with professional and clinical explanations of Andy's stuttering while demanding to know which therapeutic approach was to be used. He himself suggested that a Wolpean approach (systematic desensitization) be used. It was readily apparent that Bill was unwittingly sabotaging any attempt to get at the dynamics underlying the process by which the family functioned while proving his intellectual prowess and placing himself in competition with this therapist.

Whatever gaps of verbal communication occurred were filled in by Diane, who declared that "there's nothing wrong with this family," and who was also apparently unaware of the dynamics of family therapy. As the therapist, I was beginning to feel overwhelmed by the degree of intellectualization, rationalization, and resistance to further probing, but shared these feelings with them. Although this acknowledgment was met with further resistance, their defensiveness soon dissipated as I attempted to explain what was happening.

It was further apparent that Bill, Diane, and Dan were a coalition fending off Andy and his stuttering behavior, but no attempt was made at the time to confront them with that reality, for fear of arousing further resistance and perhaps enmity toward me. Their own fragile family network, and my lack of rapport with them, also dictated otherwise.

To counteract what I believed to be a deteriorating clinical relationship, information about the onset and perpetuation of stuttering behavior was presented. Although Bill continued in his attempt to impress me with his knowledge and expertise, he also appeared willing to listen to what I had to say.

It should be noted that Andy's intermittent participation and sharing of his feelings about stuttering were characterized by nearly total fluency. Dan was less verbal and responded to me with a minimum of language. There was also virtually no verbal interaction between them.

Toward the close the session, I was convinced that Bill and/or Diane would be unwilling to continue in family therapy, particularly when Bill asked what I was going to do for Andy. When we scheduled our next appointment, both Bill and Diane appeared generally impassive. Nonetheless, the entire family surprised me with their arrival at the session the following week.

Apparently, Bill and Diane felt they had benefited from the previous session and were delighted with Andy's fluency then and increased fluency during the interim. Despite their more positive attitude about participating further in family therapy, Bill and Diane continued to erect psychological barriers to my inclusion in the family network. Only Andy and Dan appeared willing to accept my participation, with their own sharing of typical family interactions at home. This included Dan's expressed resentment toward his parents' preoccupation with Andy and his stuttering, and Andy's feeling that the only real attention he received from his parents was in relation to his stuttering.

These disclosures were met by defensive protestations from Bill and Diane, who declared their nonpartiality in relating to Andy and Dan. Moreover, Bill continued to try to impress me with his academic and professional knowledge while still maintaining that it would be best for Andy to have individual speech therapy from me. Throughout the session it was also apparent that Andy's fluency was directly related to the degree of parental concealment of feelings. That is, the more Bill and Diane attempted to conceal by intellectualizing, the more dysfluent Andy became; and the more they shared feelings (which was minimal), the more fluent he became, with associated reduction of his secondary features. When this was pointed out to Bill and Diane, it was still difficult for them to take even partial responsibility.

It was not surprising when the next three family therapy appointments were cancelled immediately prior to their scheduled times, and I believed I had seen the last of the family (particularly as none of the therapy fees had yet been paid). When they arrived, on time, for their sixth scheduled appointment, I shared my surprise with them. Despite defensive excuses for their therapy cancellations, Bill finally acknowledged that all had not been well in family matters.

He now began to share his concerns about what he described as his "mid-life crisis" and boredom with his apparently successful private clinical practice. My own self-disclosure of similar feelings and experiences drew him out further with his acknowledgment of intermittent difficulties in the marital relationship. This apparently triggered Diane's disclosure of similar feelings about the marriage and her personal struggles with trying to be a successful wife, mother, and career woman.

Andy and Dan, obviously moved by their parents' personal concerns, immediately moved to comfort them, with a pouring forth of tearful emotion by all. It was immediately evident that this was the caring, loving, and sensitive family I had originally hypothesized, and psychopathology was not evident per se. That it had been struggling to maintain itself and survive the turbulences of modern-day life, did not appear to me extraordinary. That the stuttering was an expression, partly at least, of the inter- and intra-conflicts also seemed consistent with the reality of the family struggles.

We are not suggesting that these struggles or Andy's stuttering immediately ceased with the revelations made during the session. However, by the sixteenth session Andy's stuttering had virtually disappeared, his relationship with Dan had improved significantly, and although Bill and Diane continued to grapple with their own personal concerns, each was able to give to the other the support needed.

At the sixteenth session, the family decided to terminate therapy with the understanding that a follow-up session six months hence would be arranged. Several days before this prearranged session Andy called to inform me of the family's decision to cancel their appointment. Totally fluent, he told me his speech was "fine" and that things were going well. I wished him and his family well and did not contact them again until one year later.

In speaking with Diane by telephone, I learned that Andy's speech was normal, and that although things were not always smooth for them, she and Bill had been in individual psychotherapy for the past four months, and "learning much." The proverbial icing on the cake for me was the information that Andy had made a successful speech for his bar mitzvah.

What is most important to understand from this description of a "stuttering family" is that stuttering in the family is not necessarily rooted in psychopathology, nor is it only an individual problem but a family one as well. That it is a problem involving unique and dynamic familial interrelationship processes is more likely. It should be further understood that family therapy is not a panacea for treatment even for those children who stutter mildly or moderately.

Although this author has had success in treating several other "stuttering families," there have been some who were unresponsive to a family systems approach. Certainly, one might argue that such families are unresponsive because of deep-seated psychopathology. We tend to believe, rather, that it may be the unique features, processes, and complex inter- and intrapersonal relationships that dictate failure or success in a family therapy approach.

An individual counseling approach   The decision to forgo family therapy for individual counseling would be determined by consideration of the following criteria: (1) severe degree of secondary stuttering characteristics; (2) presence of family and/or individual psychopathology; (3) no apparent family dysfunction; (4) confirmed or established self-image as a "stutterer"; and (5) refusal by the family to be involved in family therapy.

Individual counseling for young children takes many shapes and forms, and to describe the vast number in use would go beyond the scope of this book. It would be most appropriate, however, to discuss a few within the context of the theories described elsewhere in the book and in particular as they might apply to the stuttering child.

Based on the criteria listed above, it is immediately obvious that the therapist is presented with a challenge perhaps more formidable than that in the case of Andy. Not only is family resistance more pronounced, but so are the factors that perpetuate the stuttering behavior, in particular, the confirmed self-image problem.

Nondirective client-centered counseling   Charles Van Riper (No. 18), in a concise and provocative essay, describes vividly how the therapist can enter the life space of the stuttering child in order to understand exactly what the child is experiencing and feeling. Using nonverbal monitoring, Van Riper makes a strong case for its use over typical verbal mirroring with stuttering children who may be too threatened by verbal interaction. Although the therapeutic outcome is not discussed, the process is one that allows the child and the therapist to experience together all of the hidden fears and avoidances associated with the child's unique stuttering pattern.

We believe that this working-through process can also be facilitated with verbal mirroring as long as the therapist is sensitive to the child's terror in communicating verbally. It is possible to integrate both verbal and non-verbal mirroring or reflection within the context of play therapy, which we do not view as a separate and distinct form of treatment. In very young children, play is more likely to be the chief medium of communication. Here, again, the major determining therapeutic factor is the client-therapist relationship, through which the shame, guilt, anxiety, preoccupation, and low self-esteem associated with the stuttering behavior can be resolved.

At this point in our discussion it is appropriate to recall the basic principles of play therapy first described by Axline (1969).

1. The therapist must develop a warm, friendly relationship with the child, in which good rapport is established as soon as possible.

2. The therapist accepts the child exactly as he is.
3. The therapist establishes a feeling of permissiveness in the relationship so that the child feels free to express his feelings completely.
4. The therapist is alert to recognizing the "feelings" the child is expressing and reflects those feelings back to him in such a manner that he gains insight into his behavior.
5. The therapist maintains a deep respect for the child's ability to solve his own problems if given an opportunity to do so. The responsibility to make choices and to institute change is the child's.
6. The therapist does not attempt to direct the child's actions or conversation in any manner. The child leads the way; the therapist follows.
7. The therapist does not attempt to hurry the therapy along. It is a gradual process and is recognized as such by the therapist.
8. The therapist establishes only those limitations that are necessary to anchor the therapy to the world of reality and to make the child aware of his responsibility in the realtionship. (p. 73–74)

We agree with Van Riper though, that play therapy in and of itself will not necessarily be productive in the modification or elimination of the stuttering pattern and the enhancement of a nonstuttering self-image. Perhaps with the mildly stuttering child who is not yet embedded in the stuttering morass, we may find traditional play therapy to be the approach of choice.

The decision to use a traditional play therapy approach, or a modified verbal and nonverbal client-centered procedure, or a nonplay face-to-face client–therapist communicative interactional approach will certainly be determined by the age, intelligence, emotional attitude, and maturity of the child, as well as by the severity, nature, and degree of the stuttering behavior. Further, the wise therapist must be acutely aware of the role other members of the family play, although not directly involved in the therapy, during the course of therapeutic intervention. Of particular importance to the therapist is the possibility that one or several family members may be wittingly or unwittingly sabotaging the therapeutic effort, which brings us to the issue of parent counseling.

Parent counseling Parent counseling has long been a favorite strategy used in conjunction with traditional symptomatic or interpersonal approaches with stuttering children. It is useful to summarize Bloodstein's review (1981), which includes several important aspects regarding the efficacy of parent counseling in the treatment of early childhood stuttering. Among the various major admonitions to parents typically are (1) encouraging them "to refrain from reacting negatively to the speech difficulties in any way, and to see to it as far as possible that the special interruptions are not brought to the child's attention by others" (p. 353); (2) attempting to improve the parent–child relationship; and (3) helping parents to eliminate those conditions or factors that exacerbate the stuttering behaviors, such as unrealistically high levels of aspiration.

Bloodstein cites the use of desensitization therapy as described by Van Riper (1972) in order for the child to cope better with environmental pressures at home, which presumably would be effective when the therapist is unable to work directly with the parents. He also describes the study by Egolf et al. (1972), which involves the parent directly in the therapy process, thereby teaching the parent a different and more positive way of dealing with the child.

We believe that traditional parent counseling, whether used independently or in conjunction with speech therapy for the child, is most likely to be, more or less, an information-giving process that would provide us little knowledge of the dynamic relationships between and among all family members. This is not to suggest that such an approach should be abandoned, as some "stuttering families" are not so dysfunctional as to require more than definitive advice and practical ways to cope with the stuttering child. We do believe, though, that if we are to counsel only the parents, we must refrain from placing them in the role of having caused the stuttering, but rather in the role of agents who can positively contribute to the overall well-being of the child and the elimination of stuttering.

Unfortunately, much of what we are suggesting is difficult to accomplish in the school setting. Even with the advent of PL 94–142 there has not been the full commitment of involving parents directly in the rehabilitative process, much less in the educational one. Too often, the parents of stuttering children who need to be involved most in their therapy are the ones most resistant to participating. Until the helping educational professions together formulate a more definitive philosophy and policy regarding the participation of the family in the child's overall education, we will continue to employ what could be considered a piecemeal approach. Unfortunately, again, our educational system does not appear motivated to initiate such a radical departure from traditional policies.

Individual counseling for the older child   The criteria we have established for our decision to counsel young children would apply to older children and adolescents, but it is possible to go beyond the individual counseling techniques and use an approach that would be more appropriate for older children and adults as well. For this reason we avoid redundancy and present such an approach.

Stuttering in the Older Child and the Adult

It is obvious that older stuttering children and stuttering adults do not share all of the features that characterize their respective problems or for that matter their personalities and needs. In examining these differences, it is readily apparent that the older child (1) still lives at home; (2) is still in the process of self-image formulation; (3) is still involved in all of the conditions and problems associated with the prepubescent or pubescent periods; (4) is limited in choice-making decisions of life; and (5) is still in the process of shaping an overall and distinctive personality pattern. The adult, meanwhile, typically (1) is likely to be functioning independently and no longer living at home;[1] (2) has a firmly established self-image; (3) is coping with problems and issues of school, career, and interpersonal relationships with other men and women; (4) is free to make choice-making life decisions; and (5) has a fixed personality pattern.

Regardless of the differences enumerated, it is possible to formulate an eclectic counseling approach suitable for either population and yet specialized to meet the needs of the stuttering individual.

Cognitive stuttering therapy A rationale for stuttering therapy based on the requirement that stuttering individuals learn to accept responsibility for their communicative behavior was originally introduced by Rubin and Culatta (1971) and later developed by Culatta and Rubin (1973). Among the major principles initially proposed, they note that (1) speech therapy should be cognitive and direct without regard to time or symptom; (2) those who stutter must acknowledge their ability to be fluent at least some of the time and have the ability to be fluent all of the time; (3) the individual can have control over his or her own dysfluency and fluency; (4) stuttering is viewed as an offensive and unpleasant behavior by most listeners and particularly the therapist, who must not conceal this same attitude; (5) stuttering is self-reinforcing and provides a payoff to the individual, which must be dealt with directly in therapy; and (6) the individual misevaluates his or her ability to be fluent on the abstract as well as concrete levels and is given direction to change this concept.

Culatta and Rubin have enumerated eleven principles that underscore their therapeutic approach. They are presented in the sequential order in which they must be mastered: (1) communicating verbal content in terms of fluency and not dysfluency; (2) belief in the physical ability to be fluent; (3) self-acknowledgment of responsibility for fluency previously achieved; (4) self-acknowledgment of the individual's own reason for stuttering and objectifying it; (5) recognition that it is valid to question reasons for dysfluency and to evaluate the stuttering objectively; (6) assuming direct responsibility for fluency achieved during therapy; (7) consciously manipulating fluency; (8) predicting the nature of speech subsequent to either fluent or nonfluent speech, in order to demonstrate control; (9) demonstration of control over dysfluency and fluency upon request; (10) lengthening fluent and dysfluent responses; and (11) consciously controlling fluency and dysfluency over longer periods of time.

The program developed by Culatta and Rubin appears to have a direct relationship to the cognitive-behavioral approach introduced by Ellis at the annual meeting of the American Psychological Association in Chicago in

---

[1] In present-day America, this is not necessarily the case, as economic conditions have dictated otherwise. This obviously presents us with issues we will discuss later.

1956 and later developed by him (Ellis and Harper 1961). Although Ellis focuses on emotional disturbance, which we believe does not necessarily apply to most who stutter, his theory is nonetheless quite relevant with regard to stuttering behavior in general. As stated in the preface to one of his contributions, ". . . people largely control their own destinies by believing in and acting on the values or beliefs that they hold. . . . [P]eople do not directly react emotionally or behaviorally to the events they encounter in their lives; rather, people cause their own reactions by the way they interpret or evaluate the events they experience" (Ellis 1977, p. 3). Ellis further believes that basic irrational beliefs that characterize most instances of emotional disturbance are essentially absurd and self-defeating and that the purpose of a cognitive-emotional therapeutic process "is to induce the person to recognize the absurdity of his beliefs, to relinquish them, and to adopt new, more adaptive ones" (p. 3).

Moleski and Tosi (1976) compared the use of rational-emotive therapy to Wolpe's systematic desensitization therapy in the treatment of stuttering and found rational-emotive therapy to be more effective in reducing stuttering behavior as well as accompanying anxiety and negative attitudes toward stuttering. They do not indicate, however, if any changes occurred with respect to self-image. It is also important to note that the authors assume stuttering to be an emotional disturbance.

Regardless of the apparent differences between Culatta and Rubin's and Ellis's principles and therapeutic approaches, one major similarity is fundamentally clear—the notion that the individual need not continue to indoctrinate himself or herself with attitudes inculcated over a period of time, and can choose a different manner of behavior through a logical thought process.

In Chapter 1, on counseling, we discussed the use of contracting as a means of assisting the client in fulfilling goals established in therapy and practicing new modes of behavior outside the clinical environment. Shames and Florence (1980) introduced the use of contracts in their behavioral approach to stuttering therapy. Goldberg (1981) has made contracts a fundamental part of his behavioral-cognitive stuttering therapy program (BCST), taking the stuttering individual through fifteen major steps, beginning with extended prolongation of fluent speech and continuing through generalization of normal fluency.

The Institute for Rational-Emotive Therapy in 1984 developed a Rational-Emotive Therapy Self-Help form to be used by clients as part of homework assignments in which they record those things they feel most upset about on a particular day or throughout the week (see Figure 1). Such a qualitative rating scale can be a useful tool in assisting stuttering persons to develop a more realistic attitude about their stuttering.

We see the use of contracts as an effective means by which the client not only makes a rational commitment to change an undesirable behavior (stuttering) or attitude but as a self-reinforcing instrument for establishing permanent change.

A cognitive-emotional counseling approach Goldberg (1981) has developed a systematic approach to fluency training based on the principles originally outlined by Rubin and Culatta and later by Shames and Florence. Goldberg's program is structured within an operant conditioning model that includes fluency shaping activities that inhibit stimulus anticipation and enhance stimulus and response generalization. He develops fifteen strategic principles, which he employed with children as well as with adults:

Principle 1: Clinical program flexibility—This allows for varying the program based on the variables of (a) age of client, (b) severity of disorder, (c) degree of commitment by the client, (d) extent of family as well as other environmental support, (e) clinical setting, and (f) amount of time available for therapy.

Principle 2: Establishing clear role relationships—The therapist serves as a change agent who is responsible for educating and guiding the client as well as providing techniques and support for the production of fluent speech.

Principle 3: The stimulus of anticipation—The therapist reinforces the individual's awareness of the occurrence of stuttering and through prolongation focuses the individual's attention on the specific word being spoken, thereby reducing or eliminating all stuttering behaviors.

Principle 4: Reinforcing desired behaviors—The therapist modifies the frequency and severity of disfluent speech through the application of contingencies, which in turn will reinforce the occurrence of fluent speech.

Principle 5: Teaching the individual to speak fluently—The individual is taught how to be consciously fluent through an understanding of *why* fluent speech can be attained.

Principle 6: Direct work on fluent speech—By teaching the individual to speak fluently, secondary characteristics of stuttering are eliminated.

Principle 7: Developing understanding through demonstration—The individual is helped to understand that he or she has the ability to choose to be fluent. Discussion of avoidances, resistances, and self-perpetuating negative attitudes is conducted in conjunction with direct action.

Principle 8: Use of small sequential steps—Maximizing new and positive minimal changes will minimize the possibility of failure.

Principle 9: Automatic speech through repetition—By practicing through repetition, effortless, automatic fluent speech is achieved.

Principle 10: Reinforcing increases in fluent speech—Negative behaviors must be eliminated by ignoring or punishing them and positive behaviors such as small increases in fluent speech must be reinforced.

Principle 11: Early generalization—Employing discriminative stimuli for fluent speech in various environmental situations early in therapy will enhance generalization of fluent speech.

Principle 12: Stressing positive changes—The therapist encourages client-initiated discussions on how it feels to speak fluently while deemphasizing discussion of negative aspects.

Principle 13: Positive aspects of stuttering—The client learns how to par-

RET SELF-HELP FORM

Institute for Rational-Emotive Therapy
45 East 65th Street, New York, N.Y. 10021
(212) 535-0822

(A) ACTIVATING EVENTS, thoughts, or feelings that happened just before I felt emotionally disturbed or acted self-defeatingly: _____

(C) CONSEQUENCE or CONDITION—disturbed feeling or self-defeating behavior—that I produced and would like to change: _____

(B) BELIEFS—Irrational BELIEFS (IBs) leading to my CONSEQUENCE (emotional disturbance or self-defeating behavior). Circle all that apply to these ACTIVATING EVENTS (A).	(D) DISPUTES for each circled IRRATIONAL BELIEF. Examples: "*Why* MUST I do very well?" "*Where is it written* that I am a BAD PERSON?" "*Where is the evidence* that I MUST be approved or accepted?"	(E) EFFECTIVE RATIONAL BELIEFS (RBs) to replace my IRRATIONAL BELIEFS (IBs). Examples: "*I'd* PREFER *to do very well but I don't* HAVE TO." "*I am a* PERSON WHO *acted badly, not a BAD PERSON.*" "*There is no evidence that I* HAVE TO *be approved, though I would* LIKE *to be.*"
1. I MUST do well or very well!		
2. I am a BAD OR WORTHLESS PERSON when I act weakly or stupidly.		
3. I MUST be approved or accepted by people I find important!		
4. I am a BAD, UNLOVABLE PERSON if I get rejected.		
5. People MUST treat me fairly and give me what I NEED!		
6. People who act immorally are undeserving, ROTTEN PEOPLE!		
7. People MUST live up to my expectations or it is TERRIBLE!		
8. My life MUST have few major hassles or troubles.		
9. I CAN'T STAND really bad things or very difficult people!		

(OVER)

10. It's AWFUL or HORRIBLE when major things don't go my way!		
11. I CAN'T STAND IT when life is really unfair!		
12. I NEED to be loved by someone who matters to me a lot!		
13. I NEED a good deal of immediate gratification and HAVE TO feel miserable when I don't get it!		
Additional Irrational Beliefs:		
14.		
15.		
16.		
17.		
18.		

(F) FEELINGS and BEHAVIORS I experienced after arriving at my EFFECTIVE RATIONAL BELIEFS: _____

I WILL WORK HARD TO REPEAT MY EFFECTIVE RATIONAL BELIEFS FORCEFULLY TO MYSELF ON MANY OCCASIONS SO THAT I CAN MAKE MYSELF LESS DISTURBED NOW AND ACT LESS SELF-DEFEATINGLY IN THE FUTURE.

Joyce Sichel, Ph.D. and Albert Ellis, Ph.D.

ticipate actively and consciously in specific behaviors that result in fluent speech.

Principle 14: Fluency and Environmental Support—The outside environment becomes as important as the clinic environment for the positive reinforcement of fluency by significant others in the client's life.

Principle 15: Establishing commitment through fluency contracts—Through the use of contracts the client is forced to cope with resistances to becoming fluent and held self-accountable for the efforts at the development of fluent speech.

Goldberg's program is a very positive approach to the elimination of stuttering behavior in individuals of all ages. Although it includes a form of directive counseling for clients and parents, it does not fully address the resistances those who stutter demonstrate, nor does it completely manage the self-image problem. Regardless of fluency achieved, the individual may persist in the belief that he or she is still a "stutterer."

The author recalls a classic example of such a case—a twenty-nine-year-old man who learned to be completely fluent in all speaking situations and with all people, yet who maintained "but I still *feel* I stutter." Six subsequent months of client-centered counseling failed to effect any major change in his attitude and he resisted psychiatric referral. Therapy was terminated, the man continuing to be obsessed with his stuttering.

Though the preceding example may not be typical of denial of fluency, which in this case was apparently rooted in deep psychopathology, variations on the theme are not uncommon. We would agree also with most other writers who believe that elimination of the stuttering symptom will not necessarily be replaced with other debilitating symptoms. Yet we do maintain that stuttering that has its origin in childhood and persists into adulthood carries with it entrenched attitudinal patterns that are not readily dislodged regardless of the fluency achieved.

We believe that by combining the cognitive approach proposed by Goldberg with an application of the client-centered counseling approach outlined in Chapter 1, we can best deal with the multidimensional nature of the stuttering problem. The ten intervention factors are as follows:

1. *Developing the appropriate attitudes necessary for active listening.* We must be prepared and open to understand the means by which the stuttering individual copes with his or her stuttering reality. No judgment is made in the beginning regarding the client's perhaps distorted view of self and/or perception of reality, in general, although the client is aided in listening to his or her own communicative message.

2. *Viewing the client as a person.* We share with the client the belief that stuttering is not something one is but, rather, represents one behavior, albeit negative, among many positive behaviors. The client is helped to understand that despite the pronounced nature of stuttering, we all have our own distinctively negative attributes, but these are only one part of who we are.

3. *Being aware of the obstacles to active listening.* We must be prepared to acknowledge and understand our own feelings that become activated by who the client is, what is being communicated, and how it is being communicated. It means listening to our own negative attitudes toward stuttering and not denying that listening to its unpleasant features bothers or disturbs us. It also implies our acknowledgment of our negative reactions to the client's negative distorted attitudes.

4. *Viewing ourselves realistically.* We must not confuse the struggles of any particular stuttering individual with our own life struggles and perhaps negative self-concept, and must be prepared to separate out the client's possible projections on us. It means avoiding the role of rescuer, which takes away the importance of our client's active role as choice maker. It also implies tolerating our client's impatience with us when we refuse to take responsibility for the client's fluency. Only when we serve as objective facilitator can our client make full use of his or her own potential for change.

5. *Valuing client choice.* Because some clients may demonstrate resistance to achieving fluency and/or unwillingness to make the necessary commitment to such change, we must understand that any dramatic change in behavior is often fraught with anxiety or even terror. Such feelings should not be viewed as psychopathological necessarily, as the implication of achieved fluency carries with it not only dramatically different perceptions by others of our client but the client's own perception of what these changes may mean for him or her in all aspects of life. We as therapists may lead our client to the proverbial waters but the client must make the decisive choice to drink. Only if the individual is provided an opportunity to explore these resistances and their implications can the full realization of self-choice become apparent and real.

6. *Using client–therapist contracting.* The contracting procedures described in Goldberg's model need no repetition, except that they must be complemented by continual analysis, review, and modification through the interpersonal counseling process. Here, again, as therapists we must avoid cajoling and judgment making, which would only alienate the client from the particular contract and from us. We proceed at the client's pace with the mutual understanding that any obstacle to progress and contract elaboration is the responsibility of the client. Rationalization, avoidances, and resistances are fully discussed so that the client is made fully aware of what he or she is choosing or not choosing.

7. *Using confrontation.* Confrontation can be most effectively utilized when a stuttering client attempts to hide behind irrational verbal statements of cognitively distorted thinking with respect to descriptions of self, avoidance of fluency, or maintaining the status quo. Sharing with the client our inability to understand the incongruency of his or her expressed communicative message or attitude places the responsibility directly on the client to clarify exactly what meaning is intended or what feeling is being experienced. Though a direct challenge to the client, discomforting as it may be, it nonetheless may be carried out gently, caringly, and objectively.

8. *Acknowledging the value of therapist self-disclosure.* Therapist self-disclosure can be an effective means of reinforcing positive behavioral change, developing positive self-image, and extinguishing or neutralizing self-defeating behaviors and attitudes. It aids the client in the realization that he or she is not alone in personal life struggles, albeit different ones from the therapist's. The client, therefore, can feel comforted in knowing that he or she is not "sick" or "stupid" when attempting to hide behind the rationalizations, illogical thinking, and misperceptions often associated with stuttering and the fear, embarrassment, and struggles that also accompany it.

To self-disclose does not mean preoccupying the client with the struggles of our own personal lives as a means of working out our own unresolved problems. It does, however, provide a more supportive, safe, and accepting clinical environment in which the client is freer to explore the self-perpetuating behaviors that contribute to stuttering.

9. *Blending symptomatic strategies with counseling.* Use of Goldberg's BCST model does not always imply the necessity for intensive counseling because the instrument itself allows for some degree of informational counseling. But when a client presents us with complex cognitive and emotional struggles, we are required to follow a plan that includes a continual interweaving of both strategies. Even minimal positive changes in fluency should be further reinforced by some discussion of the client's reaction to his or her accomplishment. There may be times also when we wish to focus our attention more on one strategy than another, but we always allow for the inclusion of the other, depending on the level of progress of the client. We do not offer a rigid procedure to follow because unique client needs and our own objective and subjective analyses would dictate a flexible approach.

10. *Attending to body language and paralinguistic cues.* The nonverbal and nonlinguistic features of communication will assist us in providing further clues to our client's struggle with fluency and attitudinal change, particularly when the messages are inconsistent with the verbal message given.

The client–therapist relationship   Regardless of the therapeutic approach used in stuttering therapy, we would agree with Cooper (1974) that the therapeutic relationship "facilitates the client's adaptation of more accurate perceptions which enable the stutterer to achieve maximum success . . ." (p. 81). We would add that because each therapeutic relationship differs by the very nature of the individuals involved, there can be no definitive rule governing its ongoing development. It does imply, however, mutual adaptation to moment by moment changes in behavior, attitude, and circumstances, thereby enjoining us as therapists to be flexible in all our responses rather than following any one predetermined course of action.

We do not wish to imply that we dispense with the overall therapeutic model we have chosen to use but, rather, that we make it relevant to the contracts we have negotiated with our clients. If contracts are be broken, so be it, as long as both participants explore together the reasons and then renegotiate new ones.

One further caution we need to acknowledge as therapists is that because most of the available evidence suggests little or no presence of pronounced psychopathology in most stuttering individuals, we should adhere to a well model in our approach. That is, we must view each relationship in such a way as to facilitate learning in both of us.

Finally, the relationship requires that we diligently avoid the use of the term *stutterer*, which contradicts the very mutual nature of the relationship and what we wish to accomplish in therapy. This may not be easy because the term has been well inculcated in us both personally and professionally. Those of us who resist this change in our belief system can only ask the questions: Why must we persist? and Of what value is continued use of the term?

Special conditions for family therapy Family therapy as a viable mode of treatment for stuttering adults would be applicable only when the individual's most frequent interpersonal involvement is with other members of the family, regardless of whether the child lives at home. It is conceivable that if family patterns in the past have been an influential part of the stuttering process, they will continue to be so. The choice by the individual to remain living at home, ostensibly for economic reasons, may also be indicative of separation and bonding needs not yet resolved.

Certainly we must not assume that these needs are necessarily related to the stuttering dynamics, but an initial family assessment would help clarify the issue. Then it would be possible for us as therapists to determine the efficacy of continued family therapy, individual cognitive-emotional therapy, or both. Whatever the therapeutic strategy, the final choice must be made by the stuttering individual.

RESEARCH CONSIDERATIONS

Within this chapter we have presented rationales to explain etiology and therapeutic models deemed appropriate for children and adults who stutter. We do not believe that the vast amount of research has yet corroborated a definitive etiological theory, a characteristic stuttering personality, or even the most effective treatment model. We have posed as many questions as we have attempted answers, hoping to stimulate further debate and investigation.

A Proposal For Investigation

We believe that before we can ascertain which therapy model can stand the most rigorous scientific test, we will need to determine first which factors contribute to the developing stuttering pattern. We have suggested that although constitutional factors have some experimental support, these factors must be viewed in the light of subsequent family dynamics. It would seem appropriate, then, to consider a well-established test instrument that can be used to differentiate stuttering from nonstuttering families. For such a purpose we recommend the Taylor-Johnson Temperament Analysis (Taylor and Johnson 1977).

The T-JTA   The Taylor-Johnson Temperament Analysis (T-JTA) is designed to "ascertain and evaluate the significance of certain personality traits which influence personal, social, marital, parental, scholastic, and vocational adjustment" (p. 1). It provides in visual form an evaluation describing an individual's feelings about himself or herself at the time of answering the 180-item inventory.

Most important from our present perspective is that the scale is not designed to measure serious abnormalities or disturbances but, rather, to measure several "important and comparatively independent personality variables or behavioral tendencies" (p. 1). A unique feature of the test is the Criss-Cross ratings procedure that allows individuals to respond to the items as they apply to themselves or as they apply to others, such as a spouse, parent, sibling or offspring.

The analysis also includes the delineation of nine major traits and four major trait patterns:

1. Nervous (vs. composed)
2. Depressive (vs. lighthearted)
3. Active-social (vs. quiet)
4. Expressive-responsive (vs. inhibited)
5. Sympathetic (vs. indifferent)
6. Subjective (vs. objective)
7. Dominant (vs. submissive)
8. Hostile (vs. tolerant)
9. Self-disciplined (vs. impulsive)

a. Anxiety pattern
b. Withdrawal pattern
c. Hostile-dominant pattern
d. Emotionally inhibited pattern

Finally, the test meets stringent reliability and validity criteria.

We believe the T-JTA can provide us with definitive information regarding interpersonal family dynamics as they may or may not relate to the stuttering process within the context of the family system.

REFERENCES

ACKERMAN, N. W. Family psychotherapy: Theory and practice. *American Journal of Psychotherapy*, 20 (1966), 405–414.

ANDREWS, G., CRAIG, A., FEYER, A. M., HODDINOTT, S., HOWIE, P., and NEILSON, M. Stuttering: A review of research findings and theories circa 1982. *JSHD*, 48 (1983), 226–246.

ANDREWS, G., GUITAR, B., and HOWIE, P. Meta-analysis of the effects of stuttering treatment. *JSHD*, 45 (1980). 287–307.

ARONSON, A. *Clinical Voice Disorders*, 2nd ed. New York: Thieme, 1985.

AXLINE, V. *Play Therapy*. New York: Ballantine, 1969.

BARBARA, D. A. *Stuttering: A Psychodynamic Approach to Its Understanding and Treatment*. New York: Julian, 1954.

BLOODSTEIN, O. *A Handbook on Stuttering*. Chicago: National Easter Seal Society, 1981.

BLUM, A. A neurofunctional theory of stuttering. Unpublished paper, 1984.

BRUTTEN, E. J., and SHOEMAKER, D. J. *The Modification of Stuttering*. Englewood Cliffs, N. J.: Prentice-Hall, 1967.

COOPER, E. Integrating relationship and behavior therapy procedures for adult stutterers. In L. L. Emerick and S. B. Hood (Eds.). *The Client–Clinician Relationship*. Springfield, Ill.: Chas. C Thomas, 1974.

CULATTA, R., and RUBIN, H. A program for the initial stages of fluency therapy. *JSHD*, 16 (1973), 556–568.

EGOLF, D. B., SHAMES, G. H., JOHNSON, P. R., and KASPRISIN-BURELLI, A. The use of parent–child interaction patterns on therapy for young stutterers. *JSHD*, 37 (1972), 222–232.

EISENSON, J. Personal communications, 1984.

———. (Ed.). *Stuttering: A Second Symposium*. New York: Harper & Row, 1975.

———. A perseverative theory of stuttering. In J. Eisenson (Ed.), *Stuttering: A Symposium*. New York: Harper, 1958.

ELLIS, A. The basic clinical theory of rational-emotive therapy. In A. Ellis and R. Grieger (Eds.), *Handbook of Rational-Emotive Therapy*. New York: Springer-Verlag, 1977.

———. Rational-Emotive Therapy. In V. Binder, A. Binder, and B. Rimland (Eds.), *Modern Therapies*. Englewood Cliffs, N.J.: Prentice-Hall, 1976.

ELLIS, A. and HARPER, R. A. *A Guide to Rational Living*. Englewood Cliffs, N.J.: Prentice-Hall, 1961.

FARBER, S. L. Genetic diversity and differing reactions to stress. In L. Goldberger and S. Breznitz (Eds.), *Handbook of Stress: Theoretical and Clinical Aspects*. New York: Macmillan, 1982.

GLAUBER, I. P. The psychoanalysis of stuttering. In J. Eisenson (Ed.), *Stuttering: A Symposium*. New York: Harper & Row, 1958.

GOLDBERG, S. A. *Behavioral Cognitive Stuttering Therapy*. Tigard, Oreg.: C. C. Publications, 1981.

GOLDIAMOND, I. Stuttering and fluency as manipulatable operant response classes. In L. Krasner and L. P. Ullman (Eds.), *Research in Behavior Modification*. New York: Holt, Rinehart & Winston, 1965.

HAHN, E. F. *Stuttering*. Stanford, Calif.: Stanford University Press, 1956.

HAMILTON, V. An information processing model. In L. Goldberger and S. Breznitz (Eds.), *Handbook of Stress: Theoretical and Clinical Aspects*. New York: Macmillan, 1982.

INSTITUTE for RATIONAL-EMOTIVE THERAPY. *RET Self-Help Form*. New York, 1984.

JOHNSON, W. *People in Quandries*. New York: Harper & Brothers, 1946.

JOHNSON, W., AND ASSOCIATES. *The Onset of Stuttering*. Minneapolis, Minn.: University of Minneapolis Press, 1959.

KIDD, K. K. A genetic perspective on stuttering. *Journal of Fluency Disorders*, 2 (1977)259–269.

KOPP, G. A. Metabolic studies of stutterers: I. Biochemical study of blood composition. *Speech Monographs*, I (1934), 117–132.

KORZYBSKI, A. *Science and Sanity*. Lancaster, Pa.: Lancaster Press, 1933.

LUDLOW, C. L., and COOPER, J. A. Genetic aspects of speech and language disorders: Current status and future directions. In C. L. Ludlow and J. A. Cooper (Eds.), *Genetic Aspects of Speech and Language Disorders*. New York: Academic Press, 1983.

MOLESKI, R., and TOSI, D. J. Comparative psychotherapy: Rational-emotive therapy versus systematic desensitization in the treatment of stuttering. *Journal of Consulting. Clinical Psychology*, 44 (1976), 309–311.

MORGAN, R. F. (Ed.). *The Iatrogenics Handbook*. Toronto: IPI Publishing, 1980.

MURRAY, H. L. and REED, C. G. Language abilities of preschool stuttering children. J. Fluency Dis. 2, (1977) 171–76.

NELSON, M. O. Stuttering and the Control of Speech: A Systems Analysis Approach. Cambridge: Cambridge University Press, in press.

ORTON, S. T. Studies in stuttering. *Archives of Neurology and Psychiatry*, 18 (1927), 671–672.

RIEBER, R. W., ET AL. *The Neuropsychology of Language*. New York: Plenum, 1976.

RUBIN, H., and CULATTA, R. A point of view about fluency. *Asha*, 13 (1971), 380–384.

SCHWARTZ, M. F. *Stuttering Solved*. New York: McGraw-Hill, 1976.

SHAMES, G. H., and FLORENCE, C. L. *Stutter-Free Speech*. Columbus, Ohio: Chas. E. Merrill, 1980.

SHAMES, G. H., and SHERRICK, C. E., Jr. A discussion of nonfluency and stuttering as operant behavior. *JSHD*, 28 (1963), 3–18.

SHEEHAN, J. G. Conflict theory and avoidance reduction therapy. In J. Eisenson (Ed.), *Stuttering: A Second Symposium*. New York: Harper & Row, 1975.

———. Theory and treatment of stuttering as an approach-avoidance conflict. *Journal of Psychology*, 36 (1953), 27–49.

SHEEHAN, J. G., and COSTLEY, M. S. A reexamination of the role of heredity in stuttering. *JSHD*, 42 (1977), 47–59.

SPEECH FOUNDATION of AMERICA. *Counseling Stutterers*. No. 18. Memphis, Tenn.

STOCKER, B. and PARKER, E. The relationship between auditory recall and dysfluency in young stutterers. J. Fluency Dis 2, (1977) 177–87.

TAYLOR, R. M., and JOHNSON, R. H. *Taylor-Johnson Temperament Analysis Manual*. Los Angeles: Psychological Publications, 1977.

TOMATIS, A. *L'Oreille et le Language*. Paris: Editions du Seuil, 1963.

TRAVIS, L. E. *Speech Pathology*. New York: Appleton-Century, 1931.

VAN RIPER, C. *Speech Correction: Principles and Methods*, 5th ed. Englewood Cliffs, N.J.: Prentice-Hall, 1972.

———. *The Nature of Stuttering*. Englewood Cliffs, N.J.: Prentice-Hall, 1971.

———. The severe young stutterer. In *Counseling Stutterers*, No. 18. Memphis, Tenn.: Speech Foundation of America.

WEST, R. An agnostic's speculations about stuttering. In J. Eisenson (Ed.), *Stuttering: A Symposium*. New York: Harper, 1958.

WESTBY, C. E. Language performance of stuttering and nonstuttering children. J. Commun. Dis. 12 (1979) 133–45.

———. The phenomenology of stuttering. In R. West (Ed.), *A Symposium on Stuttering*. Madison, Wis.: College Typing Co., 1931.

WILLIAMS, D. E. Stuttering therapy for children. In L. E. Travis (Ed.), *Handbook of Speech Pathology and Audiology*. New York: Appleton-Century-Crofts, 1971.

———. A point of view about "stuttering." J. Speech Hearing Dis. 22 (1957) 390–97.

WINGATE, M. E, Speaking unassisted: Comments on a paper by Andrews et al. *JSHD*, 48 (1983), 255–263.

WOLPE, J. *Psychotherapy by Reciprocal Inhibition*. Palo Alto, Calif.: Stanford University Press, 1958.

5

PSYCHOLOGICAL CONSIDERATIONS OF LANGUAGE-DISORDERED CHILDREN AND THEIR FAMILIES

INTRODUCTION

As we take on the formidable task of exploring the many dimensions of psychogenetic and social processes in the development of language disorders in children, we need to set some limits and take some positions that may not satisfy the orientation of many workers in the field.

We have chosen to use the term *language disorder* to describe broadly a particular behavior, regardless of etiology, following Bloom and Lahey (1978). They view language along three basic dimensions. The first is language form, in which the elements of a message such as its shape and sound are combined. The second is language content, which is what individuals talk about or understand relative to the message. The third is language use, in which speakers choose to speak in a particular way, depending on the listener and the context. For our present purposes we also treat the interaction of the form, content, and use of language as a complete entity, bearing in mind that each, when independently impaired at times, may be a function of diagnostic categorization. As Bloom and Lahey have indicated, the emphasis must be on what children do and what they have trouble doing, so that interference in the language system may be better understood.

We shall not discuss the multidimensional nature of learning disability in children except to isolate the language component and explore its effects on the overall psychosocial development of the child. During our discussion, however, we must remain cognizant of the educational implications for, as well as the influence of other learning disability components on, the developing child. Further, our coverage of distinct categorical entities, such as mental retardation, aphasia, and autism, will be limited to the basic consideration of psychosocial effects only and consistent with a generic viewpoint. To do otherwise would deflect the thrust of the present chapter.

One final stipulation we have made is to treat articulation disorders as a phonological aspect of language and related to all other linguistic features. In their review of the research of children with phonological disorders, Bernthal and Bankson (1981) conclude that these children, particularly those with multiple sound errors, also have difficulties in comprehension, syntax, and vocabulary.

Although the synergistic view, which implies complex interactions and interfacing among all linguistic features, is still subject to further empirical confirmation, our search of the literature has failed to justify the separation of phonology from other linguistic aspects on the basis of psychogenetic and social processes. Regardless of the philosophical positions taken here, it is hoped that considerable debate will be provoked and further empirical research inspired.

PSYCHOGENESIS OF LANGUAGE DISORDERS IN CHILDREN

It is a truism when we suggest that parents who spend much time with and give considerable attention to their children will produce healthy, productive, communicative, and independent adults. Yet, like every maxim applied to human development and in particular communicative development, the exceptions force us to modify the original rules. So-called ideal familial circumstances do not always bring about the fully functioning adult as we would wish to predict. Similarly, we often find such adults to evolve from unstable, deficient, and uncommunicative parenting.

The genesis of human communication is too complex an act to explain by a mere collection of either independent or dependent variables; but by attempting to describe the quality of such variables and how they interrelate, we should be able to formulate postulates about its development. Toward this goal, we need to identify the most recent research findings and discuss the many relevant factors to elucidate our understanding of the problem. The most logical place to begin is with a discussion of the relationship of home environment and early language development. We shall not include children at this time who have acquired language deviations resulting from identified physical, physiological, neurological, or sensory deficits.

Home Environment and Language Development

Several of the most recent and extensive longitudinal studies investigating the relationship of home environment and early cognitive development, done in the United States and Canada, have been compiled by Gottfried (1984a,b). Citing a variety of measures employed by many authorities—including the Home Observation for Measurement of the Environment (HOME) Inventory, the Illinois Test of Psycholinguistic Abilities (ITPA) and the Bayley Scale of Infant Development (Bradley and Caldwell 1984), the Family Environment Scale (FES), the Purdue Home Stimulation Inventory (PHSI), the Test of Early Language Development (TELD), and Variety of Experience Checklist (VEC) (Gottfried and Gottfried 1984), the Reynell Developmental Language Scales (RDLS) (Siegel 1984); and the Bifactor Environmental Action Model (BEAM) (Wachs 1984)—Gottfried concludes "that assessments of proximal home environmental variables are reliable and valid indicators of the stimulation and experiences available to infants and young children" (p. 329).

He further concludes that cognitive development in young children correlates with several closely related home environment variables, among which he finds the following: (1) "Stability of home environment accounted for most of the correlations between early environment and subsequent cognitive development" (p. 336). (2) Play materials, maternal responsiveness, maternal involvement and verbal responses to infants' vocalizations were found "to have the highest and most consistent relationships" (p. 338). A meta-analysis by Glass, McGraw and Smith (1981) supports the findings summarized by Gottfried, with maternal involvement and responsivity and play materials showing the highest mean correlation with the development of cognition and language.

The effects of socioeconomic status   Although much research has revealed that children from lower socioeconomic groups demonstrate developmental lag in acquiring cognitive and language skills (Bereiter and Engelmann 1966), more recent research has identified specific factors that would account for the delay. Based on research conducted by Bradley and Caldwell (1984), Gottfried and Gottfried (1984), Barnard, Bee, and Hammond (1984), Johnson, Breckenridge, and McGowan (1984), Siegel (1984), and Beckwith and Cohen (1984), Gottfried reports that children from lower socioeconomic status (SES) families tend to receive a relatively less intellectually advantageous home environment conducive to cognitive and language development than those from higher SES families. Differences, however, were noted strictly as a function of socioeconomic factors, regardless of other factors. The inescapable finding was that "mothers of relatively higher intelligence, as measured by vocabulary, provided a more enriched environment for their children" (P. 330).

Of particular interest was the conclusion that "middle compared to lower SES mothers spoke more to their children, were socially more involved, provided more intellectual tasks in terms of play materials, and showed consistently higher levels of caregiver responsiveness" (p. 331). An additional significant finding was that crowding in the home adversely affected home stimulation in terms of quality and quantity, thereby contributing to cognitive and linguistic lag.

We should bear in mind, as we consider the merits of the conclusions drawn by the preceding studies, that several significant factors impinge on the nature of socioeconomic class. To begin with, lower SES mothers tend to be single parents, many of whom work, and who are unable to provide the necessary home stimulation and caregiving characteristics of higher SES mothers. Second, because Gottfried and Gottfried (1984) and Johnson, Breckenridge, and McGowan (1984) define intelligence as measured by vocabulary, we believe such a narrow definition fails to consider other facets of intelligence. That is, we cannot assume that lower SES mothers are necessarily intellectually inferior, but only that linguistic stimulation may be lacking because of the quantity and quality of parent–child contact.

Environmental deprivation   Abundant evidence supports the notion that early environmental deprivation is causally related to language delay. Spitz (1945, 1946a, 1946b), in his now classic study, investigated the effects of an emotionally vacant orphanage when infants were placed there at four months of age. Deprived of most human contact beyond the bare necessities of bodily needs, the infants became essentially developmentally retarded and susceptible to extreme emaciation (marasmus) and profound sadness (anaclitic depression). After two years, on follow-up, 37 percent of the children had died. Of those surviving, severe cognitive, linguistic, and intellectual and social deficits were observed. Although such catastrophic situations hopefully no longer exist, they do demonstrate how extreme disregard for infants' emotional needs can interfere with or destroy their normal development.

To a considerably lesser degree, Harlow et al. (1966) and Mineka and Suomi (1978) found short-term distress when primate infants were separated from their mothers. Although comparison of their results to those for human infants would be somewhat indefensible, Stayton and Ainsworth (1973) demonstrated that there is less short-term distress when a secure mother–child attachment is interrupted.

Bowlby (1960) attributed a variety of insults, such as linguistic, cognitive and intellectual retardation, behavioral and socialization disorders, and disturbed interpersonal relationships, to separation from parental figures. Rutter (1983), however, found that the long-term deficits described above were more closely related to the degree of privation to which the child had been exposed previously, the young age at which the separation had occurred (between ages one and four), the duration of the separation, and the quality and promptness of subsequent parenting.

Less obvious environmental deprivations occur in families where conditions are generally unfavorable for language development. These conditions include negative communicative interactions between family members, which we shall presently discuss in terms of dysfunctional family dynamics.

Bilingualism   Although early references point to bilingualism as a definitive factor in the etiology of language disorders in children, it is now believed that due to early methodological problems and cultural biases in research, positing such a relationship is not tenable. Whatever psychosocial correlates appear present in bilingual families seem more closely related to socioeconomic class.

Lambert (1977), writing on the effects of bilingualism in children, reviews the literature and suggests that bilinguals who are matched with monolingual controls actually appear to be more cognitively flexible, creative, and divergent in thought. Thus we would be hard-pressed, given the present state of knowledge on the subject, to support the view that bilingualism per se is directly related to psychosocial maladjustment and language disorder.

Dysfunctional Family Dynamics

Because language in children typically develops and evolves within the family structure and system, it is incumbent upon us to explore how dysfunctional family dynamics may interfere with and inhibit that development. Consistent with our discussions elsewhere in this text, we must consider family dysfunction along a continuum from marked psychopathology to minimal maladjustment. In so doing, however, we must bear in mind that the severity of the language disorder or delay is not necessarily contingent on the degree of psychopathology, as the child's own unique way of coping may alter the effects on him- or herself and perhaps influence the entire family system.

Unfortunately, the literature on the relationship of the language development and family systems theory is disappointingly sparse. Nevertheless, it is possible to review some findings.

Cantwell, and Baker (1977) found a high degree of behavior disturbance among children with language problems. In a later effort, Cantwell, Baker, and Mattison (1979) studied 100 speech- and language-delayed children, finding eight specifically language-disordered children who were diagnosed as having attentional deficit disorder with hyperactivity as defined by the DSM Code of the American Psychiatric Association (1980). The investigators did not find the psychiatric disorders, however, to be etiological to the language disorders.

One of the most comprehensive studies conducted was that of Stevenson and Richman (1978). In their epidemiological study of 705 children living in outer London, they found that of twenty-two children with expressive language delay, thirteen (59 percent) had behavior problems, compared to 14 percent in the total population. Similarly, children with behavior problems had more than four times the expected rate of severe expressive language delay. A follow-up study of these children one year later revealed consistency in both the behavior problem and language delay. Behavior problems were characterized by immaturity, problems in social relationships with siblings and peers, and marked dependency on the mother.

The authors caution that we not assume a cause-effect relationship between disturbed behavior and communication deficits. This should be obvious, as the children studied were three years old, thereby obscuring any evidence of family dysfunction as a causative factor contributing to language dysfunction. It is possible that in children who are both behaviorally disturbed and languaged disturbed, environmental stress may contribute to both. The evidence clearly suggests an association between behavior problems and social and family factors, and that language-disturbed children come from homes with particularly adverse conditions.

Mother–child interactions   Earlier we reviewed the literature relating home environment in general to language development in the child, and it is clearly apparent that the mother–child interaction is the predominant feature in that relationship.

Walbert et al. (1978) used the Caldwell Inventory of Home Stimulation to assess the home environments and mother–child interactions of a language-delayed group and a matched control group of normal preschool children. Their most significant findings were that mothers of normal speaking children were more responsive to, more involved with, and less restrictive of their children. The mothers of language-delayed children, although generally conscientious, tended to relate to their children similarly. Missing, however, was a "dynamic verbal interchange" or a positive reciprocal communicative relationship.

These investigators were careful to note, however, that because the children studied were beyond two and a half years, it was possible that the mothers of the language-delayed children related poorly, reciprocally, in response to the already established language delay, thereby exacerbating the language delay and the poor communicative relationship. Walbert et al. wisely avoid the temptation to assign blame for the breakdown in the communicative interaction or cite poor mother–child involvement as a causative factor in the language delay.

One major criticism is with the Caldwell Inventory of Home Stimulation that was used to evaluate the child's environment. The scale only considers the influence of the mother–infant interaction and does not measure the effects of all family interrelationships, such as the possible effects of the marital relationship, on the mother's relationship to the child. Our criticism, however, should not detract from the overall value of Walbert et al.'s significant contribution.

Olsen-Fulero (1982) has reviewed research that indicates that the mother's underlying intention gets served by the many different ways she converses with her child. Olsen-Fulero's own study demonstrates variability among mothers, especially in those behaviors most closely connected to a mother's intention. Her review demonstrates that the conversational mother who asks questions, rarely negates, and who gives few directions facilitates the child's language development. Her own findings suggest that the mother who stimulates, challenges, and encourages autonomy in the child facilitates the child's cognitive development. Her study further reveals evidence of highly individualized conversational styles among mothers who interact with their children.

One major criticism of Olsen-Fulero's work, which is also applicable to many other studies of mother—child interaction, is the small sample of children and mothers used.

Waterhouse (1982) studied twenty-one same-sex, same eye-color twin pairs and found that maternal speech patterns varied across families (mothers), reflect the child's developmental state, and reflect the mother's perception of her child. In a highly succinct and enlightening discussion, Waterhouse warns us that the complex communicative interactional process between the child and mother is confounded by too many elements to draw conclusions about causality. Covariances involving genetic/familial patterns and dynamic communicative adjustments made by both mother and child might better explain the significant relationships found between mothers' and children's language performances, according to Waterhouse.

Other writers have researched the mother—child relationship with respect to language development and have found significant correlations between language development and specific attributes of mothers' speech, but these attributes have been difficult to interpret (Furrow, Nelson, and Benedict) 1979; DePaulo and Bonvillian 1978). Söderbergh (1982) confirms earlier linguistic research in his study of three-year-old infants, finding that mother—child communication, as dialogue, may contribute to positive language development, although he is cautious about drawing any conclusions.

Brazelton (1981) used split-screen videotapes of mothers interacting with their infants during the first days and weeks of life, demonstrating a dyadic communicative interaction. Unresponsive mothers were reported to be identified prior to their infants' birth.

Lasky and Klopp (1982) found that mothers of normal language children demonstrated frequent communicative interaction in terms of expansions, reduction, imitation, use of questions, use of answers, acknowledgments, provision of information, nonverbal behaviors, and use of nonverbal deixis (pointing or glancing), whereas mothers of language-disordered children infrequently demonstrated these behaviors. As was noted by previous researchers, mothers and their normal language children seemed to be reciprocally involved in the communication process, with subtle adjustments made by the mothers in response to their children. The limited sample used in the study and the relatively older age of the infants (twenty-seven to forty-five months) prevent many definitive conclusions, particularly when we consider that the first two years are of the most crucial importance in language learning.

It appears obvious that any attempt to understand the complex dynamics of the evolving language development in the child must include the mother's or the main caretaker's stimulation. As Winnicott (1965) has implied, we cannot view the infant in isolation in attempting to assess language development. Further, just as we cannot separate the child from the mother, neither can we separate the mother from her own self- concept and the attitudes that pervade her sense as a person in relation to other aspects of her life and to other persons, particularly her spouse. Mothers do not enter into reciprocal relationships with their infants untouched by prepartum personality and emotional patterns, nor are they immune to the continuing influences of the child, spouse, and other children in the family.

The parents' interactions with the child and the effects on his or her language development will be influenced directly or indirectly by their own perceptions of themselves. So, too, will the mother alter her communication with the child in the continuing, changing relationship.

Thus what we have is a dynamic relationship in which the mother relates to her child within a complex family system, rather than in a circumscribed cocoon, a conclusion that would tax the credibility of any experimental investigation. To borrow from Winnicott, we would add that we cannot view the mother in isolation in attempting to assess language development.

Family relationships   There appears to be virtually nothing in the literature surveyed that explores the effects of family relationships, the marital relationship in particular, on the development of normal or abnormal language development. Because most children do develop language even in the midst of severely dysfunctional families, can we assume therefore that infant language development is immune to the psychopathological processes of these families? Hardly. Even the most ardent advocate of biochemical factors in the ontogenesis of schizophrenic or autistic language in children would acknowledge that aberrant family communications cannot be disregarded.

For the present, however, we are not discussing such extremes in linguistic breakdown, nor are we assuming that language disorder necessarily requires deep-rooted family pathology. We do suggest that subtle and oftentimes not so subtle variations in dyadic and triadic family interactions must be considered as possible etiological factors along with the unique constitutional or genetic correlates, whatever these may be, in the child. An even more complex consideration may well be the unique coping style of the family and its individual members, regardless of individual or family psychopathology per se.

In his extensive review of studies dealing with marital stress, means of coping, and its effect on depression, Ilfeld (1982) fails to identify what influences, if any, such factors have on children in the family. Based on his own major survey of more than 2000 households sampled from a Standard Metropolitan Statistical Area, Ilfeld found marital stressors to have a strong influence on depression in the family, but does not indicate specifically what effects there are on the children, much less on their language development.

Arrival of a child into a nuclear family that originally had consisted of two or three persons brings into play new factors and activates already present ones to challenge the new family. Although no documented evidence is available to isolate which factors would be etiological to faulty language development in the newly arrived child or for that matter the already present children, it would be helpful to identify those factors that characterize the functioning family and contribute to family and individual growth.

Fogarty (1976) has described the ideal functioning family, and we summarize his model as follows:

1. The family is adaptable to and positively responsive to any change. It readily accepts any disruption, able to move from its status quo position. This would include its response to a child with special needs.

2. No one person is seen to have an emotional problem, but whatever emotional problems are present exist in the family unit and are altered by the way family members cope.

3. There is a closeness and connectedness among all family members as well as with the families of origin.

4. Family members solve problems by dealing with them rather than avoiding or distancing themselves from them. Never is the identity of any family member distorted by or fused with another family member. That is, each is able to maintain his or her own personal integrity.

5. If a problem does arise between two family members, such as the parents, it is dealt with without the involvement of an innocent third person to judge or solve the dispute. That is, the child is not used to solve the problem that belongs to the parents.

6. Individual differences are respected, encouraged, and fostered to bring out the best in each person.

7. Each person is free to think and feel individually in relationship to self and to other members of the family.

8. Each person is clearly identified and differentiated from other persons in the family. Each person is aware of what the other person gets from himself or herself and what he or she gets and needs from others.

9. There is a recognition and awareness of "emptiness" in each other, but each is allowed the opportunity to fill his or her own void. Thus the child who may be struggling to solve a personal issue is not rescued by the values and judgments of others, but is aided to discover personal means to deal with the problem.

10. There is a positive emotional climate with the avoidance of what is "right" and what "should" be done. *Truth exists only in what is truly practiced* (italics mine).

11. Healthy family functioning is directly related to and dependent on each family member's enjoying other family members and the family as a whole. The

problem, stated or unstated, of one family member is acknowledged and respected.

12. Any one family member feels free to use any other family member for feedback and learning with no fear of embarrassment or criticism.

Whereas the reader may take issue with Fogarty's description of an ideal functioning family system as not being real, we would respond that the crucial element is the necessity for families to *strive* toward the ideal. It is the recognition of the process, not the result, that has the greatest impact.

Therapists who work with language-disordered children who have no identified organic etiological components are well aware of the wide variations among parenting and family styles. These same workers who are also knowledgeable in child development theory would attest to the considerable range of possibilities and family circumstances under which language normally develops. Clearly, even in the most dysfunctional family, children develop language. Conversely, language-disordered children frequently have been observed in apparently functioning families. Where, then, do the discrepancies lie?

We submit that professional workers are not always privy to the subtle interactional processes among family members, particularly between mother and child. Even the most carefully thought out and objectively conducted research would be challenged to identify, in the antiseptic and experimental environment, perhaps obscure elements that either contribute to or impede language development. We do not wish to infer, however, that such research is unproductive. On the contrary, there have been numerous studies that have taken investigators into the home to identify, firsthand, the positive elements that characterize language development. But even the best intentioned investigator could not possibly know what occurs behind closed doors after the investigator has left. Does this suggest that we ought to refrain from such investigations? Not at all. We believe it is practically possible to determine those interactional factors, albeit subtle or obscure, that could be revealed through blind self-rating instruments. These we shall discuss later.

The language-disordered child as the "identified symptom"   Previously, we stated that a child could embody certain types of conflict between parents or among several members of the family, and that the conflict may be manifest in a specific aberrant behavior such as stuttering. Or, when conflict may not be present, it may be a change in family circumstances that initiates negative behavior. Conceivably, it is possible that disruption of language development may result directly or indirectly from the child's reaction not only to obvious elements, such as a silent environment, family communication characterized by continual marital bickering, or unrealistic parental expectations, but also as a reaction to the arrival of a sibling, the mother needing to work, or a mother–father relationship that avoids conflict.

The author recently was referred a four-year-old child whose language was characterized by severe syntactic, semantic, and phonological delay. Formal testing could not be carried out due to his marked hyperactivity, and his language comprehension was only marginally adequate. Pediatric and neurological workups were unremarkable and the parents did not report any events indicating otherwise. Most evident during the intitial contact with the child was his inability or refusal to focus on separately introduced play materials. For example, he would manipulate several toy cars for a few moments and then search for other play items. Vocalizations during this time were characterized by holistic single- or double-word utterances, with a distinctly higher level of content than of form.

Family therapy was initiated in order to learn more of the family interactional dynamics. Included were Jason (the child), his ten-year-old brother, Gavin, and the parents, Mr. and Mrs. C. The session was essentially characterized by constant interruptions by Jason, which interfered with the communicative efforts of others. His failure to remain seated during the session taxed this therapist's clinical acumen as well as his patience, but several significant facts were learned. Mrs. C had been working a day shift as a data processor for more than four years, and Mr. C worked the graveyard shift as a security guard. The family therapy session revealed that during the afternoons, Jason was left free to do as he pleased in the home, without supervision, while his father slept. The only contact Jason had with his mother was in the late afternoon and early evening, when she felt too tired to relate to him. Other revealing family behaviors consisted of inconsistent and uncompromising differences in parental discipline; extreme guilt expressed by Mrs. C regarding her lack of attention given to Jason and her anger toward Mr. C regarding his lack of attention toward her and Jason; Mr. C's apparent indifference, defensiveness, and passivity in his relationship to all members of the family; and Gavin's unverbalized anger toward all.

The nature of the family communication can best be described as chaotic, which unsurprisingly resembled Jason's own dysfunctional behavior. Two subsequent family sessions differed little from the initial one, except that the family struggle to find some resolution of their difficulties was clearly evident. Although they aptly realized that Jason required more than traditional language therapy and that continued family therapy would indeed be helpful, they could not bring themselves to make a structured commitment to therapy.

This case study is one example of how interpersonal family communication and behavior in conjunction with individual personal attitudes and struggles can create a family atmosphere antithetical to normal language development in one family member. The example, moreover, points to the conclusion that no one factor within the family process can readily be assigned a major role in the development of a language disorder. It does suggest, however, that dysfunctional family dynamics could be manifested in the form of language dysfunction in the child.

The Relationship of Genetic and Psychosocial Influences

Definitive experimental evidence relating hereditary factors to the ontogenesis of language disorders is woefully lacking, although Ludlow and Cooper (1983) cite several descriptive case studies that have been carried out (Arnold 1961; Luchsinger 1970; Mattejat, Niebergall, and Nestler 1980; and Zaleski 1966). They conclude from the evidence from chromosomal studies that there is little scientific basis for a link between sex chromosome deficiencies and the development of language problems. Even fewer studies have attempted to establish a relationship between phonological problems and a genetic base. Ludlow and Cooper do report, however, that children who are found to have some chromosome aberration also tend to have communication impairments. They cite Annell, Gustavson, and Tenstam (1970), Haka-Ikse, Stewart, and Cripps (1978), Nielsen and Sillesen (1976); and Nielsen, Sorenson, and Sorenson (1981), who report language and phonological acquisition to be delayed in 40 to 75 percent of the cases studied.

Stark, Mellits, and Tallal (1983), based on the results of their studies, do not believe we have a means to establish a direct etiology to language disorders and suggest that family studies along with standard intelligence tests, language tests, and perceptual-motor measures would help us to define etiological correlates. In his study of environment, age, and organismic specificity and their effects on the cognitive-intellectual development of the child, Wachs (1984) suggests that organismic specificity may be a significant factor during the first two years "in terms of interpreting differential reactivity to the environment" (p. 320). Based on the results of his experimental investigation of thirty-eight infants who were eleven months of age at the beginning of the study, Wachs concludes that whereas male and female children are equally sensitive to their environment, they are so in different ways, and that there is a specificity for certain environmental dimensions. The hypothesis that different individuals, regardless of sex, will react in different ways to the environment was supported with the conclusion that "genotypically based individual differences mediate the response of the individual to the environment" (p. 321), and that a bridge may be established between biological and experiential factors.

For a more thorough description of the differential responses to the environment by different genotypes, the reader is referred to the provocative work of Bodmer and Cavalli-Sforza (1976).

It has often been said that, considering all of the negative influences that impinge on the young infant, it is amazing how so many learn to speak. Apparently, there must be enough positive influences that foster normal language development. Because the research thus far has failed to isolate highly specific psychosocial determinants, we must also continue to investigate the possibility that individual coping styles may be a significant factor in overall language development.

We are well aware that with regard to the behavior of children under severe external stress, there is enough clinical evidence to suggest wide variations of response. We are also aware that some children under minimal external stress also respond along a wide continuum. Unfortunately, the lack of systematic investigations precludes us from drawing definitive conclusions, but enough evidence exists to justify some speculation.

It is evident from our earlier discussion and review of stuttering behavior in children that there is strong evidence to suggest a genetic base for its development, but virtually no studies in the speech-language pathology literature draw such parallels in child language development. Garmezy (1983) leads us through a review of the literature dealing with the stressors of childhood, but limits his discussion to the "psychological threat posed by loss of or separation from a parent or significant caregiver" (p. 51) and the traumatic effects of war and civil discord on children. He summarizes several different studies of resilience in children, finding some congruence regardless of methodology, conditions of stress, and type of behavioral disorder. Although Garmezy does not discuss predisposing factors as such, he alludes to the growing interest in "protective" factors, discussed by Rutter (1983) in the same text.

As others have recognized, genetic factors play a significant role in establishing individual differences in the development of and susceptibility to behavior disorders in children, according to Rutter. He discusses the effects of combined or isolated chronic and acute stressors that induce disorder. He notes: "The notion here, then, is of factors which are largely inert on their own, but which serve as 'catalysts' when combined with acute stressors of some type—to use a chemical analogy" (pp. 22–23). After the work of Brown and Harris (1978), Rutter cites catalytic factors, described as 'vulnerability' variables, that tend to *increase* the effect of stressors, whereas other catalytic factors, described as "protective" variables, tend to *reduce* the effect of stressors. Much of the data reported by Rutter unfortunately applies to adults, and he wisely cautions us not to generalize too quickly to children. Nevertheless, he suggests that it would be useful to explore the effects, if any, of vulnerability and protective variables in childhood.

To parallel Rutter's concluding remarks, we believe that some children may be impeded in their language development following adverse experiences, whereas others may not. In fact, the latter may not only show resilience in not yielding "but the 'stresses' may actually have had a positive and beneficial effect" (Rutter 1983, p. 34). Such variables as age, sex, genetic background, temperament, problem-solving skills, and the nature of family interactions will all have to be considered important to explain how and why individual differences operate. Although the direct effects of adverse experiences on language development are somewhat known, it is important that we attend to indirect effects. As Rutter notes: "Thus early events may operate through their action in altering sensitivities to stress, or in modifying styles of coping which then protect from, or predispose towards, disorder in later life only in the presence of later stress events" (p. 34).

PSYCHODYNAMIC CORRELATES OF THE
LANGUAGE-DISORDERED CHILD

Our discussion so far has centered around general and specific psychoge-netic factors contributing to language disorders in children. At this point, it would be useful to consider in more detail how language deviations manifest themselves psychodynamically relative to the major linguistic dimensions of phonology, semantics, and syntax.

In addition, we must recognize the psychological effects language disorders sometimes have on the child as well as on other members of the family. Although these effects may vary relative to a known organic base, such as a childhood brain injury, mental retardation, or deafness, or relative to a functional base, such as environmental deprivation or family dysfunc-tion, we will find many similarities as well as differences. How the child and family members cope with either a developing language disability or an established disorder itself depends on the interrelationship among unique organismic factors within the child, the special circumstances of the family, and the attitudes of each family member. Because experimental evidence identifying these factors is not yet forthcoming, we have to rely on clinical evidence to postulate or at least speculate about such variables.

Specificity of the Disorder

The literature does not reveal any experimental evidence to suggest what definitive psychological effects, if any, occur in relation to specific language disorders. It is understood that original etiological-psychological factors may persist beyond the actual establishment of the disorder and be confounded by the way the child and/or family may respond to the language delay. It is also possible that the original etiological factors may no longer persist but that the language delay *does*, along with its accompanying psy-chological effects.

Most workers would agree that even the language-delayed child is saying some words by age eighteen months, and that some normal children may be saying little by three years of age. It is therefore the task of the speech-language pathologist to distinguish exactly and as early as possible those children whose language represents a significant and definitive prob-lem from those children who may be developing language somewhat later for unremarkable reasons. Moreover, it may be necessary to determine those psychological correlates that are manifestations of difficulty in concep-tualizing information, difficulty in learning the language code, difficulty in applying the code conventionally, difficulty in using the code in speaking, or a late development of cognition, conventional code, and use of the code (Bloom and Lahey 1978).

Phonological variations   Rousey, one of the earliest investigators to ad-vocate that articulation is symptomatic of a fundamental psychological disturbance, (1971) declares: ". . .errors in articulation of consonants reflect developmental failures in personality rather than reflecting stops or arrests in the normal maturation process of speech articulation" (1971, p. 820). He appears to distinguish speech production from subsequent verbal language patterns, a proposition at variance with current thinking on language theory and development.

Representing a psychoanalytic viewpoint, Rousey refers to Erikson's infantile sexuality theory in describing the clinical meanings of misarticulated sounds. He hypothesizes the following:

1. Disturbance in early and significant relationships with the father is represented by the substitution of /f/ for /θ/.
2. Deprivation disturbance in the mother–child relationship is represented by distortions and substitutions of the /l/.
3. The oral expression of aggression in the child is manifested in the substitution of /d/ for /ð/.
4. Fixation of the child at the infantile level is represented by the persistence of a frontal lisp.
5. Difficulty in early psychosexual development during the anal period is represented by the appearance of a lateral lisp.
6. Anxiety characterizes the production of a strident (whistling) /s/.
7. Early lack of impulse control and the inappropriate release of aggression are represented in both the consonantal and vowel /r/.
8. Early fixation in psychosexual development is represented by the interchange of sounds characteristic of the oral stage of development.

In a later formulation, Rousey (1974) suggests that when the individual has experienced some sexual trauma, in reality or fantasy, substitution of /v/ for /ð/ may occur. He further suggests that substitution of /w/ for /r/ represents dependence on obsessional styles of thinking.

It is important to understand that Rousey's theory that "the presence of a sound articulated correctly reflects mastery of stages of emotional development" (1974, p. viii) is based essentially on years of clinical evidence but not verified by any substantial experimental data. Although some of the experimental results reported by Rousey and his colleagues do suggest trends in support of certain aspects of his theory, he is careful to suggest that much more research must be done.

We would agree, but at the same time not ignore the wealth of clinical evidence gathered to support Rousey's intriguing theory. One, in fact, need not subscribe to classic psychoanalytic theory in order to find some substantiation for a relationship between ego and articulatory development. Indeed, it would be difficult to treat articulatory or phonological development as an entity apart from the total organismic nature of the individual. Yet, in a recent publication, which deals with the psychological factors affecting speech production, there is only a brief allusion to Rousey's theoretical development (Darby 1981). We would hope that such an omission does not represent a dogmatic bias of antipsychoanalytic psychiatry, as even the broad implications of Rousey's work cannot be ignored.

Regardless of psychodynamic theory, it is conceivable that dysfunctional family interrelationships, in which the child becomes the identified victim, may determine specific phonological errors, with or without other accompanying behavioral symptoms. Although at present it is difficult to make a strong case for a phonemic specificity, because articulatory-deficient children tend to have multiple errors, it is possible that the phonemic *pattern* represents the psychodynamic status of the child. Moreover, it might be useful to explore deviations in psychological development in terms of distinctive feature analysis. Most important is that we as professionals remain open to any possibility, regardless of previously cherished beliefs.

Syntactic and semantic variations   Although it would be tempting to speculate on a relationship between deviations in psychological development and deviations in the form and the content with which the child uses language, there is nothing in the literature investigated to support such a conjecture relative to typical language-delayed children. The difficulty in designing studies to test such relationships has been addressed by Weintraub (1981), who experimentally investigated the relationship between the use of syntax in adults and psychological defense mechanisms, and found that inferences about behavior and personality can be made from analysis of the major features of free speech. He states: ". . . We must consider . . . the fact that the frequency of occurrence of even simple grammatical structures is so dependent upon cognitive, maturational factors in preschool children that the influence of emotional variables may be extremely difficult to determine" (p. 46).

It is generally agreed by professionals in the field that autistic children demonstrate, among many other characteristics, disturbances in cognitive and linguistic processes. Although it is not our purpose here to delve into the biochemical/psychogenic conflict over etiology, we agree with Rutter (1978), among others, that many symptoms could be secondary to the primary disturbance of cognitive-linguistic impairment.

According to the DSM-III criteria established by the American Psychiatric Association (1980) for infantile autism, the child's language development is grossly defective, often characterized by echolalia, immediate or delayed, and/or reversal of first and second person pronouns, and metaphorical language. Fish and Rivto (1979) report that in some cases babbling is retarded from the start and the child is mute. In others, both babbling and the first words may develop normally or with minimal delay, only to be arrested or to regress at the end of the second year or at the beginning of the third. In those children with more developed speech, the use of complex syntax, the formation of long sentences, and the comprehension of subtle and abstract meaning are disturbed with characteristic distortions of syntax and fragmentation of speech. Fish and Rivto also note the use of idiosyncratic terms that may be understood only if the original context of the child's association is known.

Effects of the Disorder on the Child

Regardless of the type, nature, quality, or degree of language dysfunction, the child will react to the difficulty relative to his or her unique perception of it. Secondary symptoms in the form of defenses may appear to counteract the anxiety or to gain some degree of control of the anxiety. The choice of method and the quality with which the child manifests such defenses are due to a complex interaction of the child's identification with the coping style of the parent, personal developmental level, and unique coping style. Whereas many children with recognition and awareness of their phonological, syntactic, or semantic discrepancies readily cope and adapt with approximations toward normalcy, others are stuck in the mire of linguistic dysfunction. For these children, behavioral and personality changes occur that often obscure the earlier predisposing conditions associated with the development of the language disorder.

In their review of the literature, Cantwell and Baker (1977) found a tendency toward psychiatric dysfunction in speech-language–disordered children. Confirmation of this tendency was later reported by Cantwell and Baker (1977) and Baker, Cantwell, and Mattison (1979). In childhood psychosis, defensive behaviors become the most apparent characteristics of the child's illness and are basic to the actual syndromes of autism, symbiotic psychosis, and pseudoneurotic psychosis (Thompson and Havelkova 1983).

Among the specific effects of language disorders of children are changes in self-concept, somatic problems, behavior disorders, and educational problems.

Stress and coping It would be convenient to generalize that the language-disordered child will develop a distorted self-image similar to that of the stuttering child. Nothing in the literature reviewed, however, suggests such a corollary. Certainly, the child may be conscious or *made* conscious of the inability to communicate appropriately by many factors, such as parental and sibling reactions or the attitudes of peers and others. We are led to consider, then, how the unique personal coping mechanism operates relative to the degree of stress experienced by the child.

The coping process has a dual function, including the regulation of emotional distress and solving the problem (Rutter 1983). We doubt that it comes into play, relative to the child's awareness of a language deficiency, until five to seven years of age, Piaget's concrete operational stage. Among other things, the child is now able to compare personal linguistic functioning, in part at least, with that of others and experiences the anxiety that comes with being unable to command appropriate use of the language. Citing the work of Rose (1976), Maccoby (1983) speculates that because the hippocampus, which has a role in behavioral maturation, does not fully mature until the age of six years, it is possible that the child's ability to cope may be partly connected to physiological maturation. If we add temperamental differences (presently we do not know if these are genetically or environmentally determined, or both) and environmental response as one further variable, it is apparent that no simple explanation regarding the response by the child to personal language functioning is possible.

Although not referring to language disorders per se, Rutter (1983) states the overall problem succinctly: "Intuitively, it seems that the coping process itself, in terms of active problem solving and of emotional palliation, is likely to influence outcome, but empirical data on the actual importance of coping mechanisms are still lacking" (p. 34).

Somatic changes   A somatoform disorder is the physical expression and experience by the individual of an inability to cope successfully with psychosocial events. Although there is little empirical or experimental evidence to suggest that the child's inability to cope with the language deficiency will be expressed somatically, it is useful to explore the possibilities. Cantwell, and Mattison (1980) did find in their studies of forty-six children with pure speech disorders and fifty-three children with both speech and language disorders that among the major complaints were those somatic in nature. We concur with Geist (1983) that it is unlikely for a linear cause-and-effect relationship, in which a psychological conflict leads to a specific physical disorder, to exist. It is more likely, according to Geist, that a systems model in which a complex interaction of psychological, social, and physical factors takes place would prove more useful.

Billy was a six-year-old boy who had been suffering asthmatic attacks for several months. Upon intake, he evidenced severe expressive language difficulties. The family lived on a remote farm, generally removed from social contacts. Clinical testing of nonverbal performance revealed intelligence functioning to be within the norm. Cognitive receptive language was also essentially intact. Medical data, including neurologial information, were unremarkable except for the asthma. The mother reported that three years previously, at about the time Billy stopped speaking, the family was desperately attempting to save their farm from foreclosure. Although the family survived the threat to their personal and economic lives, Billy apparently was fixated developmentally in his expressive language. The mother further reported that Billy was generally ignored, except for satisfying his basic needs, during the family's struggle to maintain the farm. Hungry for attention from his mother and his father, Billy would often sit in his room picking at his toys and was generally disinterested in television. When he carried over his isolated behavior to kindergarten, his teacher initiated the referral for help.

It would be presumptuous of us to draw any definitive conclusions from this anecdote, except to suggest that while psychogenetic-social conflicts may have played a primary role in the linguistic lag, subsequent psychogenetic-social factors may have played a definitive secondary role in exacerbating the language disorder. That a somatic illness may be associated with such factors cannot be ignored.

Behavioral problems Profound behavioral changes in language-different children are most readily observed in autistic children. Based on his own empirical evidence and the research of others, Prizant (1983) suggests that the complex we know as the autistic syndrome, which includes deviant language, difficulties in social interaction, and compulsive and ritualistic behaviors such as echolalia, must be viewed in an interactive way. He further adds that the phenomena evidenced should be studied relative to cognitive processing and cognitive-linguistic development. Prizant appears to straddle the gap between viewing the communicative dysfunction as either a primary or secondary deficit, and gives the impression of favoring a type of coping mechanism used by the autistic child. Such a mechanism is not unlike that presented by Rutter (1983), which was discussed earlier.

Although qualitatively different, the performance deficit associated with mentally retarded children can be viewed as an impairment of adaptive behavior, to a certain degree. We would agree that genetic and physiological factors set limits in these children's language acquisition and usage and ultimate language repertoire. But we cannot ignore the adventitious effects on language by their response to their own deficits.

According to Beier (1964), behavioral disturbance tends to occur more frequently in the mentally retarded than in the general population, but the degree to which the retarded child can respond to his or her own awareness of a language deficit is unclear. Certainly, the child who approximates near normal intellectual functioning is more likely to be aware of personal communicative abilities and will attempt to cope accordingly. But even with the moderately retarded child whose language is successfully remediated, it is obvious that a modicum of awareness of the deficit can be present. What effects such awareness may have on the child prior to remediation have not been revealed in the literature surveyed. One thing is certain, however, and that is that the mentally retarded child is more vulnerable to the development of unsuitable behavior than the normally endowed child, in the form of anxiety, hyperactivity, and a deficient self-concept.

Some children who are unable to acquire language capability because of known neurological etiology are commonly referred to as "congenitally aphasic" or "developmentally aphasic." They are striking in their manifestations of emotional lability, distractibility, and hyperactivity. We must be cautious, however, not to equate these children with autistic children, who present a somewhat different symptom complex.

The inability of developmentally aphasic children to process information auditorally contributes to the confusion and disorganized behavior often seen by therapists (Emerick and Hatten 1979). When we consider, then, the constellation of primary deficits that is present, it is not difficult to understand the problem such a child would have in coping emotionally. Less understood is whether or not the child's coping behavior is a manifestation of the primary deficit, a secondary one, or both, as we have seen in adult aphasia.

If we add to these behavioral responses family reactions, we are confronted with a formidable challenge to sort out those elements that are most amenable to change. Treatment of one or more features would certainly influence the impact of the disability on the child.

With respect to more typical speech- and language-delayed children seen in school, Baker, Cantwell, and Mattison (1980) found immaturity, restlessness, short attention span, excitability, tantrums, constant climbing, and solitary behavior to be characteristic of children with both speech and language disorders. It should be noted, however, that certain methodological problems in their study, such as lack of a "normal" control group of children, sampling method, and heterogenity problems (for example, mixing dysarthric with functional disorders) preclude us from making further definitive judgments. Nonetheless, it would be difficult for us to purport that speech- and language-delayed children are oblivious to their difficulties, and suggest that these children probably represent a high-risk factor for behavior disorders.

Education problems   Although it is not our intention to explore the vast domain of the learning-disabled child and his or her environment, it is generally agreed that language problems are common among children with learning problems. Because the ability to use language is critical to the development of other academic skills, it is not surprising that the language-deficient child, regardless of etiology, who enters school will demonstrate varying degrees of personality and behavioral problems such as poor interpersonal relationships, hyperactivity, aggression, anxiety, disinterest, anger, hostility, and selective attention difficulties. To what degree these characteristics are primary to subsequent academic underachievement, or are consequential to biogenetic bases for underachievement, is not yet fully understood.

Beasley's (1956) classic contribution, written more than thirty years ago, is still timely to our understanding of the child with delayed language development:

> It can be inferred that a young child who does not develop language at the usual time will bring to a language-learning situation all his previous experiences. He will have acquired certain attitudes about himself as a nonspeaker, reflecting what others think about him (funny, bad, stupid, slow, stubborn, lazy, etc.), which may act as a barrier to learning. He will also have developed certain patterns of behavior to cope with his language inadequacy, such as withdrawal, aggressiveness, apathy, or dependency, which will affect his attempts to talk. He will have been exposed to efforts employed by others to induce him to talk. These will color the way he perceives the teacher's efforts. (pp. 52–53).

Although much of what we can say, definitively or generally, about the complex internal and external forces that impinge on the child's striving toward linguistic adequacy is still within the realm of speculation and uncertainty, Beasley's elegant and lucid words deserve to be heeded. Indeed, some empirical support, although meager, for Beasley's formulations is evidenced in the Baker et al. study alluded to earlier. Evaluations by teachers of speech- and languaged-disordered children in their study revealed many adjustment problems, including a negative attitude toward authority, diminished academic achievement, and disruptive behavior. As speech-language pathologists, it is incumbent upon us to develop more precise means to intervene appropriately when dysfunctional behavior is evidenced in language-disordered children. How this may be accomplished shall be discussed later.

Effects of the Disorder on the Family

In their critical review of the literature on psychiatric disorders in children, Cantwell and Baker (1977) cautiously take the position that except in rare instances, psychiatric disorders do not cause speech and language delay. They do, however, state that in most cases psychiatric difficulties are caused indirectly by the speech and language delay.

Alluding to the methodological problems associated with the definition of psychiatric disorder, the delineation of precise types of language delays, and the determination of other related factors such as intellectual retardation and brain damage, they take the position that the parent–child interaction must be better understood. They suggest that the language-delayed child will be the most likely child in the family to "evoke disturbed patterns of parent–child interaction" because of the child's difficulty in communicating, because of individual temperament, or for other reasons. The child, in turn, will be more likely to develop emotional difficulties.

We support such a contention, but would add that a triadic or even a quadrant interaction should be considered more consistent with family systems theory. The effects of language delay on total family interaction cannot be underestimated, as any pronounced change in one family member will disrupt the equilibrium of the entire family, with each member striving to reestablish the family balance.

What is important to understand is that the family is an interaction of personalities, in which the members react to each other as individuals. Each has a particular conception of his or her role as well as a conception of the roles of all other family members. Any alteration of behavior in one member (for example, the language-delayed child) is viewed by other members in the light of their own personal perspective or temperament, which in turn will affect the original family member's perception of style. The language-delayed child will then react to the way in which he or she is being perceived. If the perception of one or another family member is imbued with negativism, the child will respond behaviorally in the way discussed earlier, and coincidentally begin to perceive himself or herself negatively. This in turn will further exacerbate the initial family attitude and response.

It should be made clear that this does not necessarily infer that the language-disordered child who reacts aberrantly does so in response to deep-rooted family psychopathology. We prefer to review dysfunctional or inappropriate family response to the child along a broad spectrum of typical family life, with the admonition that even in the best of families, members become victims of their own peculiar attitudes and temperaments. That the child and indeed the family need assistance is obvious, but that intensive psychiatric intervention is always necessary does not represent our view.

The reaction from parents   Our discussion has implied that the child's language disorder has as much of an effect on parents' reactions as the latter does on the child's response to the disorder, as well as on the disorder itself. Many of us are familiar with parents of language-disordered children who report that they had been told, "Don't worry, he'll outgrow his baby talk." Our concern about these families is not so much that the child would undoubtedly have benefited from earlier language therapy intervention, but that the family, particularly the parents, would have been spared the anxiety, uncertainty, and confusion about the child's language competency despite the earlier reassuring imperative statement.

Parents often demonstrate an uncanny intuitive ability to recognize that "something is not right" and, because of well-intended but glib statements from professionals unfamiliar with developmental linguistic processes, begin to question their own integrity as parents, which in turn may further negatively influence their child's language development and self-concept. Weintraub (1981) reminds us that the failure of parents to interpret their child's immature language usage during the course of everyday family interaction can result in both noncomprehension and misunderstanding. We would add that such breakdowns in communication will contribute further to difficulties in the child–parent relationship.

The reaction from siblings   Siblings of language-disordered children often become forgotten members of the family and, in terms of family systems theory, the "silent identified patient." That is, while the parents are preoccupied with the other child, the nonaffected siblings may either receive less attention, become the objects of unrealistic expectations by the parents, or be scapegoated by others.

Lefebvre (1983), discussing sibling reactions to a handicapped child in the family, cites several studies that describe how the sibling may be affected. Among the studies noted, that of Shere and Kastenbaum (1966) found emotional disturbance among nonaffected twins more often than among affected twins, with genetic endowment held constant. Lavigne and Ryan (1979) found more irritability and social withdrawal in siblings of handicapped children, before age five, than in siblings of chronically ill children.

Therapists frequently report overindulgence of the affected child by an older sibling who understands the affected child's deficient use of language, or the avoidance of interaction by the sibling with the child. Even occasional ridicule or teasing by the unaffected sibling will interfere with the affected child's attempts to cope and may contribute to the disruption of family relationships. We suggest that such behavior may be indicative of the unaffected sibling's feeling a threat to his or her own place in the family or to his or her own developing self-concept.

Because no studies have revealed definitively negative attitudes by siblings, we hesitate to make any generalizations about their behavior. We do suggest, however, that such investigations could be very fruitful in adding to our understanding of the psychosocial dynamics in families with language-disordered children.

Effects of Other People on The Child

Even less data are available on the negative effects that peers, teachers, and other professionals have on the child who is deficient in language. Fortunately, teachers and other professionals are more likely to have a positive effect through therapeutic and educational intervention. Nonetheless, it is useful to consider some of the evidence that suggests negative influence on the child from external sources.

The reaction from peers   Although very young children with language disorders may be relatively unaware of how they are viewed by their peers, who are also unconcerned about or unaware of the discrepancy in language development, the school-age child is increasingly sensitive to the reaction of others. Thus the language-disordered child becomes vulnerable to humiliation or shame if his or her language proficiency is inconsistent with the unwitting norm established.

Flavel (1979) has described the growing awareness of one's image as perceived by others as part of a larger developmental process that is described as "metacognition." That is, the entering school-age child is beginning to develop skills at monitoring his or her own thought processes and performance. The language-disordered child, in our view, however, may not have developed such skills, placing the child in a situation in which he or she becomes vulnerable to the growing cognitive perceptions of peers. Struggling to cope with the personal perception that "something is different," and responding to peer reaction, the child begins to behave in ways that are perceived even more negatively by peers. The child is caught in a vicious cycle of attempting to please, being unable to do so, struggling further, and incurring even further negation.

The more pronounced the language deviation, the greater the likelihood of negation, particularly in the case of the mentally retarded, emotionally disturbed, hearing-impaired, or aphasic child. Certainly, the degree to which the child responds and the quality of that response are dependent on internal factors such as temperament and individual coping mechanisms and external factors such as the family support system.

The reaction from teachers   Few workers would disagree that the teacher's attitude and behavior toward the language-disordered child may have a profound effect on the child's continuing language development.

Weinberg and Santana (1978) argue that overidentification with the child and rescuing the child from psychological and social pressures may result in insensitivity to the parents' needs and frustrations and may be in competition with them. Although these authors are referring to handicapped children in general, we believe their concerns would apply to the language-disordered child.

Writing on the language problems of disadvantaged children, Shuy (1972) describes in vivid detail how difficult many teachers find it to cope appropriately with their pupils, either through lack of training or through frustration over their inability to handle the concomitant problems associated with language delay or usage in that population. Pleading for further research in teacher attitudes in this area, Shuy urges also that special attention be given to them and that teachers be required "to develop an ability to learn how to deal with the child's language, how to listen and respond to it, how to diagnose what is needed, how to best teach alternative linguistic systems, and how to treat it as a positive entity" (p. 203).

We believe that the quality of response by the teacher to learning-disabled, emotionally disturbed, aphasic, hearing-impaired, and mentally retarded children who are linguistically impaired is no less important. Either the overestimation or underestimation of these children's capabilities will interfere with their progressive development in language and in other behaviors. We do not question the academic competency with which the teacher helps these children, but we are concerned that the teacher may not always have the self-awareness of personal deep-rooted feelings that may emerge as projections toward these children and that may interfere with their honorable intentions (see Chapter 9 for a more extensive discussion on the issue). There is little doubt in our minds that the way the teacher perceives the child and the language disability will in turn influence the way the child perceives self and the language disability. Only further experimental study of these provocative issues can bring to light the complex nature of these relationships.

The reaction from other professionals   Parents of language-disordered children or children who they believe to be language-disordered typically put great faith in the ability of professionals to provide the necessary information and expertise to help them and the children and perhaps to assuage their guilt over their own real or imagined responsibility for the disorder. Such faith is a formidable challenge to the professional, who is placed in the position of being all-knowing and is expected to answer to parental concerns that may go beyond the professional's level of competency.

The implication is that, as professionals, we must have a keen sense of our own specialized knowledge and a mature acknowledgment and acceptance of our limitations. To believe or do otherwise is to fault ourselves and certainly the already fragile family concerns. Glib, condescending, or authoritative-sounding responses to genuine and sometimes naive questions only serve to obscure the real issues, delay necessary intervention, and perhaps alienate the parents from subsequent professional assistance. In any case, it is the language-disordered child who also suffers.

In the final analysis, only appropriate referral and/or comprehensive differential assessment will address the needs expressed by the family. We must trust that such is the rule in real practice and that any exception is an isolated event to which we must direct our influence in affecting change.

INTERVENTION STRATEGIES

It is apparent to any serious worker in the field of childhood language disorders that emotional components may be difficult to separate from cognitive and symptom-based treatment strategies. In keeping within the context of the present chapter and the tone of the rest of the book, however, we shall focus only on treatment models that are essentially psychological in nature, bearing in mind their effects on cognitive and linguistic processes.

Because it is generally understood that language develops within the framework of the interpersonal relationships among family members, the mother−child relationship in particular, we believe, as Beasley (1956) has already suggested, that interpersonal relationships are as important for the child without language or with disordered language. It is important, therefore, to reacquaint ourselves with the work of Cameron (1947), who Beasley quotes, and who we believe needs to be recognized as one of the earliest writers on a pragmatic approach to language learning. Cameron states:

> Language habits creep so gradually into all reactions that no one can really say of a child's behavior, "Here at this instant role-taking in terms of language had its start." In play, language at first functions merely as a component or an accompaniment, but later and secondarily it acquires status as a semi-independent, equivalent form of behavior that allows its possessor to take roles first in words without deeds and then in fantasy as well. We have pointed out that language habits mold us into conformity with our culture, because language is a cultural product and highly conventionalized, and we have said that through language our covert symbolic behavior is also organized along social lines. On the other side of the ledger is the fact that language and organized thought are together a means of enriching our potentialities for social role-taking enormously.
>
> Talking becomes in itself not only the most effective instrument of interpersonal communication, eventually superseding all others, but also the medium through which one builds up a repertory of social roles. By learning to say what others say in context, a child learns first to express his attitudes and then, by expressing these conventional attitudes appropriately, he tends actually to acquire them as his own. (p. 95)

Intervening on the interpersonal level, however, also requires that we recognize that some language-disordered children will not be responsive to a unitary approach. As Wachs (1984) points out, similar intervention approaches are not applicable to all types of language-disordered children. It is necessary, he believes, to look at the individual characteristics of each child, relative to the child's particular earlier experience, social environment, and biological differences.

We further take the synergistic position, reviewed by Schwartz et al. (1980), that phonological deficits are one aspect of total linguistic behavior and that our counseling intervention makes no distinction based on differing forms or content of such behavior. We do acknowledge, however, that individual differences, regardless of the nature of the linguistic disorder, must be considered.

Play Therapy

We have typically seen play therapy employed with stuttering children (see Chapter 4) and with language-disordered children for the purpose of resolving the child's negative feelings about self and others. We submit that play therapy has a far greater value by enhancing the linguistic competence of very young language-disordered children.

Because play constitutes a major means by which young children formulate, develop, and solidify all parameters of the linguistic process, it makes sense that we should implement therapeutic procedures to enhance these processes. The importance of the interpersonal communicative interaction between child and parent further supports our rationale for the use of play strategies to simulate such interactions.

We do not believe that play should be used only with language-disordered children who also happen to be emotionally disturbed. On the contrary, its value can be demonstrated in very young children who are language disordered, regardless of etiology, family function, or emotional adjustment. We recognize that such a viewpoint is a departure from traditionally held beliefs about play therapy, but we believe, nonetheless, that we can justify its use in a more generic way.

A behavioral-symptomatic-linguistic approach   Earlier in this book we described how play therapy may successfully be used with young stuttering children, utilizing the model originally introduced and developed by Axline (1969). With certain modifications appropriate for use with the language-disordered child, we have developed an approach based on behavioral-symptomatic principles and the principles of transformational grammar.

1. *Establishing rapport.* Utilizing play materials both familiar and unfamiliar to the child, the therapist joins the child in play, first with those materials chosen by the child. The therapist refrains from verbalization, unless the child verbalizes first, in order to establish a situation whereby the child feels in partnership with the therapist. Any threat to the status quo of

the child can thus be minimized or averted to provide an atmosphere of safety in which intercommunication can gradually occur. Most important is that the child feels that a friendship is developing. All attempts at "teaching" by the therapist should be avoided at this time.

2. *Accepting the child as a person.* One of the most formidable tasks for the therapist is to avoid the trap of taking the position of the authority who knows what is best for the child. Such a position denies the child free expression of the self and the opportunity for verbal communication to occur and develop. Instead, the therapist must acknowledge and accept the child nonjudgmentally, with the understanding that the child has the capacity to change and learn. It means the formulation of a relationship in which mutual respect naturally develops through the interchange of two people.

3. *Providing an atmosphere for feelings to be freely expressed.* As the child gradually begins to feel secure in the relationship, the opportunity for the expression of any feeling, untouched by the therapist's judgment, occurs. It is facilitated by the therapist's own expression of feelings within the context of the play situation. It further allows the therapist a better understanding of the child's present cognitive-linguistic processing behavior. Permissiveness in the relationship is not meant to imply license for the acting-out child to damage physical surroundings or for physically abusing the therapist. The therapist must respond to this child not as a parent or as a child but as another person whose personal rights have been infringed upon. We believe it is possible to set limits within the therapeutic situation whereby the child may learn the importance of mutual respect and yet at the same time not feel constraints on the expression of feelings.

4. *Reflecting the expression of feelings and thoughts.* As the relationship develops, the child feels freer in expressing feelings and thoughts to which the therapist may respond via the method introduced by Rogers (described in Chapter 1). The therapist may also use modeling techniques as described by Courtright and Courtright (1976) and Van Riper and Emerick (1984), whereby the child's play is verbalized, using appropriate transformational forms ranging from "daddy" to "daddy's coming home." Van Riper and Emerick's description of the use of expansions, extensions, self-talk, and parallel talk is particularly pertinent, so that the child is provided the full opportunity to be exposed to appropriate language usage.

5. *Encouraging child-centered choice and change making.* As the child gradually begins to recognize that expressed feelings are being accepted and to be aware of developing language usage, he or she also develops the capacity to make choices and changes appropriate to the growing self-concept. The latter we believe also positively influences the more complex use of language as the child gains more and more control over the immediate environment, albeit the clinical one at first. With direct or indirect parental support, the possibilities for even greater positive change are enhanced. We see the developing self-concept and increased language usage as mutually interdependent, so that both must be consistently encouraged.

6. *Allowing therapy to proceed at a pace appropriate to the child.* We believe it

is inappropriate, as Van Riper and Emerick have suggested, always to correct the child's misarticulations or inaccurate use of language. We can never be certain that the child is ready to be corrected, nor can we be sure if it is an effective way to enhance proper linguistic usage. A more effective approach is the use of modeling of self-correction by the therapist, vividly described by Van Riper and Emerick. Depending on the child's response to the therapist's self-correction, it is possible to determine the readiness of the child to move forward.

7. *Using language as an integral part of interpersonal relationships.* The child soon discovers that language and the personal relationship with another person are closely interwoven. Through the clinical experience, the child recognizes, on some undefined level, the effect that each has on the other.

8. *Measuring responses and taking a leadership role.* Play therapy has often been criticized for its apparent unstructured and undisciplined process, unamenable to measurement. We would agree that total permissiveness within the play therapy situation would be counterproductive in terms of language and personal enhancement. We take the position that the therapist, like the child, must take the prerogative to lead clinical events toward a positive outcome. Children appreciate adult control and direction as long as it is done with respect for the child as a person.

We do not know if the need to learn is an innate process, but workers in our field are well aware of the pleasure evidenced by children who learn to use language more effectively under direction by the therapist. Thus play therapy may be structured in such a way as to facilitate the counting of appropriate linguistic responses in accordance with sound behavioral principles, without infringing on the clinical interpersonal relationship.

Family Therapy

A comprehensive search of the literature through computer data banks has failed to uncover any studies that describe the use of a family therapy approach in the treatment of language disorders in children. Consistent with our earlier discussions relevant to the development of language disorders in children, we maintain that family therapy can be used as a unitary or complementary method to enhance language development in the language-disordered child. Although the author has worked with some families in which therapy appeared to have little impact on the child's disordered language, he can report successes with other families.

A case in point   Jamie R, five years old at the time, was referred to me by the family pediatrician, a physician who was keenly knowledgable about developmental language stages in children. Upon initial intake, Jamie presented with speech and language characterized by vowelized articulation with concomitant unintelligible language usage. Syntactic patterning was evident, suggesting that cognitive skills were operational to a great degree. Formal nonverbal performance tasks revealed above-normal intelligence, and informal play did not indicate the presence of emotional dysfunction.

Jamie was one of six children, the nearest in age of whom was Jill, eleven years of age. Two other siblings were older adolescents, and the other two were in their twenties. Only one of them did not live at home. Mrs. R was a full-time homemaker and Mr. R was an airline executive.

The initial family therapy session, which included Jamie, Jill, and Mr. and Mrs. R, provided an opportunity to obtain the background history, including medical information. The only remarkable data to come forth revealed that Jamie was considered and treated essentially as the "baby" in the family, doted on from the earliest age by all family members except by Mr. R, who was often away for days at a time on business trips. A live-in Spanish-speaking maid, who also cared for Jamie while Mrs. R attended classes at a local junior college, was said to speak often to Jamie in Spanish. Jamie reportedly understood a considerable amount of the second language, but apparently did not attempt to use it expressively.

It was hoped that the entire family could return for the second family therapy session, but conflicting schedules made that impossible. The maid, Juanita, however was now included. Although indications were apparent during the initial family therapy session, it was now clear that virtually all the participants attempted to speak for Jamie at various times. Mrs. R acknowledged that the other children did the same.

There did not appear to be any underlying evidence of pronounced family dysfunction. This seemed to be a caring and loving family, the members of which were ready to do whatever was necessary to help Jamie. The author surmised that such was also the case for the absent siblings. Although Mr. and Mrs. R acknowledged that perhaps they had been contributors to Jamie's delayed language development, their concerns were not contaminated by defensive protestations. They appeared ready to do whatever was necessary to help Jamie.

Still puzzled by the apparent lack of extraordinarily negative etiological influences to account for Jamie's severe verbal expressive difficulties, the author probed further into the family interactional relationships. In doing so it was learned that Juanita had been with the family for only four years. Prior to that Jamie had reached or surpassed developmental milestones, including the use of two intelligible words by nine months. Also, until that time the family had had the services of a housekeeper who had been with them many years. Her untimely death brought profound sadness to the family, which to now had not completed the mourning process.

The second session was extended one hour to allow the family, particularly Mr. and Mrs. R and Jill, to experience the pain which to now had been concealed.

Apparently the family homeostasis had been severely disrupted upon the death of Mary (the housekeeper), resulting in a complex realignment of family members. It was not clear to this author whether or not Jamie actually took on the role as the identified patient to reflect the underlying family grief, but the abrupt interruption of his developing expressive language at that time could not be ignored.

Subsequent family therapy sessions, which intermittently involved other family members, were used to facilitate the grief process, provide information about language and speech development, and provide an environment in which Jamie in particular could be allowed to communicate freely, albeit unintelligibly. Family members were also provided specific guides to reinforce Jamie's correct linguistic approximations while avoiding correcting him.

To the astonishment of this author, within five months Jamie's expressive speech and language had approached 80 percent intelligibility, without the benefit of traditional speech and language therapy, though he had also been in kindergarten during that time. Termination of family therapy was naturally agreed upon and a follow-up speech and language reevaluation one year hence revealed essentially normal speech and language consistent with his chronological age. Only w/r and θ/s substitutions remained.

This case is one illustration of the exclusive use of family therapy and counseling to effect dramatic changes in a child's disordered language usage. We cannot ascertain, however, the exact elements of that process to bring about essentially normal language in the child. Obviously, all of the details described plus those operating in a concealed manner were responsible.

What is pertinent to our present discussion is that family therapy does not always require a dysfunctional family per se in order to be successful. On the contrary, disordered language development in a child could be related to very subtle familial dynamics. Also, it must be noted that other traditional strategies could certainly have yielded similar results, but without the concomitant resolution of other family issues. Most important, however, is our recognition and acceptance of the fact that it is possible for otherwise normal children to fail in their ability to acquire language normally.

Other Counseling Strategies

There is considerable literature on the use of counseling for parents of language-disordered children. Most has included the transmission of information to the parents about language development and training parents to use constructive communication strategies at home and to assist the child to practice assigned homework given by the child's speech-language pathologist.

The literature on the use of counseling with school-age children who are language impaired has been less fruitful, except in those cases in which the child is also emotionally disturbed and/or learning disabled. Unfortunately, most school speech-language pathology programs are not structured to provide, nor are school speech-language pathologists prepared to offer, counseling to the language-disordered child.

The least amount of empirical data is available regarding counseling in conjunction with the use of symptomatic strategies, but pragmatic approaches appear to be coming close to reconciling the two strategies.

Counseling the parents   To counsel parents of language-disordered children effectively, it is necessary to go beyond piecemeal handouts of information to help alleviate only the language problem. We agree with Zedler (1972) that social acceptance, feelings of personal adequacy, and encouragement of individual potentialities are as important to the child as language management and in fact are an integral part of it.

Pressman (1983), in her study of the effects of a home-based early intervention program on parents' self-confidence and children's development, found for thirty child–parent participants that the parents' self-confidence as primary teacher of the child had increased. She also found increased stimulation in the home and in the children's intellectual development as measured by their growth in language.

Although several books published within the last fifteen years have provided guidelines for the worker in special education to use with parents of handicapped children, Webster (1977) offers the practicing speech-language pathologist practical guides to developing appropriate counselor–parent relationships in working with communicatively impaired children. Molyneaux and Lane (1982) offer step-by-step procedures for working with parents of communicatively impaired children, and provide the student and professional a unique interview analysis model to evaluate the effectiveness of the counselor–parent interview. Although few references surveyed reveal precise guidelines geared to counseling parents of language-disordered children, therapists can readily apply the principles described by Webster, Molyneaux and Lane, and other researchers to whom they have referred.

Finally, the role of the speech-language pathologist as counselor-educator for parents, to promote speech-language development before an interference in the process occurs, cannot be underestimated. The American Speech-Language-Hearing Association and Rossetti (1984) have addressed the need for workers in the field to counsel with mothers-to-be whose pregnancy was labeled high risk, to follow cases through their delivery, and to conduct annual follow-ups. Rosetti's general guidelines are based on the philosophic premise of the infant's right to optimum development, the need for early intervention, the responsibility of the parent as the primary programmer, the infant's need for nurturance, and the importance of "play" to the infant's development and a healthy family environment.

Counseling the child   It is important for us to understand that counseling the school-age child or adolescent who is language delayed or language disordered does not imply that emotional disturbance must be a prerequisite condition. Language, we have seen, is learned or not learned within the context of biogenetic, cognitive, and interpersonal factors. Although we may be tempted to dismiss the language problem as an impeded stage of development, regardless of emotional components, it is more useful for us to understand the problem along a broad continuum of human development and individual coping behavior.

We would certainly agree with Wiig and Semel (1984) that counseling would benefit the child or adolescent who needs to express feelings and attitudes about his or her deficit in order to "gain insight into the bases for the difficulties he experiences in interpersonal communication and into the causes for emotional reactions and inappropriate behavioral responses" (pp. 583–584). Equally important, in our view, is that the counseling process will actually enhance the form and content of the language behavior itself, without our necessarily working on the language independently.

We do not wish to imply that such an approach should or can be applied universally or indiscriminately. Children with neurological and/or organic involvement, or even those who are severely emotionally disturbed, are much more likely to respond favorably to conventional modes of speech-language therapy. Counseling in these cases, however, as an adjunctive method would also be of value.

Following the broad guidelines outlined in Chapter 1, and applying principles already suggested for play therapy, it is possible to implement these in counseling with the language-impaired child, with due respect to differences in age abilities and severity of the problem. We must also be reminded that family therapy may be used to complement our individual counseling procedures.

Active listening provides us the opportunity to derive a clinical impression of the nature of the child's feelings, attitudes, and self-concept. Although these revelations may be not forthcoming immediately, and although the child may resist the relationship at first, patience on the part of the therapist will soon nullify the resistances. Through the process of listening with empathy, openness, and awareness, the therapist feeds back to the child that which is perceived, thereby further stimulating the child's use of language.

When the therapist views the child as a person, the therapist's respect for the child may be manifested in the way language is used to develop the relationship. Even the child whose language functioning is severely delayed will respond nonverbally or perhaps verbally in the light of the therapist's unconditional regard.

The author recently worked with a six-year-old child who was essentially nonverbal but whose evaluative and cognitive skills were close to the norm. The child entered the office while the author was munching a large, red apple. The fruit served to open up the relationship, which until then had been virtually nonexistent. Sharing the apple with the child, while imparting to her its delicious qualities, the author was able for the first time in weeks to elicit two- and three-word forms along with appropriate affectual behavior. Most important, in the light of our present discussion, was the nature of the interaction, which was based on a mutual sharing of a pleasurable experience.

Often in our work with language-disordered children, we feel that as therapists we must always make the choices and decisions that we believe to be in the best interests of the child and of therapy. Unfortunately, as we emphasize the latter, we slight the former. We miss vital opportunities for language growth when we take a directive, albeit well-intentioned, therapeutic approach in which we do not provide opportunities for the child to bring his or her own world into the clinical world. The child offers us the richness of his or her own experiences, which can be readily utilized within the context of our established strategies. Client choice and therapist choice need not be in conflict as long as the therapist can selectively determine which of the child's contributions are most compatible with the therapist's intentions. Therein lies the opportunity for a mutually satisfying therapeutic relationship, as well as a source for language enhancement.

With older children, particularly adolescents, the formulation of contracts will be necessary to reinforce clinical successes and ensure carryover into the child's daily life. Bearing in mind our previous discussion, only through a mutual give and take and respect for each other's ability and integrity can the contract become a constructive instrument to foster positive change. Although parental participation could well be encouraged, in many cases it must be consistent with the integrity of the child–therapist relationship. To do otherwise is to negate all of the efforts that have gone into establishing the relationship and to nullify the results of therapy. Whatever the arrangements made, contract negotiation is a vital opportunity to eliminate further deficient language patterns and to enhance more appropriate use of language.

Some language-disordered children, including those who are emotionally disturbed and/or delinquent, present to therapy many obstacles to language improvement. In these cases, the use of confrontation may be an effective means to help provide these children control over their own destructive, self-defeating behavior, which may be interfering with their language competency. Confrontation must occur, we maintain, in the context of a caring, nondefensive, and unconditional regard for the child, who is struggling to survive in a world he or she perceives as threatening or rejecting. Although resistances to any kind of change, language or otherwise, may tax the emotional and intellectual limits of any therapist, these must be regarded as the child's attempt, albeit ineffectual, to cope with his or her present intolerable reality. Rigid, authoritarian, and judgmental attitudes on the part of the therapist will serve only to exacerbate an already intolerable state of existence in the child and further entrench his or her negative attitudes toward other persons in the environment.

Used in conjunction with other strategies, confrontation can be a powerful tool not only to enhance the communicative therapeutic relationship but also to help the child realize how language can be used to achieve a more productive role for himself or herself in society.

Therapist self-disclosure is another technique that can be used successfully with language-disordered children of all ages. It is a way of having the child enter into the world of the therapist while losing neither personal integrity nor role identity. It is compatible with our earlier discussion that the therapeutic relationship involves mutual respect in which the child is viewed and respected as a person.

Tim was a sixteen-year-old language-disordered adolescent who came from a family in which the father had been absent for twelve years and the mother was an alcoholic. Expelled from school many times, as well as in and out of juvenile hall for petty thefts, Tim also had other severe learning disabilities. Early efforts to help Tim with his language disability were unsuccessful until he had a therapist who was able to relate to him on his level. Sharing feelings of her own childhood struggles with Tim was instrumental in forming a therapeutic relationship in which Tim was finally able to trust an adult and start on the long road toward educational and emotional adjustment, including functional language usage. Certainly, the therapeutic relationship could not have been sustained by the use of therapist self-disclosure alone, but through the judicious consideration and use of other techniques we have described, positive change was possible.

Therapist sensitivity to the language-disordered child's body language and paralinguistic behavior is especially important, particularly with the child who is essentially nonverbal. It is a valuable opportunity to discover cognitive processes concealed by the absence of verbal language. Although the therapist's verbalization of the nonverbal message may not always be on target, more important is the realization by the child that the therapist is trying to understand. Indeed, the child will at least be exposed to verbal language stimulation and be brought into the communicative relationship.

The child who is also cognitively affected presents us with a more complex but hardly a hopeless challenge. Even this child, who may be neurologically, developmentally, or mentally impaired, will nonetheless communicate nonverbal messages that the therapist may need to decipher. In these cases it is necessary for the therapist to respond both nonverbally and verbally if only to discover what the child is communicating. Even a minimally appropriate nonverbal or, better, verbal response by the child can be the beginning of a fruitful communicative relationship leading to more productive language processing and functioning in the child.

We do not believe that counseling alone will bring about linguistic changes in all language-disordered children, or even that enhancement of the child's self-image, personal adjustment, or emotional behavior will automatically produce age-appropriate language functioning. Conversely, achievement of normal language functioning will not necessarily produce emotionally well-balanced behavior. Empirical studies have yet to isolate all of the parameters that operate in the complex cognitive-emotional-linguistic relationship. For these reasons we must not neglect the use of traditional symptomatic strategies that have become refined, particularly over the last twenty-five years.

It appears obvious to this author, however, that a pragmatic approach to language therapy would be most compatible with the interpersonal counseling approach outlined here. Which shall receive most emphasis depends on several important conditions, including academic preparation of the therapist; sufficient intellectual competence of the child (although it should be noted that moderately low-level mentally retarded children are responsive to counseling methods); cooperation of the parents; degree and quality of neurological competence; and acceptance by and cooperation of school personnel. In the final analysis, however, the therapist must not only weigh these conditions but also consider unforeseen circumstances that may arise during therapy. Independent of all conditions, the therapist should feel free to be flexible and respond appropriately to the changing needs of the child.

CONCLUSION

We have attempted in this chapter to draw together the vast body of information provided by experts from many fields in order to arrive at a more complete understanding of the role of interpersonal family dynamics in the genesis of childhood language disorders. Although definitive empirical research has not yet confirmed much of the clinical evidence available, we cannot ignore the significance of what has already been learned. Even more tenuous is our knowledge and understanding of all of the variables that are inherent in the therapeutic process, yet that in some way account for real positive change in the acquisition of language in the language-disordered child.

Finally, we have suggested that the establishment of an interpersonal therapeutic relationship may be fundamental to the language therapy process. How much of the process must involve counseling strategies alone or how much should depend on more traditional approaches is yet to be determined. We have attempted at least to provoke further discussion and more carefully controlled research on the matter.

REFERENCES

AMERICAN PSYCHIATRIC ASSOCIATION. Identity related disorders. In *Diagnostic and Statistic Manual of Mental Disorders (DSM-III)*. Washington, D.C., 1980.

ANNELL, A. L., GUSTAVSON, K. H., and TENSTAM, J. Symptomatology in schoolboys with positive sex chomatin (the Klinefelter syndrome). *Acta Psychiatrica Scandinavica*, (1970), 71–80.

ARNOLD, G. E., The genetic background of developmental language disorders. *Folia Phoniatrica*, 13 (1961), 246–254.

AXLINE, V. *Play Therapy*. New York: Ballantine, 1969.

BAKER, L., CANTWELL, D. P. Psychiatric disorder in children with speech and language retardation. *Archives of General Psychiatry*, 34 (1977), 583–591.

BAKER, L., CANTWELL, D. P., and MATTISON, R. E. Behavior problems in children with pure speech disorders and in children with combined speech and language disorders. *Journal of Abnormal Child Psychology*, 8 (1980), 245–256.

BARNARD, K. E., BEE, H. L. and HAMMOND, M. A. Home environment in a healthy, low-risk sample: The Seattle study. In A. W. Gottfried (Ed.) *Home Environment and Early Cognitive Development: Longitudinal Research.* Orlando, Fla.: Academic Press, 1984.

BEASLEY, J. *Slow to Talk.* New York: Teachers College, Columbia University, 1956.

BECKWITH, L., and COHEN, S. E. Home environment and cognitive competence in preterm children during the first five years. In A. W. Gottfried (Ed.), *Home Environment and Early Cognitive Development: Longitudinal Research.* Orlando, Fla.: Academic Press, 1984.

BEIER, D. Behavioral disturbances in the mentally retarded. In H. A. Stevens and R. Heber (Eds.), *Mental Retardation: A Review of Research.* Chicago: University of Chicago Press, 1964.

BEREITER, C., and ENGELMANN, S. *Teaching Disadvantaged Children in Preschool.* Englewood Cliffs, N.J.: Prentice-Hall, 1966.

BERNTHAL, J., and BANKSON, N. *Articulation Disorders.* Englewood Cliffs, N.J.: Prentice-Hall, 1981.

BLOOM, L., and LAHEY, M. *Language Development and Language Disorders.* New York: John Wiley, 1978.

BODMER, W., and CAVALLI-SFORZA, L. *Genetics, Evolution and Man.* San Francisco: Freeman, 1976.

BOND, C. R., and MCMAHON, R. J. Relationships between marital distress and child behavior problems, maternal personal adjustment, maternal personality, and maternal parenting behavior. *Journal of Abnormal Psychology*, 93 (1984), 348–351.

BOWLBY, J. Grief and mourning in infancy and early childhood. *Psychoanalytic Study of the Child.*, 15 (1960), 9–52.

BRADLEY, R. H., and CALDWELL, B. M. One hundred seventy-four children: A study of the relationship between home environment and cognitive development during the first five years. In A. W. Gottfried (Ed.), *Home Environment and Early Cognitive Development: Longitudinal Research.* Orlando, Fla.: Academic Press, 1984.

BRAZELTON, T. B. The first four developmental stages in attachment of parent and infant. Paper delivered at the Twelfth Annual Margaret S. Mahler Symposium, Philadelphia, May 1981.

BROWN, G. W., and HARRIS, T. *Social Origins of Depression: A Study of Psychiatric Disorder in Women.* London: Tavistock, 1978.

CAMERON, N. *The Psychology of Behavior Disorders.* Boston: Houghton Mifflin, 1947.

CANTWELL, D. P., and BAKER, L. Psychiatric disorder in children with speech and language retardation: Critical review. *Archives of General Psychiatry*, 34 (1977), 583–591.

CANTWELL, D. P., BAKER, L., and MATTISON, R. E. The prevalence of psychiatric disorders in children with speech and language disorder: An epidemiologic study. *Journal of American Academy of Child Psychiatry*, 18 (1979), 450–461.

COURTRIGHT, J., and COURTRIGHT, I. Imitative modeling as a theoretical base for instructing language-disordered children. *Journal of Speech and Hearing Research*, 19 (1976), 655–663.

DARBY, J. K. (Ed.), *Speech Evaluation in Psychiatry.* New York: Grune & Stratton, 1981.

DePAULO, B. M., and BONVILLIAN, J. D. The effects on language development of the special characteristics of speech addressed to young children. *Journal of Psycholinguistic Research*, 7 (1978), 189–211.

Diagnostic and Statistic Manual of Mental Disorders: DSM-II 1968 and DSM-III 1978. Washington, D.C.: American Psychiatric Association. 1980.

EMERICK, L., and HATTEN, J. *Diagnosis and Evaluation in Speech Pathology.* Englewood Cliffs, N.J.: Prentice-Hall, 1979.

FISH, B., and RIVTO, E. R. Psychoses in childhood. In J. D. Noshpitz (Ed.), *Basic Handbook of Child Psychiatry*, Vol. II. New York: Basic Books, 1979.

FLAVEL, J. H. Metacognition and cognitive monitoring. *American Psychologist*, 34 (1979), 906–911.

FOGARTY, T. F. System concepts and the dimensions of self. In P. J. Guerin (Ed.), *Family Therapy: Theory and Practice.* New York: Gardner, 1976.

FURROW, D., NELSON, K., and BENEDICT, H. Mothers' speech to children and syntactic development: Some simple relationships. *Journal of Child Language*, 6 (1979), 423–442.

GARMEZY, N. Stressors of childhood. In N. Garmezy and M. Rutter (Eds.), *Stress, Coping and Development in Children*. New York: McGraw-Hill, 1983.

GEIST, R. Conditions with physical presentations and their psychosomatic relationships. In P. D. Steinhauer and Q. Rae-Grant. (Eds.), *Psychological Problems of the Child in the Family*. Basic Books Inc: N.Y. 1983.

GLASS, G. V., McGRAW, B., and SMITH, M. L. *Meta-Analysis in Social Research*. Beverly Hills, Calif.: Sage, 1981.

GOTTFRIED, A. W. (Ed.). *Home Environment and Early Cognitive Development: Longitudinal Research*. Orlando, Fla.: Academic Press, 1984a.

———. Home environment and early cognitive development: Integration, meta-analysis and conclusions. In A. W. Gottfried (Ed.), *Home Environment and Early Cognitive Development: Longitudinal Research*. Orlando, Fla.: Academic Press, 1984b.

GOTTFRIED, A. W., and GOTTFRIED, A. E. Home environment and cognitive development in young children of middle socioeconomic-status families. In A. W. Gottfried (Ed.), *Home Environment and Early Cognitive Development: Longitudinal Research*. Orlando, Fla. Academic Press, 1984.

HAKA-IKSE, K., STEWART, D. A., and CRIPPS, M. H. Early development of children with sex chromosome aberrations. *Pediatrics*, 62 (1978), 761–766.

HARLOW, H. F., HARLOW, M. K., DODSWORTH, R. O., and ARLING, G. L. Maternal behavior of rhesus monkeys deprived of mothering and peer associations in infancy. *Proceedings of the American Philosophical Society*, 110 (1966), 58–66.

ILFELD, F. W., Jr. Marital stressors, coping styles, and symptoms of depression. In L. Goldberger and S. Breznitz (Eds.), *Handbook of Stress: Theoretical and Clinical Aspects*. New York: Macmillan, 1982.

JOHNSON, D. L., BRECKENRIDGE, J. N., and McGOWAN, R. J. Home environment and early cognitive development in Mexican-American children. In A. W. Gottfried (Ed.), *Home Environment and Early Cognitive Development: Longitudinal Research*. Orlando, Fla. Academic Press, 1984.

LAMBERT, W. The effects of bilingualism on the individual: Cognitive and socio-cultural consequences. In P. Hornby (Ed.), *Bilingualism: Psychological, Social and Educational Implications*. New York: Academic Press, 1977.

LAVIGNE, J. V., and RYAN, M. Psychological adjustment of siblings of children with chronic illness. Pediatrics, 63 (1979), 616–627.

LASKY, E. Z., and KLOPP, K. Parent–child interactions in normal and language-disordered children. *Journal Speech and Hearing Disorders*, 47 (1982), 7–18.

LEFEBVRE, A. The child with physical handicaps. In P. D. Steinhauer and Q. Rae-Grant (Eds.), *Psychological Problems of the Child in the Family*. New York: Basic Books, 1983.

LUCHSINGER, R. Inheritance of speech defects. *Folia Phoniatrica*, 22 (1970), 216–230.

LUDLOW, C. L., and COOPER, J. A. (Eds.). *Genetic Aspects of Speech and Language Disorders*. New York: Academic Press, 1983.

MACCOBY, E. E. Social-emotional development and response to stressors. In N. Garmezy and M. Rutter (Eds.), *Stress, Coping and Development in Children*. New York: McGraw-Hill, 1983.

MATTEJAT, F., NIEBERGALL, G., and NESTLER, V. *Speech disorders in children of aphasic fathers: A developmental psycholinguistic case study. Praxis der Kinderpsychologic and Kinderpsychiatric*, 29 (1980) 83–89 (in German).

MINEKA, S., and SUOMI, S. J. Social separation in monkeys. *Psychol. Bulletin*, 85 (1978), 1376–1400.

MOLYNEAUX, D., and LANE, V. W. *Effective Interviewing: Techniques and Analysis*. Boston: Allyn & Bacon, 1982.

NIELSEN, J., and SILLESEN, I. Follow-up until age two through four of unselected children with sex chromosome abnormalities. *Human Genetics*, 33 (1976) 241–257.

NIELSEN, J., SORENSON, A. M., and SORENSON, K. Mental development of unselected children with sex chromosome abnormalities. *Human Genetics*, 59 (1981), 324–332.

OLSEN-FULERO, L. Style and stability in mother conversational behavior: A study of individual differences. *Journal of Child Language*, 9 (1982), 543–564.

PRESSMAN, S. The effects of a home-based early intervention program on parents' self-confidence and children's development. Unpublished dissertation, 1983. Rutgers University.

PRIZANT, B. M. Language acquisition and communicative behavior in autism: Toward an understanding of the "whole" of it. *Journal, Speech and Hearing Research*, 48 (1983), 296–307.

ROSE D. H. Dentate gyrus granule cells and cognitive development: Explorations in the substrates of behavioral change. Unpublished doctoral dissertation, Harvard University, 1976.

ROSSETTI, L. A longitudinal study of developmental status of high risk infants. Paper presented at the annual meeting of the American Speech-Language-and Hearing Association, San Francisco, November 1984.

ROUSEY, C. *Psychiatric Assessment by Speech and Hearing Behavior*. Springfield, Ill. Chas. C Thomas, 1974.

———. The psychopathology of articulation and voice deviations. In L. E. Travis (Ed.), *Handbook of Speech Pathology and Audiology*. New York: Appleton-Century-Crofts, 1971.

RUTTER, M. Some issues and some questions. In M. Garmezy and M. Rutter (Eds.), *Stress, Coping and Development in Children*. New York: McGraw-Hill, 1983.

———. Diagnosis and definition of childhood autism. *Journal of Autism and Childhood Schizophrenia*, 8 (1978), p. 139–161.

SCHWARTZ, R., LEONARD, L., FOLGER, M., and WILCOX, M. Early phonological behavior in normal-speaking and language-disordered children: Evidence for a synergistic view of linguistic disorders. *Journal of Speech and Hearing Disorders*, 45 (1980), 357–377.

SHERE, E., and KASTENBAUM, R. Mother–child interaction in cerebral palsy: Environmental and psychosocial obstacles to cognitive development. *Genetic Psychology Monographs*, 73 (1966), 255–335.

SHUY, R. Language problems of disadvantaged children. In J. V. Irwin and M. Marge (Eds.), *Principles of Childhood Language Disabilities*. Englewood Cliffs, N.J.: Prentice-Hall, 1972.

SIEGEL, L. S. Home environmental influences on cognitive development in preterm and full-term children during the first five years. In A. W. Gottfried (Ed.), *Home Environment and Early Cognitive Development: Longitudinal Research*. Orlando, Fla: Academic Press, 1984.

SÖDERBERGH, R. Linguistic effects by three years of age of extra contact during the first hour post-partum. In C. E. Johnson and C. L. Thew (Eds.), *Proceedings of the Second International Congress for the Study of Child Language*, Vol. 1. Washington, D.C.: University Press of America, 1982.

SPITZ, R. A. Anaclitic depression: An inquiry into the genesis of psychiatric conditions in early childhood, II. *Psychoanalytic Study of the Child.*, 2 (1946a), 313–341.

———. Hospitalism: A follow-up report. *Psychoanal. Study of the Child*, 2 (1946b), 113–117.

———. Hospitalism: An inquiry into the genesis of psychiatric conditions in early childhood. *Psychoanalytic Study of the Child.*, 1 (1945), 53–74.

STARK, R. E., MELLITS, E. D., and TALLAL, P. Behavioral attributes of speech and language disorders. In C. L. Ludlow and J. A. Cooper (Eds.), *Genetic Aspects of Speech and Language Disorders*. New York: Academic Press, 1983.

STAYTON, D. J., and AINSWORTH, M. D. S. Individual differences in infant responses to brief, everyday separation as related to other infant and maternal behaviors. *Developmental Psychology*, 9 (1973), 226–235.

STEVENSON, J., and RICHMAN, N. Behavior, language and development in three-year-old children. *Journal of Autism and Childhood Schizophrenia*, 8 (1978), 299–313.

THOMPSON, M., and HAVELKOVA, M. Psychoses in childhood and adolescence. In P. D. Steinhauer and Q. Rae-Grant (Eds.), *Psychological Problems of the Child in the Family*. New York: Basic Books, 1983.

VAN RIPER, C., and EMERICK, L. *Speech Correction: An Introduction to Speech Pathology and Audiology*. Englewood Cliffs, N.J.: Prentice-Hall, 1984.

WACHS, T. D. Proximal experience and early cognitive-intellectual development: The social environment. In A. W. Gottfried (Ed.), *Home Environment and Early Cognitive Development: Longitudinal Research*. Orlando, Fla: Academic Press, 1984.

WALBERT, M., INGLES, S., KRIRGSMAN, E., and MILLS, B. Language, delay and associated mother–child interactions. In M. Lahey (Ed.), *Readings in Childhood Language Disorders*. New York: John Wiley, 1978.

WALLERSTEIN, J., and KELLY, J. The effects of parental divorce: Experiences of the preschool child. *Journal of the American Academy of Child Psychiatry*, 14 (1975), 600–616.

WATERHOUSE, L. H. Maternal speech patterns and differential development. In C. E. Johnson and C. L. Thew (Eds.), *Proceedings of the Second International Congress for the Study of Language*, Vol. 1. Washington, D.C.: University Press of America, 1982.

WEBSTER, E. *Counseling with Parents of Handicapped Children: Guidelines for Improving Communication.* New York: Grune & Stratton, 1977.

WEINBERG, N., and SANTANA, R. Comic books: Champions of the Disabled Stereotype. *Rehabilitation Literature*, 39 (1978), 327–331.

WEINTRAUB, W. *Verbal Behavior: Adaptation and Psychopathology.* New York: Springer-Verlag, 1981.

WIIG, E. H., and SEMEL, E. *Language Assessment and Intervention for the Learning Disabled.* Columbus, Ohio: Chas. E. Merrill, 1984.

WINNICOTT, D. W. The theory of the parent–infant relationship. In *The Maturational Processes and the Facilitating Environment.* New York: International Universities Press, 1965.

ZALESKI, T. Familial appearance of delayed development of speech. *Otolaryngologia Polska*, 20 (1966), 367–371.

ZEDLER, E. H. Social management. In J. V. Irwin and M. Marge (Eds.), *Principles of Childhood Language Disabilities.* Englewood Cliffs, N.J.: Prentice-Hall, 1972.

6

PSYCHOLOGICAL CONSIDERATIONS OF VOICE-DISORDERED PEOPLE AND THEIR FAMILIES

Part I: The Psychology of Voice Disorders in Children

PSYCHOGENESIS OF VOICE DISORDERS

Specific acoustical and physiological features of voice disorders in children cannot readily be assigned their etiological origin. They are probably the least understood of all the various communicative disorders. This should not be surprising, as the human voice is the major entity through which personality is expressed. Yet the relationship between the two has mystified us for centuries and has defied the best of scientific investigations.

Nevertheless, in this chapter we join the ranks of others who have attempted to make sense of that relationship. We also offer another perspective toward understanding its complexity. Our emphasis shall be only on etiological correlates that are essentially psychosocial, but in its manifestation, the voice disorder will also be discussed in terms of its organic as well as psychological features.

ETIOLOGICAL CONSIDERATIONS

Children with voice disorders do not fit neatly into the etiological categories that have been proposed by various investigators. More than sixty years ago Sapir (1927) described the cultural and social factors that influence the vocal dynamics and quality in individuals. Crucial also to our understanding of how these forces affect vocalization is the recognition of the uniqueness of the vocal tract structure. We should not be surprised by Formby's findings (1967) that mothers were able to distinguish the voices of their own babies from others soon after birth. Other investigators, namely, Wasz-Hockert et al. (1968) and Valanne et al. (1967), studied infant vocal cries and found differentiations among cries of the newborn. Also demonstrated was the ability for mothers to identify their own infants by the cry. Ostwald (1963) demonstrated differences between infants relative to their early cries by means of spectrographic analysis. He demonstrated too how listeners could recognize cries distinguished by need and alarm.

Moses (1954) vividly describes the vocal changes that occur as a function of the relationship between "genotypical" actions and traits and the "phenotypical" responses from others. That is, there is a relationship between the fundamental constitution and the way in which the child is attended to and protected.

Murphy (1964) discusses the origin of voice disorders in children relative to emotional conflict and confusion and in particular to the parent–child relationship. In an unpublished study cited by Aronson (1980), Barker and Wilson (1967) found that of 153 children with voice disorders, extreme family conflict was found in 65 percent of their homes; and for 97 children who were considered to have normal voices, family conflict was found in only 35 percent of their homes.

Numerous therapists have described children who have lost temporary use of their voice as a result of isolated traumatic experiences, such as automobile accident, tonsillectomy, death in the family, or witnessing a violent event. Case (1984) discusses the complex interaction between the nervous system (the limbic system mainly) and endocrine function and how internal or external environmental stimuli may disturb organismic homeostasis; that is, the balance among all functions of the human body. The reader is provided numerous references to explain the psychophysiological dynamics of emotion, but we caution that the relationships between these processes and vocal function are not yet entirely clear (Goodstein, 1958; Phillis, 1970; Scherer, 1972).

There appears to be little disagreement in the literature surveyed that emotional stress can affect musculoskeletal tension to induce aberrant changes in vocal usage (Aronson 1980; Murphy 1964; Luchsinger and Arnold 1965; Greene 1980; Case 1984; Wilson 1979; Boone 1983) and

Perkins (1983). We thus turn to a discussion of how family dynamics may have a significant bearing on the genesis of voice disorders in children.

Dysfunctional Family Dynamics

According to Van Riper and Emerick (1984), imitation and feelings of inadequacy are significant factors that may account for the development of voice disorders. To these factors we would add not only the dynamics of the parent–child relationship but also the interplay of all members of the family. Inherent in these relationships may be the seeds for the development of voice disorders that are expressions of anger, anxiety, depression, conflict, and unsatisfied needs. Consistent with our previous discussions of family systems theory, now applied to the voice-disordered child, the cause must be searched for, not within that child's intrapsychic conflict or stressful condition but by looking at the possible dysfunctional ways in which the entire family operates. Thus the child becomes "symptomatic" as a result of his or her position within the dysfunctioning family system, thereby satisfying the successful emotional functioning of all other family members.

We might question why the organism selects an abnormal vocal behavior to represent a particular dysfunctional family system. As Aronson (1980) suggests, it is possible that the child is "predisposed by personality or physiology to hyperact through a particular organ system" (p. 132). Or it is conceivable that the child's psychological and physiological adaptive mechanisms are being overloaded, forcing the emergence of vocal symptoms. One is reminded of our discussion of the etiology of stuttering. Constitutional factors appear to be taking on greater respectability today and they may well be important factors to consider in their applicability to voice disorders.

What is important for us to understand is that as tension increases in a family it may either be experienced as internal anxiety by one member or lead to conflict between two members. If a father is silently angry toward his wife, the child may express the rage through provocative vocal outbursts, perhaps leading to the development of vocal nodules. In this case, the child is manifesting the essence of a marital relationship that Kerr (1981) describes in several ways: one parent has distanced himself from the other, one parent is in conflict with the other, one parent has compromised her behavior to preserve harmony in the relationship, or both parents have united over common concern for the child—or, we would add, any combination of these may occur.

Stress in Typical Families

A constant theme throughout this book has been the notion that even the most typical family may contain roots for or manifest behavior, producing stress. This may lead to the inception of, among other things, communicative disorders. Thus, for the voice-disordered child, we might expect the same conditions. In those families, however, that are functioning well, stress is not dealt with by them as an abstract entity but as a real thing, thereby helping to minimize its effects on all family members. Children are unlikely to develop voice disorders in such families. In other words, the stress is less likely to be consolidated in voice-disorder symptoms. The likelihood of the development of such symptoms in the dysfunctional family is obviously greater in that the child, or for that matter any other family member becomes the unwitting victim of the unresolved family conflicts and resulting stress. It would be easy for us to cite the many family instances in which yelling and screaming are common modes by which parents communicate, and where the child adopts a similar means to communicate, with such vocal misuse leading to hoarseness. Such antecedent and resultant events need little further explanation except that voice disorders in children do not typically follow such an obvious pattern.

Voice disorders in children are more likely to represent individualized reactions to a multitude of possible stress situations in which the vocal behavior expressed by the child is a unique form of coping strategy. Conversely, not all children will necessarily respond in the same way to identical stress-producing situations. Shipp and McGlone (1973) have suggested that voice tremors that are supposed to disappear under stress may not exist at all. Siegman (1982) points out: "Whatever the explanation, individual variations in response to stress complicate matters enormously for anyone trying to develop a theoretical model of the effects of stress behavior" (p. 315). It is generally recognized, however, that under stress, the voice will manifest definitive emotions as well as undergo various changes, resulting in either somatic or psychogenic voice disorders. Murray, Carr, and Jacobs (1983) describe the therapeutic management of functional aphonia in five adolescents. The persistent pattern for at least four of these young people was the presence of a stressful family environment as well as maladaptive patterns in school.

There have been some attempts to measure microtremors in the voice by means of a stress-measuring device, the Psychological Stress Evaluator (PSE) (Holden 1975). Although used most extensively as a lie detection instrument, it has also been used to assess the vocal effects of stress associated with emotional disturbance. In his review of the literature on the subject, however, Scherer (1981) cautions us that the PSE is not refined enough to justify its proponents' claims of success.

Relationship of the Somatic to Psychogenic Voice Disorders

It is not too difficult to determine and identify the presence of organic vocal pathology through typical laryngoscopic or nasolaryngeal fiberoptic examination. What is more difficult and challenging is how to manage the apparent absence of an organic or somatic condition. In such cases we have tended to lump them into categories—"psychogenic," "functional," "psychosomatic," "nonorganic."

Aronson (1980) prefers the term *psychogenic*, which he believes is less ambiguous and more definitive than the term *functional*, but he does not dispense with the latter completely. He states: "A psychogenic voice disorder is broadly synonymous with a functional one but has the advantage of stating positively, based on an exploration of its causes, that the voice disorder is a manifestation of one or more types of psychologic disequilibrium—such as anxiety, depression, conversion reaction, or personality disorder—which interfere with normal volitional control over phonation" (p. 131).

Although we essentially agree with Aronson's definition, we would dispense entirely with the term *functional* to designate any form of voice disorder that has not been designated as organic. Our reason is that functional refers to an action or a process that may be operational in either organic or psychogenic voice disorders; that is, complex physiological actions involving muscular and chemical activity in conjunction with specific anatomical structures. Although we would agree with Murphy (1964), who also finds difficulty with the word, that "terms are only abstractions of the real processes" (p. 4), it is important to be able to describe precisely and behaviorally what has been abused laryngeally and how vocal structures are being misused.

For purposes of our continued discussion, then, we will refrain from extensive categorization of voice disorders. We prefer to describe them relative to both their organic and nonorganic components and their mutual psychological processes.

PSYCHOGENIC CORRELATES

Although some voice disorders may be organic or physiological in origin, they may be maintained because of psychogenic or environmental factors. Similarly, there are voice disorders that are psychogenic in origin and result in organic disorders.

Monday (1983) divides functional (psychogenic) voice disorders into two categories—functional dysphonia, where there is no organic lesion on the phonatory system, and functional laryngeopathology, where vocal abuse may lead to lesions. Examples of this second category include vocal nodules, secondary laryngitis, vocal polyps, and contact ulcers. Although the psychogenic correlates of each of the major categories may be similar, it is useful to discuss them separately so that distinctive characteristics may be differentiated.

Organic Voice Disorders

The incidence of vocal nodules in school-age children is somewhat high according to some researchers. (Warr-Leeper, McShea and Leeper, 1979). (Although there is some debate regarding the incidence and prevalence of voice disorders in children [Moore 1982], we do not believe discrepancies to be pertinent to our discussion.) Silverman and Zimmer (1975) found that 23.4 percent of 162 children in kindergarten through eighth grade exhibited chronic hoarseness, and vocal nodules were diagnosed in 77.7 percent of the children by an otolaryngologist. The incidence was higher in the primary grades, and occurred more in boys than in girls. This study suggested possible causes to be psychological factors, vocal misuse, and upper respiratory infection. The authors note that high expectations of performance had been expressed by parents and teachers, and a competitive spirit was apparent among the children. The children's voices were generally loud and strained, as were those of their siblings and vocal models.

Several studies cited by Aronson (1980)—namely, Wilson and Lamb (1973), Mosby (1967), Glassel (1972), and Toohill (1975)—revealed a wide and consistent array of psychological correlates in children with vocal nodules including poor personality adjustment, problems with aggressive or assertive behavior, emotional conflict, feelings of inadequacy, and need for loud, incessant talking. Indications of problems with their parents were also revealed. In the ten-year review of public school voice clinics, reported by Miller and Madison (1984), there was no attempt to gather data on the family background of those children seen for reported voice problems. Of the 249 students examined at the school voice clinics, 40 percent were diagnosed as having vocal nodules, 94 percent of which were bilateral. Particularly interesting were concomitant problems of upper respiratory ailments, including allergies and middle ear difficulties.

Organic voice disorders such as contact ulcers and paralysis were found to be of low incidence in the literature currently surveyed. In their survey of the literature, Baker et al. (1983) report the case of a ten-year-old male with Gilles de la Tourette's syndrome, but they can offer neither a totally psychogenic or organic explanation relative to etiology.

Relationship of etiology to family response It is obvious that there is no one psychological common denominator to explain the occurrence of somatic voice disorders in children. One would have to make a case-by-case analysis in order to search for pertinent etiological factors. Explanations of factors that might maintain the problem are no easier to make. Most investigators would agree, however, that vocal abuse and misuse in conjunction with other factors would account for most of the somatic disorders described here. Case (1984) lists several forms of vocal abuse along with etiological factors that we have selected as pertinent to children. Among them are (1) yelling and screaming; (2) using hard glottal attack; (3) calling to others from a distance; (4) speaking at inappropriate pitch levels; (5) speaking excessively or abusively during upper respiratory illness or allergy; (6) vocalizing under conditions of muscular (and we would add psychological) tension; (7) vocalizing animal and toy noises; (8) participating in games involving yelling and cheering; and (9) excessive arguing with peers and family members. What is not clear is why many children who do vocalize in any one or combination of these ways do not develop and maintain a vocal pathology. We may need to consider specific predisposing constitutional factors and family influences.

It is of interest to note that several writers have reported that parents of children with diagnosed voice problems are generally unconcerned. Warr-Leeper, McShea, and Leeper (1979), in their study, reveal that parents typically felt that their children's voice problems would not interfere with their education and were insignificant. The study also showed that family physicians did not usually recognize voice disorders as a problem in children. In a larger study involving 1962 children (Sentura and Wilson 1968), only 17 percent of the children were taken for a laryngoscopic examination by their parents, following letters describing their children's voice problems and recommending referral.

Several reasons are probable for this apparent lack of concern: (1) unlike articulation and other speech and language problems, voice problems do not generally interfere with intelligibility or communicative competence; (2) wider variations of voice usage and voice quality are more acceptable to listeners; articulation and language usage allows for little deviation before calling attention to itself; (3) parents are less well educated about the nature of voice disorders and are more likely to take on the unconcerned attitudes of their family physician; (4) public school therapists oftentimes shy away from voice therapy intervention; (5) aberrant vocal qualities in children may reflect deep-rooted unconscious conflicts in family relationships and/or in individual family members.

Relationships among use, abuse, and misuse   Because voice disorders do not usually have much of a conscious impact on the bearer and/or related family members, they are less likely to cause secondary psychological reactions directly. More likely, children with somatic voice disorders will tend to make involuntary secondary physiological adjustments to compensate for the initial interference to laryngeal functioning. Such compensatory adjustments may include chronic throat clearing, speaking at a different pitch or loudness level, and faulty realignment of the vocal and resonance tract, thereby exacerbating an already unbalanced use of the voice. Notwithstanding the initial psychological, physical, or environmental conditions that may have induced the vocal pathology in the first place, continued misuse and abuse is likely. In the case of vocal nodules, a condition that was originally unilateral could bilateralize, or the pathogenesis from the acute to the chronic stage may change.

The complex interplay of all the forces described results in a vocal prototype characterized by constriction of the laryngopharyngeal cavity, as well as by excessive medial compression of the vocal folds. Asymmetrical and asynchronous vocal fold vibrating may occur, resulting in breathiness and hoarseness or "roughness." As long as the primary conditions responsible for the voice disorder persist, it is unlikely for the disorder to change except through appropriate intervention.

Genesis of Nonorganic Voice Disorders

The paucity of substantial research to document definitive factors responsible for the development and maintenance of somatic voice disorders in children has been noted. Even less is known about the genesis of nonorganic voice disorders. Murphy (1964) appears to be one of the major original and yet definitive sources to which we must turn. Framing the disorders within the context of the parent–child relationship, he views these vocal symptoms as reflections of underlying conflicts and serving particular purposes. That is, they are viewed as secondary gains. He states:

> Finally there are occasional vocal disturbances originally produced by personal stresses, which tend to persist even after the initial discomforts have been modified or resolved. A voice disorder can become self-perpetuating. A reasonable conclusion in such a case is that a kind of "physiological perseveration" is occurring. It is also likely, though, that subtle psychological determinants are at work: the voice disorder may be serving attention-getting needs; it may be a major feature of the body image; it may serve as a focus for scapegoat behavior; other secondary gains, such as hostility satisfaction, may be present. (p. 36)

Murphy's explanation would be consistent with our understanding of family systems theory, which includes the interactional processes among all family members. The child's voice disorder, then, may represent psychological disequilibrium either in the child or in the family as a manifestation of unsatisfied needs in one or in all.

Although representing a psychoanalytic viewpoint, Erikson (1963) suggests eight stages of life, three of which are pertinent to our present discussion. Failure in the second stage (ages one to three years) results in the child feeling inadequate, having self-doubt, and inhibiting learning basic skills like talking. Failure in the third and fourth stages (ages four to five and six to seven years, respectively) results in guilt, infantile jealousy, avoidance of strong competition, feelings of mediocrity, slavish behavior, and a sense of futility. Whereas we might readily have applied Erikson's theory to our discussion of childhood language disorders earlier, it appears applicable to what several major writers have already described in children with nonorganic as well as organic voice disorders (Aronson 1980; Wilson 1979; Murphy 1964). We must resist the temptation, however, to overgeneralize our case, as the vast majority of the children who function psychologically in the way we have described do not develop either organic or nonorganic voice disorders. We are also familiar with children who present aberrant vocal symptoms but do not fit neatly into any of the psychogenic categories or dysfunctional families we have suggested. We could argue that such a reality can be attributed to our inability to isolate the concealed or subtle psychodynamics that have escaped our attention. Regardless, our task is to view each child and his or her family objectively and without preconceived biases.

Mutational voice   Puberty is a time of marked psychosocial and physiological changes, including acoustical and physical changes of the larynx.

Generally, the adolescent is able to adapt to the laryngeal changes even though the male voice drops approximately one octave and the female voice drops three or four semitones. In some instances, persons, particularly boys, do not readily adapt or are not able to reconcile the physiological changes to the psychosocial changes. In such cases the voice may be characterized by abrupt pitch breaks that persist for months or by persistent mutational falsetto, which Kaplan (1982) defines as "psychological failure of the adolescent's voice to descend or maintain its descent to a normal adult pitch at puberty" (p. 82). The resulting high-pitched falsetto voice is described by Aronson (1980) as "weak, thin, breathy, hoarse, and monopitched, giving the overall impression of immaturity, effeminacy, and passiveness" (p. 146).

Whereas endocrinological dysfunction may explain the persistence of the falsetto voice in some cases, its etiology is generally seen as psychogenic (Kaplan 1982; Case 1984; Aronson 1980; Wilson 1979). Unfortunately, the research evidence does not definitely describe its psychosocial dynamics and therefore we must rely only on clinical evidence to support a psychogenic origin. Although Case (1984) describes poor self-concept and insecurity in personal relationships as factors, and Aronson (1980) alludes to weak male identification and "a neurotic need to resist the transition into adulthood" (p. 147), we still cannot be certain that such psychological factors are primary to the disorder or secondary to it, or both.

The author had occasion, several years ago, to evaluate a fifteen-year-old boy with pronounced falsetto. The initial interview revealed a young man who was effeminate, had few friends, and who essentially had avoided any participation in typical male activities. He had been under intensive psychoanalytic treatment during the previous three years for what had originally been diagnosed as a "gender identity disorder." His parents, both holding Ph.Ds in their professions, had also been in psychoanalysis because of, according to their analyst, "their role in the etiology or perpetuation of their child's arrested psychosocial development." A family interview revealed that the boy had never been seen for an endocrinological examination, which I immediately recommended. The endocinological report revealed that their son was suffering from a severe reduction of testosterone, which was viewed as the primary source of the boy's problems. A follow-up contact made two years later revealed a young man who had made dramatic changes in his psychosocial adjustment toward a firm male identity along with a strong bass-baritone voice. His parents, too, were functioning at the peak of their professional and personal lives.

With regard to this particular case of mutational voice, we do not imply that there were no pertinent psychological factors operating. More likely, there was a complex interplay of both metabolic and psychological elements that had not been appropriately considered. We would add further that psychotherapeutic intervention was indeed appropriate, but perhaps not to the extent with which it was used.

We shall leave to the reader the ethical, medical, and psychological implications of this case, but remind ourselves of the danger of making any overgeneralizations in differential vocal assessments and of being aware of our own theoretical biases.

Conversion or hysterical dysphonia Although typically occurring in middle-aged women, conversion dysphonia has also been present in children. We would define it essentially as the partial or complete loss of voice without any apparent structural lesion, or as a peripheral physiological dysfunction whereby psychological conflict or disturbance is converted into acutal physical symptoms. Rammage, Nichol, and Morrison (1983) view it as a delayed shock reaction to emotional trauma. They also describe its occurrence following a throat virus or upper respiratory infection. The onset may be either sudden or gradual and intermittent, according to Wilson (1979). In the view of Steinhauer and Berman (1983), a conversion neurosis is more likely in children with histrionic personalities in which behavior is intense, theatrical, and demanding constant attention. Their relationships are described as demanding and superficial, and the child tends to be highly excitable, irrational, and manipulative. The end result is the alienation of others and interference with their interpersonal feelings.

In terms of family systems theory, we would view conversion dysphonia as a symptom not only of a deep personal emotional conflict but also as a misguided, unwitting attempt to change an existing intolerable familial situation. The differential voice assessment of such a disorder presents a formidable challenge to the voice therapist in that predisposing, precipitating, and perpetuating factors will need to be identified. In a public school situation this presents a considerable challenge because the school speech-language pathologist is unlikely to have access to the family environment of the child.

With respect to specific vocal symptoms, the child may present with a breathy, rough, or diplophonic voice, but abduction and adduction are normal in deep inhalation and coughing and swelling, respectively (Greene 1980). That is, the larynx may function adequately for biological purposes but not for vocalization. We will discuss the therapeutic implications of this behavior later with reference to both children and adults with conversion dysphonia.

Susan, twelve years old, was thrown from her bicycle after colliding with a moving automobile. Hospital intake revealed mild abrasions and contusions but no evidence of cerebral concussion or limb fracture. The morning following a precautionary one-night stay in the hospital, she presented with aphonia characterized by whispering only. Laryngoscopic examination revealed no visible organicity except for mild inflammation of the vocal folds due to, according to the laryngologist, a mild respiratory infection. Following two weeks of no change in her vocal behavior, she and her family were referred for a family therapy consult. Only after several family therapy sessions was it revealed that Susan's relationship with her mother had been fraught with considerable anger and resentment and that both of them had been competing for the attention and affection by the only male person in the family—a passive husband and father. (It should be noted that Susan was also being seen during this time for individual voice therapy, which also had, for the several sessions, been unsuccessful in relieving the voice symptoms.)

Only when family communication was opened up, honestly and straightforwardly, did Susan's symptoms begin to diminish. Susan's parents were readily amenable to marriage counseling for themselves, and Susan was referred for individual psychotherapy.

This anecdote is a graphic example of how intrapersonal family conflict may play a significant part in the genesis of a psychogenic voice disorder. It must be understood, however, that such family dynamics will certainly not always result in the symptomatology described, but that the interplay of several distinctive and unique personal factors will determine a particular psychopathology.

Implications of use, misuse, and abuse   Although it is clear that a direct relationship may be drawn between misuse and abuse of the voice and the development of vocal fold pathology, it is not clear how aggravation of the laryngeal mechanism may bring about vocal dysfunction in the absence of organicity. In Senturia and Wilson's 1968 study, twenty-nine of ninety-two children whose larynx could be visualized revealed no discrete lesions, yet they were found to abuse their voices in any one of several ways, including screaming, yelling, excessive speaking and throat clearing, and singing. For reasons unknown, these children were apparently impervious to the development of pathology per se. We can only speculate that constitutional resilience might explain its absence. Regardless of such a variable, we support Aronson's statement that "abuse or misuse . . . is an intermediate link in the chain of causes that begins with an emotionally determined impetus to vocalize aggressively" (1980, p. 134). What, then, are the psychotherapeutic implications? Let us examine these now.

COUNSELING STRATEGIES

It is important to make clear at the onset of our discussion that while traditional modes of voice therapy have been found to be effective in the treatment of voice disorders in children, we nevertheless insist that the interpersonal relationship established between the therapist and the child is crucial to fundamental changes in vocal behavior. As Cooper (1973) has pointed out, it is not so much a therapeutic method used that counts as how the therapist uses it. Regardless of the method used, therapists cannot avoid, nor should they, having a direct impact on the emotional attitudes and behaviors of their young clients. Not only, then, must we be fully cognizant of what we do and how we do it but also keenly aware of the effects and implications of our treatment.

Neither can we ignore the continuing influences and effects of the family and school environment on the child and his or her relationship to it, as such effects may well determine the therapeutic outcome. It is, therefore, unfortunate that many of us, particularly those of us who practice in a school setting, are unable to have substantial contact with the family in order for us to provide a more comprehensive approach. These limitations, however, need not preclude our best attempts to discover through differential assessment the factors underlying the child's voice dysfunction and to make do with whatever information is available to us.

It is obvious that no one approach is applicable to every child who presents with a voice disorder, nor do we know which technique works best; but we agree with Aronson (1980) that we must avoid treating voice disorders as "mechanical problems" only, particularly when emotional stress is a factor, and "voice therapy has to be tailored to the individual" (p. 194). It seems reasonable, then, to combine, if necessary, the best strategies available to us, to emphasize those with which we feel most personally compatible, and finally, to be open to learn those about which we know least.

Counseling with Parents

We have already described how parents are often unconcerned with the identification and possible consequences of vocal dysfunction in their children. We would hope that such an attitude would not deter us from educating them as to the nature of their child's voice disorder.

If the child is to be helped most successfully, it will necessitate the full cooperation of the parents to ensure carryover of whatever changes we are to effect in vocal or personal behaviors. Thus one of our primary goals in counseling the parents is first to provide them with information. This may be accomplished during traditional parent counseling or in family therapy, depending on the unique circumstances and needs of the family. Generally, we tend to favor a family therapy approach, if possible, so that all members of the family learn together. Reality often dictates otherwise, however, as we have discussed earlier.

We have developed a series of guidelines that the voice therapist might find useful as a point of departure:

1. *A description of the anatomy and physiology of the vocal tract geared to the intellectual level of family members.* This may vary, depending on the understanding of each member. Simple visual aids are particularly useful.

2. *An explanation of the actual organic conditions, if present.* If there is no existing organic condition, describe in the simplest way possible how hyperfunctional use contributes to aberrant vocal quality and how an organic condition may develop.

3. *A description of various forms of vocal misuse.* These, which we described earlier, may be elaborated upon, depending on their relevance to the particular child and family.

4. *An explanation of the various environmental circumstances that may contribute to such misuse.* It is helpful to begin with a general explanation and gather from the family factors pertinent to their own life circumstances. Caution should be exercised so as not to inject blame, which could be counterproductive to continued parental support.

5. *A description of basic principles of vocal hygiene.* These have been developed by Boone (1983, pp. 205–207) and are applicable to both children and adults with voice disorders. It is important, however, that the counseling therapist not overwhelm the family with all of the significant do's and don'ts, but determine those factors that in the family's view appear most pertinent. Neither the parents nor the child can be expected to make all of the changes deemed necessary by the therapist immediately, and should be given continued support for even modest modifications.

6. *An explanation of the overall means and goals of voice therapy if indicated.* Determination of the effective means toward these objectives must be discussed openly, with the parents and the child (if old enough) participating in the decision. General therapeutic approaches might include

   a. Family therapy only
   b. Family therapy with individual symptomatic therapy
   c. Parent counseling only
   d. Parent counseling with individual symptomatic therapy
   e. Individual symptomatic therapy only
   f. Family therapy with individual counseling therapy
   g. Parent counseling with individual counseling therapy
   h. Combined individual, symptomatic, and counseling therapy
   i. Individual counseling therapy only

It is important to recognize that special or unique circumstances will often dictate the method or methods of choice and that one method may not necessarily be more appropriate than another. Regardless of choice, we believe, that parent cooperation in any effort is important and necessary if permanent positive vocal changes in the child are to occur.

7. *An explanation of the role of parental assistance with the child's home practice.* Closely related to our discussion above, we believe it is unwise only to "send something home with the child" unless the parents or at least one parent is made fully aware of exactly how parent participation can best be utilized. In rare instances only (we hope) we would refrain from involving parents in the home practice, particularly if we believe they are inadvertently sabotaging our best therapeutic efforts because of deep-rooted individual or family psychopathology.

Generally speaking, and regardless of therapeutic approach, it is wise to keep parents informed throughout the voice therapy period. It is also hoped that the quality of parent education would not be adversely affected by dissimilarities of clinical settings. We would take issue with those who claim that the school setting cannot provide the quality of service that so-called clinical settings can provide. Therapeutic outcome, we believe, is determined essentially by the expertise of the clinical speech-language pathologist regardless of therapeutic environment, as has been demonstrated in the study by Cook, Palaski, and Hanson (1979).

Family Therapy

We have already discussed how environmental stresses may lead to both organic and nonorganic voice disorders. It would seem, therefore, that family therapy would be the appropriate treatment because the family environment would most likely be the major source of the life stress. There are several advantages to this approach:

1. The voice disorder as the identified symptom may more readily be traced directly to actual family dysfunctional processes.
2. The family can learn to tune in objectively to how the child is using or misusing the voice.
3. The family members can learn how to modify their own behaviors in order to effect positive vocal usage in the child.
4. The family can also learn how to help the child directly to use the voice more effectively.
5. The family is better able to effect changes in the extrafamilial environment, which may have been contributing to vocal misuse.

Neutralizing the symptoms and the behavior   Although typical family therapy focuses on modifying family homeostasis and interactional relationships among all family members in order to neutralize one member's symptom and behavior, the voice-disordered child may require a somewhat different approach. It requires that attention be given immediately to the child's actions that are directly associated with the faulty vocal condition. The therapist attempts to elicit from the child as much information as possible regarding the need to use the present vocal pattern and also regarding the child's perceptual attitudes. The therapist must preface these attempts by encouraging all family members to share their feelings without judging the feelings of others and to be prepared to listen as openly as possible. Although an outburst of hostility may create a delicate situation, it is important for feelings to be expressed and at the same time to protect the person who does so, particularly the child.

We must remember that while vocal symptoms may be maintaining and perpetuating dysfunctional family patterns, and destructive in and of themselves, they do not lend themselves easily to direct intervention. For these reasons, it is more appropriate to identify the intrafamilial relationships and interactions.

Modifying family homeostasis   In our other discussions of family therapy we have cautioned the therapist not to get immersed in the content of what is being expressed by family members but to heed the actual process that is taking place. This process includes how people communicate with each other—their vocal tone, body language, and degree of participation. It tells us how parents relate to each other, how each or both relate to the child or other children, and how children relate to each other. In essence, we are given a mirror image of what actually takes place at home.

In a child-centered family in which a child has the voice disorder, it is important that the therapist is a leader, who, in Minuchin's (1974) terms, must "join and accommodate" the family so as to create a therapeutic system. The therapist first accepts the family as it is, agreeing with the family's concern for the child, thereby gaining the trust necessary to instigate changes later. The therapist then considers the various combinations of relationships and how the elements intrinsic to them may have produced and perpetuated the voice disorder. Particular attention is directed to the latter in order to determine how it has operated as a homeostatic factor to maintain family dysfunction. Next, the therapist attempts to learn from family members specific circumstances and conditions that appear to bring about or are associated with an increase of vocal misuse and abuse. These may range from overall family life stress to sibling competition or to specific instances of marital discord.

The therapist might then program changes to help the family or specific family members to cope with the stressors or in some cases might recommend marital couple therapy. Thus, for example, it might be more constructive to help the parents to argue their conflicts in a more congruent way, thereby reducing their loud verbal outbursts. Reduction of the latter may eliminate their need to admonish their child for "screaming all the time." Whether the therapist acts to handle the dyadic relationship between two siblings, mother–child, or father–mother or triadic relationships among mother–child–father, modifications of behavior are directed to the way they interact and the context in which these interactions take place.

Recommending changes in the style of family relating does not mean altering family values to suit our own perspectives. As therapists, we need to draw upon the unrealized strengths, love, and caring that already exist to restore a healthy balance. The following case study illustrates how several of these principles may be applied.

Craig was ten years old when bilateral vocal nodules were first discovered by the family physician. Referral to a laryngologist confirmed the diagnosis. Gentle family prodding by the public school speech-language pathologist led to the initial examination after a vocal assessment had been made. There was no way of knowing how long the condition had persisted, as the family had just moved to California from the East Coast.

The laryngologist preferred taking a conservative approach by recommending voice therapy rather than surgery, but provided the family little information other than the admonition to "help him to use his voice more softly." Craig's conscientious school therapist, however, made certain that the family was fully informed about the condition, and they learned specific ways to help him at home. Craig was enrolled in voice therapy for two one-half-hour sessions a week.

Craig's vocal behavior was characteristic. As an outgoing child he screamed and yelled incessantly while playing with his friends in and outside school. According to his parents (Peter and Fay), he never stopped talking at home, and they were obviously perturbed by his shrill voice. His voice quality was generally hoarse.

After two months of voice therapy, during which time no substantial changes in vocal behavior or in vocal quality were evident, his therapist arranged for a parent conference. Skilled in parent counseling, she learned that Peter and Fay had made a diligent effort to follow her vocal hygiene advice, but that Craig was unresponsive to their well-meaning intentions. Clinically, his therapist had helped him to obtain a balanced and healthy use of the voice, but none of this had carried over elsewhere. Recognizing that elements in the family environment were hindering all therapeutic efforts, she recommended a family therapy consultation. Somewhat hesitant at first, Peter and Fay finally agreed.

During the first meeting, their futile attempts to help Craig at home were confirmed. It was also obvious to the family therapist that their efforts were consistent with an overall pattern of rigid expectations in all aspects of behavior—everyone must eat dinner at 6:00 P.M. sharp, homework must be finished before dinner, Craig must clean his room every Saturday morning, and so forth. Peter and Fay's expectations for themselves were no less compelling. Also apparent was Fay's passive toleration of these expectations, which were rooted in Peter's strong convictions. To him, it was important that "things must always go smoothly." The family therapist also noticed how Peter needed to maintain control over the course of the session and resisted the therapist's own attempts to enter into the family process. Only when such behavior was pointed out to Peter did Fay and Craig begin to express themselves openly. Peter had much difficulty in listening to Fay's deeply felt complaint that she felt stifled by what she considered to be a "cold, clockwork atmosphere" at home but that she too contributed to such an environment. Craig complained that "home isn't fun" and that he didn't like being told "what to do all the time."

It was immediately apparent to the therapist that what had first seemed like unwitting collusion between Fay and Peter was in actuality a bond between Fay and Craig, with Peter attempting to maintain control over everything and everyone. Subsequent sessions confirmed this, and more.

It seemed clear to the therapist that although Craig's voice disorder was serving as a symptom to identify the underlying family conflict characterized by discontent, hidden anger, and resentment, Peter had also been the unidentified victim, caught up in his own unresolved conflicts with his own family of origin. Reared in a family that was obviously even more stifling, rigid, and demanding, Peter had been carrying the burden of such an influence.

Fay, on the other hand, raised in a family with two older brothers where she had been expected to assume the typical passive female role, fit the model in her present marriage but not without feelings of underlying resentment and rebellion. Her and Peter's conflict thus was based on each striving to satisfy in their own way unrealized needs. Craig's persistent yelling and aggressively verbal behavior was seen by the therapist as a manifestation of the silent rages felt but unexpressed by both Fay and Peter. Craig, in a very real sense, was "crying out" not only the inner family turmoil but *for* family harmony.

It was the therapist's major task to help Fay and Peter relate to each other realistically and in the present, uncontaminated by their own past family patterns. As expressed anger began to emerge and individual frustrations came into focus, Craig's vocal behavior began to change with a reduction in vocal misuse. It was deemed important that Craig continue to be present and participate in the process, as he, too, needed to express his own frustrations and at the same time be privy to the unraveling conflicts. Individual voice therapy was also resumed in order to enhance healthier vocal usage and help give Craig the sense of being part of the process toward overall family adjustment.

No doubt, the inherent mutual love and caring in this family were significant elements in the establishment of family harmony and growth and in the ultimate disappearance of the vocal nodules and abusive vocal behavior.

Individual Counseling Approaches

Family therapy alone may not always be possible, necessary, or in fact, the most useful method of treatment. For that matter, neither may direct vocal rehabilitation be the most effective approach. Unique, individual circumstances such as family cooperation, motivation of the child, and therapist competence will determine choice of treatment. Even among the various counseling approaches, no one approach would be deemed most effective. It would also be dictated by the demonstrated needs and special circumstances of the child, family, and therapist. In fact, it may be possible to combine them or even integrate one or the other with symptomatic strategies.

Play therapy   According to Hejna (1960), among the basic principles underlying nondirective play therapy is the child's inherent need for continual growth and aspiration for self-realization. As children explore their immediate environment, they find pain, pleasure, punishment, approval, failure, and success. Some, who feel so frustrated or punished that they withdraw, feel discouraged or angry but have no viable outlet to express themselves. With respect to voice disorders, Hejna views play therapy as a natural method of releasing the child from inner frustrations, anxieties, tensions, and insecurities. As we have noted elsewhere in reference to the work of Axline (1969), play is a natural medium for self-expression whereby the child is given the opportunity to play out inner feelings of tension, insecurity, and so on. By their expression, such feelings are brought to the surface. Thus exposed, the child faces these feelings, learns to control them, and finally abandons them.

If the voice problems are caused or maintained by any of these emotional factors, then the vocal behavior may automatically change. If the voice problems create feelings of inferiority, play therapy might enhance feelings of greater confidence and self-acceptance and the motivation to change vocal behavior (Hejna 1960).

In a case study described by Mosby (1970), supportive play therapy along with traditional voice therapy was used with a ten-year-old boy who had been resistive to traditional voice therapy techniques. Psychotherapy was used as a means to discover the child's underlying aggressive behavior and sought to teach him adequate coping mechanisms. Apparently Mosby's approach was successful in inducing calmer feelings, decreasing vocal misuse, and reducing the vocal nodules.

Because dysfunctional vocal behavior often is manifested in the child's typical play activities, the eight basic principles of play therapy as described by Axline (1969) are particularly applicable. The therapist

1. Establishes warm, friendly rapport with the child in an environment characterized by soft vocalization.
2. Accepts the child completely even if vocalization is still abusive.
3. Establishes a feeling of permissiveness so that the child feels free to express feelings, thereby minimizing the need to misuse the voice.
4. Recognizes and reflects the child's feelings, which also would reduce vocal misuse.
5. Maintains respect for the child.
6. Allows the child to lead the way.
7. Does not hurry therapy, so that a more balanced vocal pattern will emerge slowly but definitely.
8. Establishes only those limitations necessary to help the child be aware of responsibilities first to self and then to others.

Operationally, play therapy may be modified to suit the particular voice disorder and varying psychological constellation of the child. Thus muteness or vocal abuse will necessitate establishing differing clinical environments so that the child will be motivated to attempt a new mode of vocalization. In play therapy, as we view it, etiology is not as important as the behavioral manifestations of the child. Yet it is possible to change the latter without necessarily working directly on the symptomatology. On the other hand, the therapist should not feel constrained to adhere only to the classic principles of play therapy but also include symptom management if deemed relevant in particular cases.

Regardless of emphasis, the therapist should avoid a hodgepodge approach and have a carefully thought-out plan, including short- and long-term goals. Any modification of the plan and objectives are acceptable because we can never be certain that any of our clients will progress in a predictable manner. Conceivably, what may have been play therapy to begin with could evolve into direct intervention strategies.

Direct counseling   Although direct vocal rehabilitation, which is both educational and therapeutic, may typically be effective in the treatment of voice disorders, those disorders that contain pronounced psychogenic components are less amenable to long-term change. For these reasons a psychotherapeutic approach would perhaps be a more suitable procedure. Yet we would not recommend its use with children indiscriminately even under the guidance of psychotherapeutically trained therapists. Several, sometimes overlapping, criteria would in part dictate and qualify such an approach. They include the following:

1. *Age*: Mental age of the child would be a prime determinant, as some ten-year-olds, for example, might be more receptive than some twelve-year-olds.
2. *Psychological impact of the disorder*: Some children have a strong adverse reaction to the disorder itself and will need emotional support to assist in coping with and changing the disorder.
3. *Adverse familial influences or lack of parental support*: Persistently negative factors within the home environment may not be amenable to change, thus the child will have to develop ways to tolerate and counteract these influences.
4. *Presence of underlying dysfunctional psychological processes*: Pronounced stress, anxiety, poor self-esteem, and conflict associated with vocal misuse and abuse may need to be addressed before traditional strategies can be productive.
5. *Failure of traditional or symptomatic strategies*: Psychotherapeutic management, when all other strategies have been nonproductive, would appear to be appropriate even in the apparent absence of psychogenic factors.

The issue of psychotherapy has received considerable attention in the literature, with most authorities generally agreed that it should be conducted by professional psychotherapists when the voice disorder is dominated by psychopathology. Whereas some writers believe that counseling should be used only to obtain information and reduce severe distress, others prefer a total hands-off approach.

This writer's own perspective is based more on the appropriate qualifications and training of the therapist than on doctrinal or parochial professional territories. As far as voice-disordered children are concerned, we are not troubled by voice symptom removal per se, even when it is a manifestation of underlying psychological processes. We do believe that it be done by a therapist who is at least cognizant of and familiar with psychopathology. After all, are any of us so bold as to prefer operating in ignorance, or would we rather function with the fullest awareness possible?

The point we wish to make is that a voice disorder is not a distinct entity but a manifestation of the total being of an individual. We need at least to recognize the psychological and behavioral implications of any attempted modification of vocal function. The problem often is that in our enthusiasm to do well, we focus on the "it" rather than on the person.

Perhaps the hesitancy of some speech-language pathologists in taking on voice-disordered children is not so much a reflection of their fear of working with these children but more an expression of an intuitive awareness of their own lack of expertise in complex psychological processes. Nevertheless, it would be useful to describe in some detail how counseling may be used by a therapist who is versed in psychological and psychotherapeutic processes.

The child with a voice disorder, be it organic or nonorganic, is in a real sense crying out for self-expression, as alluded to by Aronson (1980). We have applied several principles throughout this text that may be useful in guiding our management of these children:

1. *Learning from the child the particular circumstances, personal and environmental, in which vocal misuse and abuse occurs.* The child is encouraged to share with the therapist all information deemed appropriate, including data that at first may appear irrelevant.

2. *Developing the interpersonal relationship.* An immediately effective way to reduce abusive vocal behavior is through the natural and nonjudgmental communicative relationship that should be free to develop between the therapist and the child.

3. *Giving information about the voice and its function.* Gearing information to the intellectual ability of the child, it is possible for the therapist to provide information about vocal anatomy and physiology through visual aids. At this time, it may be appropriate to describe to the child how the voice is currently being used.

4. *Helping the child take responsibility for vocalization.* Treating the voice as a separate entity is dispelled as the child is helped to understand personal control over vocalization. The child is taught that the voice itself is not expected to change so much as the *way* in which the voice is used.

5. *Dealing with emotional issues that relate directly or indirectly to vocal misuse.* As the interpersonal relationship develops, the child becomes freer in sharing feelings to which the therapist responds empathically. (See Aronson's summary of Rogerian principles related to communication [1980].)

6. *Allowing the child to progress at his or her own pace.* As therapists, we sometimes rush the therapeutic process in our fervor to "correct the prob-

lem." This should be avoided because it very likely represents projection on our part, related to satisfying our own personal needs for "saving," rather than objectivity about the child's needs. It is important however, also to be sensitive to resistances, denial, and uncooperativeness, which must be handled gently yet firmly. The child does not behave in the way described merely to spite the therapist but is actually communicating significant personal material that begs for clarification and understanding.

7. *Straying from direct discussion or management of vocal function.* During the course of the ongoing interpersonal relationship, the therapist may need to be more attentive to the self-expression of the child rather than to the way in which the voice may be used, misused, or abused. The therapist will have to determine how much of this can be dealt with, given his or her personal qualifications and counseling competencies. If outside referral is deemed necessary, particularly if powerful psychopathological issues begin to emerge, related or not to the voice disorder, the therapist may need gradually to terminate the relationship or change its clinical character. Regardless of the decision, the child should not be left to feel rejected.

8. *Helping the child communicate more congruently or with straightforward messages.* Oftentimes, the voice-disordered child has resorted to abusive vocal behavior because of the frustration in not being able to communicate clearly with those surrounding him or her. The therapist can help the child identify those feelings and attitudes held and encourage their outward expression. Thus, instead of the child needing to scream at home in order to gain attention, it is possible to learn to say directly to parents, for example: "I really need your attention."

9. *Helping the child recognize other personal needs, hopes, and desires that are not being satisfied.* The therapist can discuss with the child unsatisfied wishes that may in reality fall within the realm of possibility. The child must also be helped to understand desires that cannot realistically be fulfilled given the existing environmental circumstances and limitations inherent in being a child.

10. *Transferring interpersonal communication from the clinic to the real world.* As the child begins to gain a fuller understanding of self, and uses the voice in a more open and balanced way clinically, the therapy session should be extended into various environmental situations in which new vocal behaviors and attitudes may be practiced. If screaming on the playing field has previously been a problem, it might be appropriate for the therapist and child to toss around a football, keeping a fair distance, in order for verbal communication to occur appropriately.

11. *Taking permanent responsibility for change.* For any vocal change to take place, the child must ultimately take full responsibility for controlling the voice in and outside formal therapy. The child must learn to take charge of any vocal situation and thereby eliminate the victim's role as a vocal misuser and abuser.

The foregoing guidelines are not exclusive to the many excellent principles and approaches that have already been enumerated and discussed in the literature and that have been successfully implemented (Boone 1983; Case 1984; Wilson 1979; Aronson 1980). The therapist may readily combine several strategies geared toward the individual child, including symptomatic methods. Let us consider, then, how we may integrate a symptomatic with a counseling approach.

A counseling and symptomatic approach combined   We previously inferred that it is wiser for the speech-language pathologist to counsel the voice-disordered child only when psychopathological processes are either directly or at least indirectly related to the disorder itself. When such a relationship exists, it would in fact be almost impossible to ignore either the vocal symptom, the child's reaction to it, or the interpersonal components. Some therapists have successfully used techniques that are simultaneously psychotherapeutic and symptomatic. LaGuaite (1976) used hypnosis successfully to reduce vocal abuse in voice-disordered children. Greene (1980) has provided both general and specific methods of achieving relaxation as a means of modifying the stressors associated with vocal hyperfunction. Wilson (1979) has applied the communication-centered speech therapy approach of Low, Crerar, and Lassers (1959) to group therapy with voice-disordered children.

The author has found that a contractual therapeutic arrangement is most conducive to a positive outcome, regardless of the methodological emphasis. That is, we are asking the child to change something but it entails awareness, motivation, cooperation, and practice.

Children generally appreciate the responsibility given to them consistent with directing their own vocal behavior and its modification. Although able to move at their own pace, they are also encouraged to move ahead forthrightly. Should commitment by the child to the therapeutic process lag, it is necessary for the therapist to discuss the problem openly, help the child with his or her own resistance, and try to modify the circumstances that may be hindering progress.

Sometimes the child may feel that the personal efforts to change vocal behavior are "not worth it," "too hard," "no fun," or "make me feel funny." As therapists, we must remind ourselves that these verbal expressions may be the outward manifestations of underlying feelings associated with self-concept, personal worth, or interpersonal conflict and as such demand our attention. At times, it may be necessary to support the child's need for "time-out" in order to discuss the issue further or to allow the child time to think more about it.

The author has found no single explanation for the inertia that may arise in therapy. He has, in fact, found such children to have parents who either rigorously supervise home practice or who take little or no interest in the child's voice therapy. Regardless of the degree of parental "cooperation," it is still the child who must ultimately be the sole agent for positive vocal change.

We are all familiar, however, with children who may be too immature to take the kind and type of responsibility suggested here. Contractual therapy in these cases may be contraindicated, yet at the same time we would not want to be party to continued dependency and immaturity. We would attempt, however, to strike a balance between a more directive therapeutic approach and the encouragement of more mature behavior. Some form or degree of parental cooperation will likely be necessary, but it is not our role to take responsibility for total personality enhancement and growth.

CONCLUSION

There appears to be sufficient evidence to suggest that voice disorders in childhood are often the manifestation of interpersonal as well as intrapersonal relationships. A specific disorder itself is rooted not so much in differential organic or nonorganic components, but in the individual child's emotional state. It is also clear that the child's actual vocal quality may reflect a particular emotional state.

The presence of such nonlinear relationships presents a considerable challenge to the voice therapist, who must be well versed in traditional vocal management techniques and sophisticated in psychotherapeutic counseling. These requirements become even more vital as we turn to our discussion of voice-disordered adults.

Part II: The Psychology of Voice Disorders in Adults

PSYCHOGENESIS OF VOICE DISORDERS

Disraeli said, "There is no index of character so sure as the voice." But is such a statement as irrefutable as it first seems? We think not. In a provocative essay, Quan (1985) has noted:

> In a purely biologic and physiologic position, the voice is controlled by muscle contractions, neural transmission, aerodynamic processes and physical reso-

nance characteristics. In some way we control what we do to our voices, thus matching it to the way in which we want to appear to others. On the other hand, the psychological position speaks of an inadvertent connection between the way a person uses his or her voice and their concomitant personality type. In the first example given of the purposeful control of voice, the character of the individual may not coincide with the vocal qualities that the person is choosing to emit. Thus the voice does not act as an "open window to the soul." In fact, it may even be very deceptive in personifying an opposite impression. On the other side, psychosomatic diseases have been identified as manifestations of the person's "true self." Under unconscious control, the voice may in fact show character that lies within. (p. 1)

In attempting to unravel the "several semantic and methodologic obstacles" inherent in the relationship between "normal voice and normal personality," Aronson (1980) has listed the following:

1. The difficulty in defining personality
2. Validity and reliability problems associated with personality tests
3. Poor definitions of voice variables
4. Alterations of research methodologies

To this list we would add the following two points: the psychoperceptual abilities of listeners are contaminated by their preconceived biases, thereby interfering with objectivity. And speakers who use their voice in a certain manner may be compensating by using a voice that differs characteristically from the original personality stereotype. Thus those individuals who are essentially introverted in nature may tend toward a voice that acoustically is resonant, firm, strong, and convincing, whereas those who are essentially extroverted in nature may tend toward a voice that acoustically is thin, weak, and unconvincing.

Unfortunately, we do not yet understand the complex nature of compensatory vocal adjustments and thus we are often misled by predetermined stereotypic judgments. It appears, then, that for the moment we must study each individual's unique vocal and nonvocal personality. Such a study has special therapeutic implications, as we shall see later.

In Part I of this chapter we briefly alluded to the complex relationship between voice and personality relative to the development of voice disorders in children. In adults, not only are these relationships more complex but they are manifested in a greater variety of disorders that often defy even the most astute of professionals.

As both Moses (1954) and Murphy (1964) have variously described the essence and nature of voice disorders, the development of the speaking voice is influenced not only by the speaker's feeling and attitudes about self but also by how the speaker perceives the listener's reaction to the voice. These factors combine and affect the speaker's vocal self-image, personality, lifestyle, and in some cases the vocal disorder itself. The symptoms of voice disorders develop via a process of adjustment in which the speaker is attempting to balance personal inner drives, private environment, and outer realities.

Clinically, there is considerable evidence to suggest that stress within the individual may manifest itself vocally but also differently, as each individual has a unique means of coping both psychologically and physiologically (Scherer 1981a&b). It has been postulated by Moses (1954) that the process of living involves tension from which the organism seeks release in order to reestablish homeostasis. But if the release does not occur and if homeostasis is not established, the organism will search for other avenues of release. A crucial role in the reestablishment of homeostasis belongs to the vocal mechanism, as a medium of communication. Moses expresses little doubt that the vocal mechanism is affected by tension release through the development of psychological maladjustment. But this in turn may result in misuse, abuse, or loss of control over the vocal mechanism. Although we would not argue that all voice disorders necessarily have their genesis in psychopathological sources, emotional stress would seem to be a common denominator in most disorders of the voice. More important, then, might be our attempt to understand more fully the ongoing psychodynamic factors that characterize perpetuation of the disorder.

Gutwinski-Jeggle (1983) suggests that most voice disorders are not the result of physiological or medical problems, but a manifestation of disturbance in relationships with significant others. If the client is unresponsive to traditional methods of therapy, we must look at the voice problem as symptomatic of the dysfunctional relationship or as an unconscious way of coping with other problems.

ETIOLOGICAL CONSIDERATIONS

The physiological ramifications of stress resulting in various voice disorders, such as vocal nodules, contact ulcers, vocal polyps, spastic dysphonia, nonspecific laryngitis, and conversion dysphonia, have been described by many investigators and therapists. Yet objective measurements of stress have proven difficult to establish. There are, however, several tools available that allow the therapist or researcher valid measurements of stress and to relate these to vocal production.

Simonov and Frolov (1973), in the Soviet Union, devised a method based on spectrographic analysis that allowed them to differentiate degree of emotional stress in 85 percent of their subjects. Their studies with Soviet cosmonauts established a relationship between heart rate (beats per minute) and changes in the human voice resulting from emotional stress. In a later article by Simonov, Frolov, and Talebkin (1975), the investigators relied upon EEG measurements to determine emotional reactions. Increased heart rates were associated with increased states of stress and vocal change. Again we must refer to the excellent review by Scherer (1981), who reports that there is considerable evidence to support the hypothesis that "for fairly high levels of stress and for a majority of subjects studied, fundamental frequency of the voice rises and the proportion of energy above 500 Hz in the spectrum increases" (p. 183). The difficulty in any type of systematic research, according to Scherer, is that we must study individual differences and different types of stress if we are to understand specific coping mechanisms.

The relationship between emotion and its acoustic correlates as expressed in the voice has challenged psychologists, physiologists, and voice pathologists for many years. Scherer (1981b) brings to our attention the current state of research on this complex relationship. Although it may be assumed that the human voice is affected by specific emotional conditions, we have yet to establish definitive associations between voice and the various milieus in which it is used. It would be impractical within the context of the present volume to discuss all of the research that has been done in the area. It is important, however, to recognize that until we have established definitive relationships between emotion and its vocal correlates, our efforts to establish relationships between emotion and correlates of vocal pathology could well be hampered. Regardless, we should not be prevented from forming associations between psychogenic factors and specific vocal pathologies. In doing so, we hope to avoid the dichotomy that continues to separate so-called nonorganic from organic voice disorders.

Vocal Nodules

We have already discussed the psychogenic correlates of vocal nodules in children and considered the psychodynamics of vocal misuse and abuse in that disorder. Vocal nodules is also one of the most common voice disorders in adults and is similarly imbued with complex psychogenic and psychodynamic components. Clinically, common personality factors have been found in such individuals. Although Aronson (1980) views the etiology and pathology as essentially comparable for both children and adults, he suggests that there are some differences. According to Aronson, the incidence of vocal nodules is more common in women than in men. These women "are talkative, socially aggressive and tense, and suffer from acute or chronic interpersonal problems that generate tension, anxiety, anger or depression" (p. 136).

Greene (1980) has found that given the pronounced anxiety aspect of the personality structure of individuals with vocal nodules, there may be psychosomatic components. No systematic research is offered, however, to support that contention. The term *psychosomatic* is still fraught with controversy and problems of definition, so we will refrain from further discussion at this time. Based on her extensive clinical experiences, though, Greene has found that those with vocal nodules may not necessarily be neurotic but, rather, well adjusted. They tend to have the competitive spirit of the business executive, singer, and actor. She describes the personality type as productive, responsible, reliable, and generally gregarious.

Earlier in our chapter we referred to Case (1984) and his comprehensive list of specific types of vocal abuse and related causal factors. It is useful now to include from them a list of those factors which are more applicable to adults with vocal nodules. These include

1. Singing in a manner inappropriate to the actual vocal equipment
2. Speaking in a noisy environment
3. Coughing and excessive throat clearing
4. Strenuous grunting while straining and exercising
5. Smoking excessively
6. Speaking excessively or abusively during menstrual periods
7. Arguing intensively
8. Talking in nightclubs and other noisy surroundings

Although we might be tempted to paint a psychogenic portrait characteristic of adults with vocal nodules, there does not appear to be enough definitive evidence in the literature to support such a contention. Furthermore, other important factors must be considered. Based on their study of the incidence, histology, and pathogenesis of vocal cord polyps, Kambic et al. (1981) believe the distinction between vocal nodules and polyps to be a "matter of opinion." Studying 591 patients, they found that smoking and increased industrialization and air pollution, along with an excessive amount of vocal use and faulty vocal techniques, to be the major culprits.

From a therapeutic viewpoint, it would be valuable to explore and understand the precipitating factors, both internal and external, that have contributed to the inception of the problem. It is also necessary to investigate and analyze the ongoing dynamic processes that perpetuate the disorder even after surgical intervention. These would include both the physiological or mechanical adjustments made by the individual to compensate for the perceived aberrant vocal quality and the psychological means by which the individual copes with the disorder. Brodnitz (1981), in his brilliant essay, emphasizes the importance and significance of clients' own psychological reactions to their disordered voices, but we shall say more about this later.

One element is obvious to us. As in children with vocal nodules, we need to understand the stressors that continue to operate in adults with a similar condition.

Contact Ulcers

Contact ulcers, like vocal nodules, are characterized by both an organic change and psychogenic factors. It appears, however, to be more prevalent in men, with many writers confirming environmental stress as a major etiological factor. Such patients have been found to be highly competitive, compulsive, and aggressive. Case (1984) describes them "to be in their early forties, highly vocal and dynamic in verbal interactions, hard driving, perfectionist, verbally aggressive, and in professions that involve considerable vocalization" (p. 141). The author has found them characteristically holding back from expressing feelings openly, tight-lipped and -jawed, and maintaining a rapid and never-ending flow of speech. They tend to resemble the Type A personality described elsewhere by Friedman and Rosenman. According to Landes (1977), American men's propensity to favor the lower pitch range in order to appear more masculine may account for the hyperfunctional abuse of the voice.

There have been negligible attempts to describe contact ulcer as a psychosomatic syndrome, and although a vast body of information has been published citing relationships between gastrointestinal ulcers and stress, these findings are still inconclusive. Greene (1980) cites a study by Cherry and Marguiles (1968), who studied three patients suffering "from pharyngo-oesophagitis due to peptic acid reflux" (p. 152). They suggested that it is possible for a backward flow of peptic acid to seep into the posterior larynx resulting in inflammation and ulceration. Other clinical workers have reported the appearance of contact ulcers in association with either acute or chronic upper respiratory infections.

Although the relationship among all these factors remains yet unclear; the speech-language pathologist is challenged to discover as many as possible of those elements in order to plan an appropriate regimen of therapy. Of particular importance is the necessity to understand the coping mechanisms, both psychological and physiological, which may be maintaining the vocal disorder and how these relate to vocal misuse and abuse.

Conversion Dysphonia

Probably no other voice disorder fits the classic definition of "functional" better than that of conversion dysphonia, except that organicity is sometimes found. Bridger and Epstein (1983) define "functional" generally as a "complaint due to disordered function rather than structure" (p. 1145). We would define conversion dysphonia as a symbolic representation of psychological conflict or stress manifested through the motor or sensory activity of the vocal tract, mainly the larynx. Sometimes referred to as hysteric dysphonia, the person with conversion dysphonia is generally middle aged, exhibiting excessive tension in the laryngeal area and having frequent sore throats or laryngitis (Bridger and Epstein 1983; Kaufman and Blalock 1982). According to Monday (1983), it appears to occur more often in women and may be associated with a precipitating unpleasant or traumatic event. Vocal abuse or misuse may not necessarily be a contributing factor, although the patient may not have a positive attitude toward vocal usage.

Greene (1980) has probably painted one of the most complete psychological portraits of such patients. They are frequently persons who demonstrate loneliness, guilt, or remorse; they develop self-pity and then vocal failure. Sometimes a fear of cancer leads to an obsessive concern over the vocal mechanism. Tension is evident in facial and postural features, and the person appears fidgety and restless and speaks rapidly. Shoulder, neck, and scalp tension produce headaches. There are sometimes gastrointestinal symptoms manifested in indigestion, poor appetite, and constipation. In extreme cases there may be anorexia in which the person restricts the taking of food severely with the idea of relieving some former digestive trouble.

Greene also describes the presence of endocrinological factors, such as menstrual pain, headache, and general malaise in persons with conversion dysphonia. Persistent anxiety resulting in overwhelming fatigue may be accompanied by insomnia.

According to Aronson (1980), the "conversion" may be into muteness, aphonia, or dysphonia. In its extreme form (conversion muteness) the characteristic findings are "chronic stress, primary and secondary gain, indifference to their symptom, other manifestations of conversion, poor sex identification, suppressed anger, immaturity and dependency, neurotic life adjustment, and mild to moderate depression" (p. 142). There appear also to be preexisting conscious and unconscious conflicts about verbal expression of anger, fear, or sadness and a halt in communication with those individuals who are of significance to the client.

Rammage, Nichol, and Morrison (1983) have also suggested that conversion dysphonia may be a delayed shock reaction to trauma. The symptoms of a rise in vocal pitch accompanied by voice breaks often appear more acute when discussing stressful events. The dysphonic individual appears less disturbed than the aphonic one and homeostasis is easier to restore. Rammage, Nichol, and Morrison also report that the individual's dysphonia often follows an actual illness such as a throat virus or upper respiratory infection. A significant corollary is that the voice symptoms appear to serve as a secondary gain. Hinsie and Campbell (1970) define it as

> secondary advantages accruing from an illness, such as gratification of dependency yearning or attention seeking . . . there are certain uses the patient can make of his illness which have nothing to do with the origin of neurosis but which may attain the utmost practical importance . . . obtaining financial compensation . . . but has acquired the unconscious meaning of love and protecting security as well. . . . (p. 316)

The following case study is a classic example of secondary gain in relationship to conversion dysphonia:

George T, a fifty-five-year-old investigator for a major insurance company, did not lose his laryngitis following a bout of the flu. Soon the laryngitis was accompanied by dysphonia characterized by a high pitched, straining or squeezed quality. Even though the vocal fold inflammation soon disappeared, the dysphonia persisted. His laryngologist, sensitive to Mr. T's associated depression, recommended psychiatric evaluation. After several psychotherapeutic sessions, it was learned that Mr. T had been seeking an early retirement from his firm but was being denied a full retirement compensation until age sixty-five unless a physical disability was present. The case history also revealed that Mr. T had never been married and had been living with two older, also unmarried, sisters for many years. The psychiatrist found Mr. T to be depressed, anxious, and enraged at his employer, whom he had "put out my life for." Expression of his rage and his hurt did not appear to have any effect on the dysphonia but in fact exacerbated it, resulting in intermittent whispering. Continuing psychiatric treatment, his psychiatrist also recommended that he receive voice therapy.

The voice evaluation confirmed that which had already been discovered. It was also possible to obtain a clear resonant voice with vowels through digital manipulation of the larynx and by having Mr. T cough or laugh aloud in a rapid CV sequence (ha, ha, ha, ha, ha). This could not be carried over into single words, although he apparently assiduously practiced obtaining clear phonation on various CVC combinations. While voice therapy was essentially symptomatic, Mr. T felt the need to express long repressed feelings of regrets, anger, and frustation with his life and deep feelings of inferiority. Both his psychiatrist and voice pathologist kept in constant touch, each sharing with the other information that was emerging in the two therapies.

After six months, following the initial psychiatric consultation, Mr. T abruptly terminated psychiatric treatment but continued in voice therapy. Still unresolved were deep feelings of self-effacement and anger. It was felt by both therapists, though, that voice therapy that combined symptomatic and psychotherapeutic management would be less threatening and more productive.

During the next two months of voice therapy, Mr. T was able to achieve a clear voice and balanced vocal usage on single words and short phrases. As he was appearing gradually to move toward his pre-flu voice, however, he announced he no longer desired any form of therapy.

This case study is revealing in that it reflects the complex interplay of many factors that relate to its genesis and perpetuation. The case also presented a challenge in differential assessment as several of the vocal symptoms were not unlike those associated with spastic dysphonia.

Spastic Dysphonia

The ideopathic etiology of spastic dysphonia has been a source of debate for years. The proponents for an organic basis contend that spastic dysphonia patients are not neurologically normal, but their abnormalities are not necessarily the cause of the spasticity. Aronson and DeSanto (1983) and Dedo and Shipp (1980) suggest that the majority of research done over the past twenty years points to some central nervous system involvement either directly or indirectly. Unfortunately, no conclusion has been reached about precise location. Shipp et al. (1985) report one case study that suggests neurological etiology above the larynx.

Although spastic dysphonia is often categorized separately from other voice disorders, Brodnitz (1976) considers the disorder to be a conversion syndrome in the vast majority of cases. In defense of his proposition, Brodnitz notes that most of these patients could sing normally, were able to isolate the onset of dysphonia as acute emotional trauma, and exhibited severe neurotic characteristics. Although there is little evidence to support the view that psychotherapeutic intervention, much less traditional therapy, has had any substantial beneficial effects, there may yet be undetermined psychodynamic forces at work. According to Izdebski and Dedo (1981), the progression of the disorder often leads the patient to withdraw from social situations and occupations, thus resulting in severe psychological consequences. Shipp (1985) has indicated that in selected cases there is probably a mechanism triggered by stress that may result in a neuromuscular imbalance involving the vocal folds.

Supporting the viewpoint of a disorder that is essentially organic in nature, Stoicheff (1983) has indicated that these patients show no remission of symptoms. It has also been determined that the onset is progressive rather than sudden, and that tremor is present in some patients. Believing spastic dysphonia to be among the most devastating and least understood voice disorders, Stoicheff theorizes the possibility of differing etiologies for the condition. He cites the inconsistency of vocal recovery postoperatively of recurrent laryngeal nerve (RLN) sectioning.

For the last ten years Dr. Herbert Dedo, who pioneered the technique, has used RLN in treating spastic dysphonia. He and his associates report that 92 percent of their patients undergoing RLN section maintained satisfactory reduction of spasticity (Dedo and Izdebski 1983). They note, however, that RLN section should not be regarded as a cure but as a means by which the communicative functioning of most patients can be enhanced. They used subjective patient self-assessments as indices of improvement.

Aronson and DeSanto (1983) have contended, however, that according to their own postoperative evaluative technique, 64 percent of their patient population failed to meet criteria for "successful" treatment. They relied upon pre- and postoperative evaluations by a speech-language pathologist. To substantiate these findings further, Sapir and Aronson (1985) conducted a study investigating therapist reliability in rating voice improvement after RLN section and found a high degree of reliability among different raters. They concluded that patients are not reliable sources of information on the voice effects of surgery. They also determined that future judgments of voice after RLN section should be based primarily on therapist judgment rather than on patient self-assessment.

The problem of spastic dysphonia takes on less clarity when we review the study by Aronson and Hartman (1981). They attempted to distinguish among three different types of spastic dysphonia. They found bodily tremor, diffuse neurological signs, and patterns of life stress associated with onset of the disorders classified, along with essential tremor. While the authors claim their results are inconclusive, they suggest that although psychogenic factors may not be necessarily responsible for vocal stoppages, they "well may serve to precipitate or exacerbate an incipient neurologic disorder" (p. 59).

There is little question that regardless of etiology or premorbid personality, the distress brought about by the disorder may have a profound effect upon the person's career and marital and social lives. Emotional responses may range from anger to withdrawal and, in extreme cases, definitive personality changes may occur. Although surgical intervention appears to be the major treatment of choice, there is sufficient evidence to suggest some form of psychotherapeutic aid, even though the latter has not been found to be a panacea of treatment.

Laryngectomy

In the last two decades, numerous advances have been taken place to assist our understanding of the anatomic-physiological factors and modes of treatment for laryngectomy. As a life-saving procedure for carcinoma of the larynx, the far-reaching psychological ramifications for the individual so afflicted has received less attention. Fontaine and Mitchell (1960) are among the earliest writers to refer to the emotional and sexual problems brought on after laryngectomy. Yet few authorities following this study have referred to the profound psychosocial implications of such a tragedy.

It has been well documented that heavy cigarette smoking and excessive intake of alcohol are the two most critical agents responsible for the development of cancerous lesions in the larynx. It has been further suggested by other investigators that tobacco and alcohol abuse are addictions that have associated features of personality disturbance, anxiety, and depression (Wallen and Webb 1975). These may be a response to an inability to cope effectively with life stresses. Discovery by such individuals that they have cancer and must have laryngeal amputation in order to survive is likely to have some profound effect on them, although there has been little research to document this.

Weisman (1979) and Weisman and Worden (1976–77) found that among cancer patients in general, those who were more emotionally disturbed tended to be withdrawn and disengaged from others. Less disturbed patients characteristically confronted the problem by accepting the situation, taking firm action and seeking medical help. Although not referring to cancer of the larynx specifically, Weisman has described four psychosocial phases related to the stage, treatment, and progression of cancer: existential plight, accommodation and mitigation, recurrence and relapse, and deterioration and decline.

It would appear obvious that removal of the larynx will have a profound psychological impact, although the effects may differ with respect to the sexes. For the male, amputation is akin to castration, which could be equated to the loss of manhood, as the larynx, next to the penis, represents malehood both symbolically and figuratively. For the female, loss of the larynx could well represent disfigurement and the associated distortion of the persona or self-image. In their study, Weinstein, Vetter, and Sersen (1964) found that women between the ages of twenty and seventy years rated the tongue as their most important organ, but no distinction was made between that and the larynx. We contend that the two would be equivalent, as both organs are integral for purposes of communication in the human species.

Most important in our roles as speech-language pathologists is how we attempt to aid such individuals in coping with their loss and the implications of readjustment. We have referred elsewhere to Tanner's incisive essay on loss and grief as they relate to the communicatively disordered, but he makes only fleeting reference to amputation as an aspect of loss of self (1980). Surprisingly little data are available in the literature surveyed about the mourning process in families where laryngectomy has occurred, but as we shall discuss presently, an explanation is possible.

Several excellent sources are available relative to pre- and postoperative counseling with laryngectomized individuals and their families (among them, Salmon 1979; Reed 1983; and Keith et al. 1977, and Kommers, Sullivan, and Yonkers (1977) view the laryngectomees home environment as a crucial determinant toward maximizing rehabilitation success), but most are essentially information rather than psychodynamically oriented. Providing information is extremely important, however, a proper interpersonal counseling relationship with the patient and the spouse could help resolve many of the problems that arise, particularly postoperatively.

In a retrospective study by Kommers and Sullivan (1979), answers to a comprehensive questionnaire given to forty-five wives of laryngectomized individuals indicated a definite "need for improved family counseling both before and after surgery" (p. 411). Of those wives interviewed, 60 percent reported shock, fear, panic, and denial upon first learning of cancer, and 50 percent noted that their husband's personality or attitude had changed immediately following surgery. They were either depressed or irritable. Although not addressed specifically, the mourning period appeared not to be prolonged. A possible explanation for this may be that with the acquisition of alaryngeal speech, considerable psychological readjustment is likely to occur.

This should not nullify the need for family counseling or family therapy to help the client and spouse work through the myriad of personal, family, and social problems that could ensue. Salazar-Sanchez and Stark (1972) used a crisis intervention model involving a speech pathologist and social worker, applying interventive and preventive strategies with laryngectomized individuals and their families. Ideally, the speech pathologist who is skilled in counseling would be the most appropriate person to assume the major task because of the greatest frequency of professional contact.

In some cases, individual counseling for the laryngectomized patient is recommended despite the fact that alaryngeal speech may not yet be fully established. Fullest use of speech aid is well justified in such cases even if only to be employed temporarily for the purposes of interpersonal communication in therapy as well as at home and socially. (The author's position is that a speech aid should be used whenever alaryngeal speech cannot be attained or as an adjunctive aid for even proficient alaryngeal speakers.) Counseling does not have to be singled out from traditional alaryngeal voice therapy, and as we have suggested all along, should be integrated within the total therapeutic process.

Finally, we should not underestimate the value of New Voice Clubs, which can serve as powerful support groups, for the patients readjusting and reentering into life. Whatever the therapeutic support, either formal or informal, the individual can be helped to find a new meaning in life despite the specter of cancer to which he or she may yet be vulnerable.

PSYCHOTHERAPEUTIC TREATMENT STRATEGIES

It appears appropriate and logical following our previous discussions that a psychotherapeutic approach to the treatment of voice disorders in adults is in order. Perhaps "psychotherapeutic" is not the best word to describe exactly how we can most effectively manage our clients. In essence, we must decide now much of a wholistic practitioner we choose to be. Or we might consider, as Brodnitz (1981) maintains, that in order for us to "normalize" vocal function it is necessary that we "respect the 'Gestalt' of the voice" (p. 24). Most important, however, is our understanding that we as voice therapists are not seeking a change in the client's essential being but only a change in which the client uses the various parts of self to vocalize. As Cooper (1973) has correctly cautioned us: all voice types in one fashion or another represent to the individual a commitment to the cultural norms of the society and/or to the stereotypes the individual has regarding the voice for a given person, position and situation" (p. 50). Thus it appears reasonable, as Cooper suggests, that vocal rehabilitation requires a variable approach with varying emphasis on either the mechanics of production or on what he describes as "vocal psychotherapy."

Because vocal change is our chief objective, much will depend on what we perceive as necessary to change and what our clients deem important to modify. The two may not always be compatible. Can we be certain that we always know best what must be changed, or can we be open to the client's personal perceptions of what can realistically be modified?

As one of the author's graduate students has so aptly put it:

. . . it may be easier for the therapist to see that certain changes can only benefit the client than it is for the client to believe such a thing, let alone to feel it on all conscious and unconscious levels. After all, a major survival activity throughout life is to "get your act together," and if this can be done while being genuine, it is certainly more powerful. But most of us rely on at least a few stopgap measures to help us present to the world what we feel is an acceptable front. This front becomes an armour defending us against the threat of being discovered to be truly what we fear we are. Creating in others a desire to shed that burdensome armour is some of the art that therapists must develop throughout their professional careers. People naturally "compensate" and it takes powerful motivation to make them want to give up that compensation." (TeSelle 1985)

We view voice therapy as a reciprocal arrangement between therapist and client whereby adaptation is made by each to suit the needs of the client as they occur during the therapeutic process. An individual counseling approach appears to be a most appropriate treatment to satisfy these requirements.

Individual Counseling

Counseling, both a therapeutic and an educational process, should be flexible enough to fit the objective reality of the clinical situation and the therapeutic relationship. Consistent with our earlier discussion in this chapter, we make no distinction between identified organicity or lack of it when psychological components are present and obvious. We do not infer that differential assessment should be omitted. On the contrary, it becomes all the more important and significant if we are to consider vocal pathology as part of a total human process.

One further consideration is pertinent to our discussion. We prefer to style our therapeutic approach to the person and not to the particular voice disorder identified. One exception to this rule, however, is the treatment of laryngectomy, which we believe to have unique characteristics so as to require special attention.

Guidelines For Intervention

We have developed several guidelines that, when considered in the context of basic counseling principles covered earlier and elsewhere, can serve to lead us appropriately toward healthier vocal usage for the person. Similarities of therapeutic guidelines for both children and adults obviously overlap, and are intentional. We have chosen as well to integrate whatever symptomatic treatment is necessary within the context of our approach but not to dwell on specifics, as they are covered elsewhere in this and other books on counseling.

1. *The case history process.* The case history may provide us with important data, but more significant is the knowledge gained through the actual interactional dialogue with the client. What is valuable is not what has

happened in the past per se, but how the client perceives what has occurred. Maintaining an open-ended discussion may also give us an immediate visual and acoustical picture of vocal usage, as well as the present feelings and self-image attitude of the client.

2. *The differential assessment.* Also interactional is the means by which we determine the effectiveness or ineffectiveness with which the client vocalizes. We also wish to discover the possible presence, if any, of pronounced organic components that may demand immediate medical attention. We prefer using the vocal analysis profile format of Perkins (1971), who considers the various components of voice as either dependent or independent functions. His discussion of the concept of constriction fits neatly with our encouragement of the client to talk about the stress associated directly or indirectly with his or her vocal usage. The performance of the oral-maxillary facial examination provides an opportunity to stimulate the expression of feelings concerning each element of the procedure. We can thus derive some notions of how our client reacts to various vocal changes that occur and those that do not. Such a process will help set the stage for the course of therapy that is to be determined.

3. *The interpersonal relationship.* As the free flow of communication between the client and the therapist develops, the client is more likely to drop the psychic defenses that may be associated with vocal abuse and misuse. Likewise, it will be easier for both to identify obvious and subtle connections between faulty vocal habits and various emotional components. This interaction also allows the therapist to learn more about the client than would ordinarily be revealed through rigid case history taking and vocal examination.

4. *The uniqueness of the individual.* The therapist needs to maintain a flexible approach that will suit the particular person being treated, and not the identified vocal disorder. For that matter, it is conceivable that one individual with vocal nodules could be more like another individual with nonorganic dysphonia than one with vocal nodules. It is also necessary for the therapist to be attuned to differing client needs, for example, financial necessity for remaining with a dead-end job or a powerful resistance to terminating a destructive and stressful marriage. It is not our role to intercede in even the consideration of such decisions but to assist the client in at least understanding the dilemma, should the issue arise, and perhaps indirectly suggest further counseling assistance. We cannot avoid the problem, however, if it relates directly to vocal management.

5. *Client responsibility.* One of the major goals in voice therapy is to educate clients that they have within themselves the ability to change many if not most of the features that contribute to vocal misuse and abuse. Client resistance to such choice making may be embedded in deep-rooted psychopathology or in needs associated with the maintenance of a particular vocal image. Regardless, we must again avoid taking the position of "rescuer" and facilitate self-direction if permanency of vocal change is to occur.

6. *Vocal personality factors.* Although the relationship between personality characteristics and vocal style is yet unclear, it is the therapist's responsibility to determine, in concert with the client, how the latter perceives self in relationship to personal vocal style. It will then be necessary to determine if the client needs to maintain a particular vocal style in order to enhance a favorable perception of self, especially if the former is faulty. The clinical challenge for change is quite formidable because it may involve a metamorphosis of individual behavior and personality. The reader is referred to a more comprehensive discussion of this issue by Cooper (1973).

7. *Therapeutic congruency.* Most therapists are well aware of voice clients who ostensibly seek help for their voice disorder but who actually have a different agenda unknown to them. Some profess the desire to follow all of the advice their therapist has to offer regarding vocal change. In actuality, though, they may put up barriers to the implementation of such changes. Others immediately ventilate pent-up feelings regarding self-esteem, life struggles, and emotional conflicts. These individuals resist taking too close a look at their problems on a deeper level and simultaneously reject management of the vocal symptoms.

Such seemingly paradoxical attitudes offer a considerable challenge to the therapist, who must now sort out with the client exactly what is actually desired. Although a nondirective counseling approach may be in order, a more direct and gently confrontive aproach could effectively be implemented. The client must be helped to decide what direction to take, with clarity and openness in interpersonal communication being maintained. Irrational and unproductive attitudes need to be exposed and recognized as inhibitors of further progress. Unsurprisingly, some such clients who are able to make this breakthrough carry these new communicative behaviors into personal relationships with significant others in their lives. Whereas dramatic changes in vocal usage may occur for a few, others may still require considerable symptomatic management.

8. *Combining symptomatic with psychotherapeutic management.* We have already implied that no one therapeutic approach is appropriate for every client, and that symptoms cannot readily be distinguished from vocal functioning or human behavior. Thus therapists need to be flexible enough to respond to whatever components arise or are evident in any one moment or extended period of therapy. Also, we must be aware that having our clients do vocal exercises necessitates an understanding of how they are responding psychologically to them. Correspondingly, any positive change in vocal behavior should be viewed in the context of the client's vocal perception of psychological behavior.

Although this overall approach may appear to resemble a potpourri of therapeutic tactics, such is not the case at all. Based on the initial assessment, voice therapy for a particular individual must have short- and long-term objectives, but be amenable to change as new data are discovered during the process. That is, therapy should be diagnostic in nature, responsive to the needs of the client, yet integrated so that both client and therapist are aware of how all elements interact. In this way "elocutionary"-type voice therapy, whereby voice is regarded as a distinct entity separate from the person, can be avoided.

9. *Contracting.* As with voice-disordered children, but perhaps even more so with adults, it is necessary for both client and therapist to be on the same track if a positive outcome is to be realized. That is, voice therapy must be characterized by a process of negotiation whereby each successive step is understood by both parties and appropriately carried out. Any obstacles to continued progress must be analyzed and removed and adjustments in therapy made, if necessary, in order for therapy to succeed.

Contracts between client and therapist will vary in their design, formality, and organization, depending on the particular therapeutic circumstances, nature of the voice disorder, and specific client needs. In most cases, the contract can be a mutually agreed-upon verbal commitment to a series of appropriate therapeutic steps. For others it must be a written commitment to meet the expectations deemed suitable by both client and therapist. Whatever arrangement is made, the contract should not be treated as an end in and of itself but as a viable means to enhance the interpersonal relationship, encourage congruency, and to ensure a positive therapeutic outcome for the client.

10. *Special counseling problems.* There are some aspects to therapy with the voice-disordered person that the therapist must be particularly conscious about. One of them involves touching the client's neck or shoulder, which for some clients could be misinterpreted as a sexual advance. In order to nullify such a perception, the therapist must explain fully the purpose of such touching or physical manipulation and ask the client permission to do so. Obviously, we need to respect the client's wishes if such actions are refused.

Transference and countertransference, if they occur, must be kept in objective perspective and should be discussed openly. Although unlikely to emerge in most cases, instances whereby dramatic positive vocal and personality changes occur may trigger them. Thus any departure from the formal clinical environment to external environments where carryover can be more objectively observed must be considered carefully.

Persistent resistance to the modification of vocal behavior despite full acquiescence by the therapist to the client's wishes must be interpreted to be deeply rooted psychodynamically. If unresolved, the therapist must take steps to recommend gently outside referral to either another therapist or psychotherapist. The therapist well grounded in theory of psychopathology will know best when and how to deal with "difficult" clients.

Some cases as in the management of the transsexual voice (Oates and Dacakis 1983) demand a joint effort between speech pathology and psychiatry, and we must therefore be ready to relinquish part of our therapeutic role in those instances. We need to appreciate the fact that we cannot be all things to all clients and mature enough to admit when we don't know. Admittedly, we may not always clearly recognize our therapeutic limits, but as long as we are vigilant in our own self-analysis while relating to clients we are operating within our ethical boundaries.

CONCLUSION

We have demonstrated that voice disorders in adults, as with voice disorders in children, cannot be separated from the person. In adults, however, the psychodynamic factors are more complex both etiologically and intrinsically to the specific disorder. Our attempt has also been to approach treatment based on the individual uniqueness of the client, and not on the disorder itself. Most important, however, is that we not neglect all of the therapeutic tools we have available to us regardless of our biases. To quote Brodnitz (1981), we need not allow the "products of our gadget-happy times . . . to interfere with the integration of vocal use as a unified function" (p. 25). Yet, at the same time, we have to recognize that even the gadgets have value in our holistic approach to the client.

REFERENCES

ARONSON, A. *Clinical Voice Disorders*. New York: Thieme Stratton, 1980.

ARONSON, A., and DeSANTO, L. Adductor spastic dysphonia: Three years after recurrent laryngeal nerve resection. *Laryngoscope*, 93 (1983), 1–8.

ARONSON, A., and HARTMAN, D. E. Spastic dysphonia as a sign of essential (voice) tremor. *Journal of Speech and Hearing Disorders*, 46 (1981), 52–58.

AXLINE, V. M. *Play Therapy*. New York: Ballantine, 1969.

BAKER, E. L., PLATT, J. A., and FINE, H. J. Tic de gilles de la Tourette: Survey of the literature, case study and reinterpretation. *Clinical Psychology Review*, 3 (1983), 157–178.

BARKER, K. D., and WILSON, F. B. Comparative study of vocal utilization of children with hoarseness and normal voice. Paper presented at the convention of the American Speech and Hearing Association, 1967.

BOONE, D. L. *The Voice and Voice Therapy*, 3rd ed. Englewood Cliffs, N.J.: Prentice-Hall, 1983.

BRIDGER, M. W. M., and EPSTEIN, R. Functional voice disorders: A review of 109 patients. *Journal of Laryngology and Otology*, 97 (1983), 1145–1148.

BRODNITZ, F. S. Psychological considerations in vocal rehabilitation. *Journal of Speech and Hearing Disorders*, 46 (1981), 22–26.

———. Spastic dysphonia. *Annals of Otology, Rhinology and Laryngology*, 85 (1976), 212–213.

CASE, J. L. *Clinical Management of Voice Disorders*. Rockville, Md.: Aspen Systems Corp. 1984.

CHERRY, J., and MARGUILES, S. I. Contact ulcer of the larynx. *Laryngoscope*, 78 (1968).

COOK, J. V., PALASKI, D. J., and HANSON, W. R. A vocal hygiene program for school age children. *Language, Speech and Hearing Services in Schools*, 10 (1979), 21–26.

COOPER, M. *Modern Techniques of Vocal Rehabilitation*. Springfield, Ill.: Chas. C Thomas, 1973.

DEDO, H., and IZDEBSKI, K. Intermediate results of 306 recurrent laryngeal nerve sections for spastic dysphonia. *Laryngoscope*, 93 (1983), 9–16.

DEDO, H., and SHIPP, T. *Spastic Dysphonia*. Houston: College-Hill Press, 1980.

ERIKSON, E. H. *Childhood and Society*, 2nd ed. New York: Norton, 1963.

FONTAINE, A. and MITCHELL, J. C. E. Oesopahgal voice: a factor of readiness. *Journal of Laryngology* 74, 870, 1960.

FORMBY, D. Maternal recognition of infant's cry. *Developmental Medicine Child Neurology*. 9 (1967), 293.

FRIEDMAN, M. and ROSENMAN, R. H. Association of specified overt behavior patterns with blood and cardiovascular findings. *Journal of the American Medical Association* 169 (1959) 1286–1296.

GLASSEL, W. L. A study of personality problems and vocal nodules in children. Paper read at the American Speech and Hearing Association Convention, San Francisco, 1972.

GOODSTEIN, L. D. Functional speech disorders and personality: A survey of the research. *Journal of Speech and Hearing Research*, 1 (1958), 359–376.

GREENE, M. C. L. *The Voice and Its Disorders*, 4th ed. Philadelphia: Lippincott, 1980.

GUTWINSKI-JEGGLE, J. Psychognen dysphonien als beziehungssturungen: Moglichkeiten and Grenzen ihrer logopadischen behendlung (Psychogenic vocal problems as relationship disturbances: Possibilities and limitations for treatment by speech therapy). *Praxis de Psychotherapic and Psychosomatik*, 28 (1983), 43–53.

HEJNA, R. F. *Speech Disorders and Nondirective Therapy*. New York: Ronald Press, 1960.

HINSIE, L. E., and CAMPBELL, R. J. *Psychiatric Dictionary*, 4th ed. New York: Oxford University Press, 1970.

HOLDEN, C. Lie detectors: PSE gains audience despite critics' doubt. *Science*, 190 (1975), 359–362.

IZDEBSKI, K., and DEDO, H. Spastic dysphonia: In J. Darby (Ed.), *Speech Evaluation in Medicine*. New York: Grune & Stratton, 1981.

KAMBIC, V., et al. "Vocal cord polyps: Incidence, histology and pathogenesis. *Journal of Laryngology and Otology*, 95 (1981), 609–618.

KAPLAN, S. L. Mutational falsetto. *Journal of the American Academy of Child Psychiatry*, 21 (1982), 82–85.

KAUFMAN, J. A., and BLALOCK, P. D. Classification and approach to patients with functional voice disorders. *Annals of Otolaryngology and Rhinolaryngology*, 91 (1982), 372–377.

KEITH, R. L., SHANE, H. C., COATES, H. L., and DEVINE, K. D. *Looking Forward: A Guidebook for the Laryngectomee*. Rochester, Minn.: Mayo Foundation, 1977.

KERR, M. E. Family systems theory and therapy. In A. S. Gurman and D. P. Kniskem (Eds.), *Handbook of Family Therapy*. New York: Brunner/Mazel, 1981.

KOMMERS, M. S., and SULLIVAN, M. D. Wives' evaluation of problems related to laryngectomy. *Journal of Communication Disorders*, 12 (1979), 411–430.

KOMMERS, M. S., SULLIVAN, M. D., and YONKERS, A. J. Counseling the laryngectomized patient. *Laryngoscope*, 87 (1977), 1961–1965.

LAGUAITE, J. K. The use of hypnosis with children with deviant voices. *International Journal of Clinical and Experimental Hypnosis*, 24 (1976), 98–104.

LANDES, B. A. Management of hyperfunctional dysphonia and vocal tension. In M. Cooper and M. H. Cooper (Eds.), *Approaches to Vocal Rehabilitation*, Springfield, Ill.: Chas. C. Thomas, 1977.

LOW, G., CRERAR, M., and LASSERS, L. Communication centered therapy. *Journal of Speech and Hearing Disorders*, 24 (1959), 361–368.

LUCHSINGER, R., and ARNOLD, G. E. *Voice-Speech-Language*. Belmont, Calif.: Wadsworth, 1965.

MILLER, S. Q., and MADISON, C. L. Public school voice clinics, part II: Diagnosis and recommendations—A 10-year review. *Language, Speech and Hearing Services in Schools*, 15 (1984), 58–63.

MINUCHIN, S. *Families and Family Therapy*. Cambridge, Mass.: Harvard University Press, 1974.

MONDAY, L. A. Clinical evaluation of functional dysphonia. *Journal of Otolaryngology*, 12 (1983), 307–310.

MOORE, P. Voice disorders. In G. Shames and E. Wiig (Eds.), *Human Communication Disorders: An Introduction*. Columbus, Ohio: Chas. E. Merrill, 1982.

MOSBY, D. P. Psychology versus voice therapy for a child with a deviant voice: A case study. *Perceptual and Motor Skills*, 30 (1970), 887–891.

———. Predominant personality characteristics of 25 children with voice disorders. Paper read at the American Speech and Hearing Association Convention, Chicago, 1967.

MOSES, P. *The Voice of Neurosis*. New York: Grune & Stratton, 1954.

MURPHY, A. T. *Functional Voice Disorders*. Englewood Cliffs, N.J.: Prentice-Hall, 1964.

MURRAY, S. C., CARR, M. E., and JACOBS, V. Functional aphasia in the child and adolescent: Therapeutic management. *Language, Speech and Hearing Services in Schools*, 14 (1983), 260–265.

OATES, J. M., and DACAKIS, G. Speech pathology considerations in the management of transsexualism: A review. *British Journal of Disorders of Communication*, 18 (1983), 139–151.

OSTWALD, P. F. *Soundmaking*. Springfield, Ill.: Chas. C. Thomas, 1963.

PERKINS, W. (Ed.). *Voice Disorders*. New York: Thieme Stratton, 1983.

————. Vocal function: A behavioral analysis. In L. E. Travis (Ed.), *Handbook of Speech Pathology and Audiology*. New York: Appleton-Century-Crofts, 1971.

PHILLIS, J. A. Children's judgments of personality on the basis of voice quality. *Developmental Psychology*, 3 (1970), 411.

QUAN, K. The relationship of voice to personality. Unpublished paper. San Francisco State University, 1985.

RAMMAGE, L. A., NICHOL, H., and MORRISON, M. D. The voice clinic: An interdisciplinary approach. *Journal of Otolaryngology*, 12 (1983), 315–318.

REED, C. G. Surgical-prosthetic techniques for alaryngeal speech. *Communicative Disorders: A Journal for Continuing Education*, 8 (1983), 109–124.

SALAZAR-SANCHEZ, V., and STARK, A. The use of crisis intervention in the rehabilitation of laryngectomees. *Journal of Speech and Hearing Disorders*, 37 (1972), 323–328.

SALMON, S. J. Pre- and post-operative conferences with laryngectomized and their spouses. In R. L. Keith and F. G. Darley (Eds.), *Laryncetomee Rehabilitation*. Houston: College-Hill Press, 1979.

SAPIR, E. Speech as a personality trait. *American Journal of Sociology*, 332 (1927), 892–905.

SAPIR, S., and ARONSON, A. Clinician reliability in rating voice improvement after laryngeal nerve section for spastic dysphonia. *Laryngoscope*, 93 (1985), 200–202.

SCHERER, K. R. Vocal indicator of stress. In J. K. Darby (Ed.), *Speech Evaluation in Psychiatry*. New York: Grune & Stratton, 1981.

————. Speech and Emotional States. In J. K. Darby (Ed.) *Speech Evaluation in Psychiatry*. New York: Grune and Stratton, 1981.

————. Judging personality from voice: A cross-cultural approach to an old issue in interpersonal perception. *Journal of Personality*, 40 (1972), 191–210.

SENTURIA, B., and WILSON, F. Otorhinolaryngic findings in children with voice deviations. *Annals of Otology, Rhinology and Laryngology*, 77 (1968), 1027–1041.

SHERRER, W. M. Diagnosis and treatment of voice disorders in school children. *Journal of Speech and Hearing Disorders* 37 (1972) 215–221.

SHIPP, T. Personal communication, 1985.

SHIPP, T., IZDEBSKI, K., REED, C., and MORRISSEY, P. Intrinsic laryngeal muscle activity in a spastic dysphonia patient. *Journal of Speech and Hearing Disorders*, 50 (1985), 54–59.

SHIPP, T., and MCGLONE, R. E. Physiologic correlates of acoustic correlates of psychological stress. *Journal of the Acoustical Society of America*, (1973), 53–63.

SIEGMAN, A. W. Nonverbal correlates of anxiety and stress. In L. Goldberger and S. Breznitz (Eds.), *Handbook of Stress: Theoretical and Clinical Aspects*, New York: Macmillan, 1982.

SILVERMAN, E. M., and ZIMMER, C. H. Incidence of chronic hoarseness among school-age children. *Journal of Speech and Hearing Disorders*, 40 (1975), 211–215.

SIMONOV, P. V., and FROLOV, M. V. Utilization of human voice for estimation of man's emotional stress and state of attention. *Aerospace Medicine*, 44 (1973), 256–258.

SIMONOV, P. V., FROLOV, M. V., and TALEBKIN, V. L. Use of the invariant method of speech analysis to discern the emotional state of announcers. *Aviation, Space and Environmental Medicine*, 46 (1975), 1014–1016.

STEINHAUER, P. D., and BERMAN, G. Anxiety, neurotic and personality disorders in children. In P. D. Steinhauer and Q. Rae-Grant (Eds.), *Psychological Problems of the Child in the Family*, 2nd ed. New York: Basic Books, 1983.

STOICHEFF, M. L. The present status of adductor spastic dysphonia. *Journal of Otolaryngology*, 12 (1983), 311–314.

TANNER, D. C. Loss and grief: Implications for the speech-language pathologist and audiologist. *Asha*, 22 (1980), 916–928.

TESELLE, N. Voice: Mirror of the soul. Unpublished paper. San Francisco State University, 1985.

TOOHILL, R. J. The psychosomatic aspects of children with vocal nodules. *Archives of Otolaryngology*, 101 (1975), 591–595.

VALANNE, E., VUORENKOSKI, V., PARTANEN, T. J., LIND, J., and WASZ-HÖCKERT, O. The ability of human mothers to identify the hunger cry signals of their own newborn infants during lying-in period. *Experientia*, 23 (1967), 768.

VAN RIPER, C., and EMERICK, L. *Speech Correction: An Introduction to Speech Pathology and Audiology*, 7th ed. Englewood Cliffs, N.J.: Prentice-Hall, 1984.

WALLEN, V., and WEBB, V. A study of background characteristics and traits of laryngectomees. *Military Medicine*, 140 (1975), 532–534.

WARR-LEEPER, G. A., McSHEA, R. S., and Leeper, H. A. The incidence of voice and speech deviations in a middle school population. *Language, Speech and Hearing Services in Schools*, 10 (1979), 14–20.

WASZ-HÖCKERT, O., LIND, J., VUORENKOSKI, V., PARTANEN T. J., and VALANNE, E. The infant cry: A spectrographic and auditory analysis. *Clinics in Developmental Medicine*, 29 Spastics International Medical Publications in Association with Heinsmann Medical, 1968.

WEINSTEIN, S., VETTER, R., and SERSEN, E. Physiological and experiential concomitants of the phantom. VRA Project No. 427, Final Report. New York: Albert Einstein College of Medicine, 1964.

WEISMAN, A. *Coping with Cancer*. New York: McGraw-Hill, 1979.

WEISMAN, A., and WORDEN, J. The existential plight of cancer: Significance of the first 100 days. *International Journal of Psychiatry in Medicine*, 7 (1976–77), 1–15.

WEISS, D. A. The psychological relations to one's own voice. *Folia Phoniatrica*, 7 (1955), 209–217.

WILSON, D. K. *Voice Problems of Children*, 2nd ed. Baltimore: Williams & Wilkins, 1979.

WILSON, F. B., and LAMB, M. M. Comparison of personality characteristics of children with and without vocal nodules on Rorschach protocol interpretation. Paper read at the American Speech and Hearing Association Convention, Atlanta, 1973.

7

PSYCHOLOGICAL CONSIDERATIONS OF SPECIAL CONGENITALLY DISORDERED PEOPLE AND THEIR FAMILIES

Part I: Cleft Palate in Children and Adults

CLEFT PALATE IN CHILDREN

Although cleft lip and palate is only one of a wide variety of craniofacial anomalies, we have chosen it for selective attention because it is the most likely to fall within the province of the working speech-language pathologist. Also it is generally the least severe of the craniofacial deformities physically and the most amenable to reconstructive surgery and habilitative intervention.

The occurrence of cleft lip and palate at birth generally requires the attention of a variety of specialists representing plastic surgery, pediatrics, otology, speech-language pathology, dentistry, audiology, and psychology. Ideally, these professionals act as a team to guide the afflicted child and the family through an oftentimes agonizing series of surgical procedures and feeding, hearing, speech-language, dental and upper respiratory problems.

Because of the interplay of many aspects of development and associated complications, it is uncertain if intelligence falls below the norm in cleft palate children. It is evident that because language generally is more slow to develop and because of the other special problems noted, generalizations about mental development may be difficult to make (McWilliams 1982).

One would expect the psychosocial problems to be a natural concomitant to all of the developmental aspects evident, and that the child's speech and language would either influence or be influenced by psychosocial factors. Let us, therefore, explore this issue.

Psychosocial Correlates

There appears to be no definitive evidence to support the view that cleft palate children are necessarily more emotionally disturbed than other children. Starr (1980) investigated the relationship between facial attractiveness and behavior in forty-nine ten-year old and older cleft lip and palate subjects and found no statistically significant relationships between the attractive and less attractive group. Starr used the six behavioral scores of the Missouri Behavior Problem Checklist to measure ratings of self-esteem and attitudes toward clefting. It was suggested that because of good lip repair, the likelihood of negative ratings by naive judges was contraindicated.

It appears, however, that physical attractiveness can be an important variable in the judgments made by others. Langlois and Stephen (1977), in their study of the effects of physical attractiveness and ethnicity on children's behavioral attributes and peer preferences, found that attractive children were perceived as being smarter and better liked than unattractive children by elementary school age peers. The effects of facial disfigurement on teachers' perception of the intellectual ability in cleft palate children were investigated by Richman (1978), who found that teachers tended to rate children with noticeable disfigurement as less intelligent than those with relatively normal facial appearance.

In a later study, Harper, Richman, and Snider (1980) studied teachers' ratings of school behavior of 124 ten- to eighteen-year-olds with two types of disability with varying degrees of disfigurement. They matched a cleft palate and a cerebral palsy group in terms of sex, age, IQ, grade level, and socioeconomic status. They also used the Missouri Behavior Problem Checklist and found cleft palate subjects to be more impulsive than the cerebral palsy subjects. Those subjects with mild physical impairment in either category demonstrated greater impulse inhibition than more severely impaired subjects. The authors caution us to reserve any definitive conclusions found because of methodological problems of sampling test standardization and teacher bias. The fact that cerebral palsied children, because of their disability, are less likely to act out also has to be considered as a contaminating factor.

Cleft palate children would certainly be more susceptible, one might believe, to the effects of the primary deformity as well as to all of the secondary consequences of the defect. Indeed, some might be emotionally disturbed, but these children are more likely to have been affected by inadequate self-coping behaviors, family responses, poor or delayed medical and nonmedical support, or any combination of the above.

Generally, however, cleft palate children are fortunate to have the advantage of multidiscipline intervention support. This would mitigate against disturbed emotional behavior and in fact would give strong impetus to their overall growth and development. Regardless of these opportunities, however, the child and the family must still endure the reality of the birth defect itself—the often frequent hospitalizations and surgeries, feeding problems, upper respiratory and hearing difficulties, speech and/or language problems, and the sometimes distorted views others have of an infant deformity.

Some mothers and fathers in particular must cope initially with the shock of who they have created. They may find it extremely difficult to admit their unspoken feelings that "you or I or we have created some sort of a monster." These self-or outer-directed recriminations only add to the frustrations these parents have in facing the reality before them. It may well be that the resultant speech or language problems, but not the cleft lip or palate per se, contribute more to adjustment problems. The initial impact of such a birth, however, cannot be ignored.

A greater incidence of mental retardation among cleft palate children has not been borne out by the empirical literature. McWilliams and Smith (1973) have reported that although intelligence may tend toward the lower end of the normal range, it does not appear as a definitive problem. If these children do test lower at the preschool level, as Musgrave, McWilliams and Matthews (1975) have found, it is more likely to be a function of the contaminating influences noted in the Harper-Richmond-Snider study and perhaps of the test instruments themselves.

Family Influences

If the child is to develop any psychosocial adjustment problems, he or she is likely to do so as a manifestation of the way the family responds to and subsequently copes with the initial physical trauma. Drotar et al. (1975) delineate five stages of adaptation by parents to the birth of a child with a deformity. These are not unlike the stages of grief described elsewhere in this text in that they include (1) the initial shock and disbelief; (2) denial; (3) anger; (4) adaptation; and (5) acceptance. How parents successfully move through these stages and what effects they have on the child is dependent on several interrelated factors, including

1. The mental health of individual family members
2. The nature of the marital relationship
3. The ability to cope with stress
4. The quality and degree of the deformity
5. The nature of and degree to which the family receives information about the deformity and its possible sequelae
6. The effectiveness of the habilitation team

Despite our clinical inclination to identify the difficulty with which families respond to the child and the deformity, the research thus far clearly indicates that parents are generally able to cope quite successfully with the many implications and complications associated with the defect itself (Tiza and Gumpertz 1962; Goodstein 1968; McWilliams 1970). Regardless of these generalizations, however, we must take care not to ignore the real concerns, anxieties, and despair presented by individual families. As Lutz (1978) advises, based on his extensive experience with cleft palate families, many are not able to cope without significant counseling assistance from professional members of the team.

Brantley and Clifford (1980) investigated maternal reactions of 200 mothers, 97 of whom had children with cleft lip/palate and 103 who had physically normal children. Using factor analyses in three factors—maternal positive affect, paternal positive affect, and parental anxiety—they found that mothers of physically normal children scored higher in terms of positive affect than mothers of the cleft lip/palate children. These findings must be interpreted cautiously because the parental assessments were retroactive and the mothers' reactions were likely to be projections on their part—that is, reactions related to their own perception of themselves as mothers. The latter reported less positive affect for both themselves and for their spouses. Although there was greater parent anxiety about the future, and although upper-class mothers of the cleft lip/palate children were more negatively affected, the mothers' projected feelings onto the fathers' were more evident when they felt that they were not in control of their own lives. The results are somewhat weakened by the lack of standardization of the assessment scale used.

Among the concerns parents do have, however, as indicated by Weachter (1959) and cited by Goodstein (1968), are (1) the appearance of the child; (2) the efficacy of surgery; (3) the development of speech; (4) spousal reactions; (5) sibling reaction; (6) family of origin; (7) mental development; (8) financial burdens; and (9) the possibility of cleft palate in subsequent children. All of these concerns, we believe, become interwoven within the various stages of adaptation, as outlined earlier, but may be minimized by the way in which families are assisted in gaining knowledge and understanding of the problems of cleft lip and palate.

Counseling The Family

Throughout this book we have insisted that providing information to the family about the nature of the communicative disorder is a fundamental aspect of the counseling process and necessary to the development of the interpersonal therapeutic relationship. It is of no lesser importance in assisting the families of cleft lip and palate children.

Lutz (1978), among others, has clearly described the immediate necessity for providing information about many aspects of the problem. Bradley (1960) questioned forty-three parents of children with cleft palate and found that these parents preferred receiving information and counseling directly from skilled professionals rather than from nonpersonal sources such as visual or auditory materials.

Spriestersbach (1961) delineates several basic concerns that parents felt were most important about which to be knowledgeable. Among them were (1) what they must do as parents; (2) information about surgical intervention; (3) cosmetic and physical aspects of the deformity; (4) prognosis related to survival; (5) understanding their own reactions to the child; (6) concomitant future difficulties; and (7) nature of speech and language problems. Lutz summarizes other important areas about which parents have concern: information about possible hearing impairment, future personality and social adjustment of the child, educational problems, vocational expectations and marriage prospects.

It is obvious that no one member of the professional team could possibly provide all of the answers to these parental concerns. On the other hand, it would make little sense for the parents to be bombarded with information from even a few of these professionals. One solution to this dilemma was found by a professional team of which this author was a member in a large midwestern city.

Serving in the roles of both speech pathologist and counselor, the author had the responsibility of gathering the impressions from other members of the team after the child and parents were initially seen by all. Although the pediatrics member was the first to provide some answers to the family's immediate concerns, the decision to pace the amount of subsequent information to be provided was left with the author. Monthly team assessments afforded families opportunities to raise pertinent issues of concern, thus saving them from professional overloading. If a major concern was related to surgical procedures, the plastic surgeon was available to give more definitive information. If any member of the team felt that the family as a whole was unable to cope, the family was referred to the author for informational counseling and, if needed, adjustment counseling. Rarely did family members report that they were at any time out of touch with the team, and although they sometimes felt overwhelmed by the input of several professional disciplines, welcomed the information that was provided to them.

This author's experiences with more than 150 families of children with cleft lip and/or palate during a period of three years tended to confirm data reported by Goodstein (1968) and others—that although parents of cleft palate children often have anxious concern about their child, their level of adjustment ultimately was not substantially different from that of parents of nonaffected children. Conceivably, the effectiveness of the team of which the author was part could explain the low level of adjustment problems, but there were plenty of instances of parents and families who needed intensive psychotherapeutic counseling. We would hesitate to state, however, that such instances would be any different for 150 families of children with no physical problems.

We cannot minimize the importance of providing families the best that modern habilitation programs have to offer. As Goodstein (1968) notes: ". . . it is important to identify those parents, who because of their own needs can benefit by special counseling help, or who, because of their own psychological inadequacies, are unable to provide emotional support for their children" (p. 208).

The use of family counseling or family therapy as the treatment of choice is not as clearly defined, particularly with very young cleft palate children, as for families of other communicatively disordered. Marital discord that is revealed after the birth of a child with cleft palate is best handled, however, within the context of couple counseling. If adjustment and attitude problems are observed in cleft palate families with other children present, we would prefer a family systems approach. Such an approach would also be beneficial for families in which the cleft palate child has been shielded from the realities of his or her condition and the suppressed feelings of the parents. That the child be able to participate actively in the therapeutic process would be a prime prerequisite.

Ricky L, aged seven, had been born with a bilateral cleft of lip and palate. In a family with two older brothers, Bobby, twelve and Micky, fifteen, Ricky had been through a series of surgical procedures that had required extensive hospitalizations complicated by severe upper respiratory infections and feeding problems.

The parents, Connie and John L, had requested a counseling consultation, ostensibly because they did not feel they could cope with Ricky's responses to the taunts of his peers at school. He was often in tears at school or at home, and Ricky's articulation and schoolwork had regressed. For Connie and John, it was an additional situation to tax their already strained limits.

Although they had had the best of what the modern team approach could offer, Connie and John had not come to terms fully with their years of struggle. After having shielded Ricky from their own unresolved grief and having insulated him from experiences they felt would aggravate his own feelings of vulnerability, they had come to realize that their own attitudes were perhaps exacerbating an already intolerable situation. Because this was an essentially functional family, the parents needed little prodding to face the issues they had concealed for so long—the harsh realities of the earlier struggles and, perhaps more important, the prospects of further cosmetic repairs.

Probably the most positive elements for productive solutions to their difficulties was the support and love they all gave to each other, the above-average intelligence of each family member, Ricky's caring and understanding teachers, a highly competent speech-language pathologist who had been working with Ricky at school, and the continued expert medical care under the supervision of Ricky's pediatrician.

Individual Counseling

A few children with cleft lip and/or palate would probably benefit from individual counseling in conjunction with speech-language therapy, as it is often the speech-language pathologist who has the most professional contact with the child. We do not wish to imply that the child need be emotionally disturbed per se for us to intervene psychotherapeutically. Often just merely the supportive, caring, and accepting attitudes expressed by the therapist may suffice to help any of those children with their associated struggles.

The therapist who has worked with the child who has difficulty in managing appropriate velar-pharyngeal competence, continues to flare the nostrils, or is unable to maintain plosian for /b/, /p/, /t/, /d/, /g/, and /k/ is well aware of the frustration and self-effacement underlying the child's attempts.

The decision to intervene psychotherapeutically will often be dictated by the child's own inclination, albeit subtle, to reveal personal concerns. Further, it would entail the support of the family; and if such intervention is to be carried out in school, it would require a liberal acceptance and approval by the appropriate administrative personnel.

We believe it is possible to weave counseling strategies among the traditional symptomatic procedures commonly employed by speech-language pathologists. Each can be mutually beneficial as long as the technique in and of itself does not become of sole importance. The therapist must be flexible enough to shift strategies in response to the changing needs of the child. Even with the young school-age child, feelings about appearance and lack of intelligibility might interfere with the implementation of speech-language techniques only. Unless these feelings are allowed to surface, they may continue to intrude upon successful resolution of the speech or voice problem.

We are not suggesting that all school-age cleft lip/palate children are necessarily aware of their unintelligibility or for that matter suffering from feelings of inferiority or rejection. As counseling speech-language pathologists, we must refrain from projecting our own sympathetic feelings and attitudes about disfigurement and hypernasal speech and voice on the child, who may be coping quite well with all of the difficulties.

Randy was an intelligent and well-liked ten-year-old who apparently had adjusted satisfactorily to his repaired unilateral cleft of the lip and palate. Although his speech was still characterized by nasal snorts and imprecise articulation, despite having had pharyngeal flap surgery, he nevertheless related well to his peers and performed successfully in school. He took in stride the knowledge that he was to have cosmetic surgery for his lip within three years and in fact looked forward to it, knowing that his appearance would most likely be improved. His supportive and caring family contributed, no doubt, to his feelings of adequacy and competence in all of his endeavors.

Randy's well-meaning school therapist had helped Randy make significant improvement in his intelligibility, and because he appeared to be "so well adjusted" felt safe in probing for possible remaining areas of concern to him. His resistance to her attempts to "counsel" and his desire to "work on my speech" was greeted, fortunately, with undefensive support by her and her realization that she had intruded inappropriately. His therapist was mature enough to acknowledge how much Randy had taught her.

We cite this example not to imply that children like Randy are totally free of any interpersonal difficulties, particularly those surrounding a repaired cleft lip/palate, but to caution that counseling may in many cases be contraindicated. In this case we do not question the counseling competence of the therapist per se but, more important, cite the value of recognizing when and when not to intervene psychotherapeutically.

Probably the greatest value in counseling parents of cleft lip/palate children and/or these children themselves is to help them cope not so much with their own reactions but with the attitudes and reactions of others. Whether expressed or unexpressed, these may present obstacles to the overall adjustment of the family and more specifically to the habilitation of the child. How well counseling is managed early in the child's life will certainly influence his or her passage through adulthood. It is to this period we shall now turn.

CLEFT PALATE IN ADOLESCENTS AND ADULTS

Those of us who work with adults who carry the literal and figurative scars of cleft lip/palate from childhood must first acknowledge that many if not most of them have blended successfully into the mainstream of society in every aspect. This does not mean that they are necessarily immune to the environmental pressures that impinge on all of us but that they have the fortitude to establish a viable place for themselves in their living environment. We need only look to those who have become productive members of the theatrical, helping, business, teaching, and legal professions to confirm our viewpoint.

Our concern here, then, is with those who have fallen between the proverbial cracks and who, because of early ineffectual habilitative management, negative family influences, other environmental factors, or any combination of these, are fixated at the inter- and intrapersonal struggles of their childhood years. Unfortunately, the lack of any substantial experimental research in the area of adolescents and adults with cleft lip/palate forces us to rely only on our own personal clinical experiences and speculative assumptions. Nevertheless, it is important that we value the insights gained from working with our adolescent and adult clients so that our understanding of the problem can enhance all of our subsequent therapeutic efforts.

Psychosocial Correlates

In this author's search of the recent literature, one study stands out as providing us with a clue to a feature that is pertinent to adolescents and adult adjustment—physical appearance and self-esteem. Starr (1982) administered the Physical Attractiveness Scale and Self-Esteem Scale to sixty-seven repaired cleft lip/palate persons age nineteen to thirty-three. Physically attractive subjects tended to rate themselves higher in self-esteem than did subjects who were less attractive. There were no differences between the two groups with regard to sex, educational attainment, or type of cleft. Starr concluded that there is a relationship between self-perception of physical attractiveness and self-esteem. He suggests that the lack of differences with respect to type of cleft could be explained by the effectiveness of plastic surgery to reduce facial disfigurement.

Our difficulty with this study is the assumption implied with the Physical Attractiveness Scale that physical attractiveness is an objectively measured variable. It would have been useful to have had independent judges rate physical attractiveness and compare those measures with the ratings of the cleft lip/palate subjects. But that would not have eliminated the problem of subjectivity. We cannot disregard, however, the importance of cosmetic appearance, which as presented in the media, is the passport to success in all areas of endeavor.

There appears to be no definitive evidence to suggest that adolescents and adults with cleft lip/palate have serious personality and social problems beyond those of a comparable non-cleft lip/palate population. We would need to make a case-by-case study in order to determine the degree to which the "deficit" itself and the attitude developed about it had influenced the personality and social development, as well as other aspects, of the persons's life.

Ralph was a self-referred, unmarried fifty-two-year-old retired postal worker who had been born with a unilateral left complete cleft lip and palate. Repair of the cleft lip and palate had taken place over several operations that began during his first year of life and ended at age twelve. He suffered a concussion at age nine when he was hit by a car. On intake he reported that there was no immediate or lasting effect on his speech and language. He also had open heart surgery when he was forty-three and again at age fifty. He was in speech therapy for most of his elementary and some of his high school years.

His decision to seek out speech therapy at age fifty-two was based on a longtime desire, and he felt now that he had retired he would have the time to do so. Although friends and relatives had told him his speech was acceptable, he felt that his "mushiness' would prevent him from finding a part-time job and expressed fear of not being understood by others. Clinical impressions revealed otherwise as his overall intelligibility approached 100 percent. Although nasal emission and hypernasality were evident, he compensated remarkably well, considering his limited velopharyngeal closure. Formal and informal psychological testing revealed above-normal intelligence but emotional insecurity, anxiety, and attitudes of inferiority and self-effacement. He saw his life as a failure, but after learning of the need to have coronary bypass surgery, decided it was time to make "something more of my life."

On the surface, Ralph appeared to have led a relatively quiet, introspective, and private life, but beneath was revealed a man who had never been able to accept the reality of his cleft lip and palate. He never thought he could do anything vocationally beyond sorting mail and had found this activity excruciatingly boring. He volunteered that his heart condition had been a message to him to live life more fully, and that although he felt that the "cards are still stacked against me" was determined to make whatever changes were necessary.

The profile illustrated by Ralph is representative of the complex psychodynamic factors that probably operate in some adults with cleft lip/palate. Certainly, as professionals, we are unlikely to have the opportunity to intervene with such individuals but should be cognizant that they do exist and recognize the reality of their suffering silence. Some cleft palate adults who ostensibly self-refer for speech therapy are actually crying out for help with their overall adjustment difficulties.

Individual Counseling

Counseling the adolescent or the adult individual with repaired cleft lip/palate is not essentially different from counseling other communicatively impaired individuals. The adult who stutters or who still maintains a deficient language pattern frequently presents the therapist with negative attitudes concerning self-worth and self-images that may be continuing to hamper that person's total life adjustment.

The individual with repaired cleft lip/palate who continues to cope unsuccessfully with listener/observer perceptions of hypernasality, oral-facial deformity, or compensatory facial distortions while speaking obviously requires counseling intervention. There are some individuals, in fact, who may struggle with their self-concept and image, although they may no longer have visual or acoustic features that call attention to the observer. These individuals apparently are still fixed in the same attitudes held at an earlier age, even though speech therapy and corrective surgery have successfully removed all signs of the original conditions.

Most important, then, for the counseling therapist is to attend to the individual's present negative attitude about self regardless of the actual physical reality. Therapists certainly have no control over how people in their clients' environments will respond to them, but cleft lip/palate individuals do have the potential to change their own attitudes toward and perceptions of themselves. It is important to acknowledge, however, situations in which a client may be prevented from job advancement because of a supervisor's unenlightened or personally distorted image of physical differences. Generally, we can do little to alter that person's projections and attitude except perhaps in only special instances. More often we can only help our client either to adjust to the present job situation, try and change it, or move to another job.

Regardless, the client must be helped to understand that he or she is not inferior and that one cannot allow the inferior attitudes of others to restrain oneself from developing the full potential of one's capabilities. After all, many of us throughout our lives are often forced to cope with situations and circumstances that seem terribly unfair, but yet we must refrain from wallowing in our self-pity if we are to effect a more positive resolution for ourselves.

Similarly, adults with cleft lip/palate must learn to separate the physical reality of the deformity from all of the other positive potentials and assets they possess. Too often such individuals burden themselves with all of their perceived liabilities, thereby obscuring all else they may have going for them in their lives. It is a task, however, that demands personal courage and tenacity because attitudes ingrained over many years resist the best of individual and therapeutic efforts.

Although there is little research evidence to support the notion of a "handicapped personality" the cleft lip/palate deformity may serve to stimulate maladjustment, which may in turn be reinforced by others in the afflicted person's environment. We must bear in mind also that the iatrogenic factor, described elsewhere, may be operating as well. As professionals, it is important that we, too, perceive our clients as persons and refrain from conceptualizations with labels. To do otherwise will only distract us from focusing on the necessary elements that will foster positive changes in our clients' attitudes and behaviors.

In addition to the psychological and interpersonal dynamics operating in adolescents and adults with cleft lip/palate are those speech and voice components that continue to interfere with communication. Although the former may appear to be the overriding issue, we must not ignore the importance of employing traditional speech and voice therapy practices to alter distorted articulation patterns and hypernasal voice.

Ralph, whom we described earlier, was able within a period of six months to improve significantly both his articulation and voice to the point where he no longer felt these interfered with his life. Although he had not had speech or voice therapy since junior high school days, his motivation and willingness to practice new patterns helped bring new meaning to his life. In his case, the counseling aspect per se appeared to play a complementary role as he made rapid and continuous progress. He became a better speaker through the interplay of successful compensatory speech and voice skills and the modification of self-effacing and self-defeating attitudes. It appears that although counseling was a contributory factor, speech and voice therapy had intrinsic psychotherapeutic value as well. To have focused merely on altering fixed attitudes would not likely have satisfied all of his goals.

CONCLUSION

Children and adults with repaired cleft lip and palate are a population who, in metropolitan areas, have had the advantage of the full range of habilitative intervention. Unfortunately, this is not the case in many of the rural areas of the United States. We still see children who have received little or only superficial medical, habilitative, and educational attention. They cannot be ignored.

Although research has failed to identify definitive problems of personal maladjustment in the cleft palate population, it has pinpointed the necessity for being cognizant of the possibility of emotional components and interpersonal problems. Although these can significantly affect the overall social, intellectual, cognitive, and communicative development of the individual, counseling alone cannot resolve all of the difficulties this population must face. Only when counseling is used in conjunction with other methods of management can the full potential for any individual with cleft lip/palate be realized.

Part II: Cerebral Palsy in Children and Adults

CEREBRAL PALSY IN CHILDREN

The profound significance of the birth of a child with cerebral palsy is well known. Cerebral palsy represents a wide constellation of neurological features characterized by paralysis, incoordination, weakness, and involuntary athetotic or spastic movements often involving the entire body, along with all of the sensory-perceptual and medical problems.

But even more significant are the severe developmental, social, and psychological implications that typically accompany and complicate the initial neurological state. Lefebvre (1983) reports 60 percent of these children to have defective vision, and 50 percent are said to have borderline or below-average intelligence. (We hesitate to fully accept the intelligence figure because intellectual growth can easily be influenced by any one or a combination of the accompanying deficits.) Lefebvre notes that nearly half of the children born with cerebral palsy are also hearing impaired, communicatively disordered, and dysphagic. Seidel, Chadwick, and Rutter (1975) found cerebral palsied children with normal intelligence to be more vulnerable to psychiatric problems than nondisabled children and those with more extensive brain damage to be three times more vulnerable to psychiatric illness. Rutter, Graham, and Yule (1970), in a carefully controlled study, found that although environmental factors such as the parents' reactions to the disability had some influence, the neurophysiological impact was much greater and revealed a distinctive primary neuropsychiatric effect.

Most important to our present discussion, however, is the recognition of the devastating and overwhelming impact, either directly or indirectly, of this complex syndrome on the emotional growth of the child. We need also to understand how the child's emotional responses may affect the condition itself. This is determined greatly by how the family and social milieu impinge on the child. As suggested by Buscaglia (1975), the person who is disabled will be influenced by society to "... limit his actions, change his feelings about himself, as well as affect his interaction with others. The degree to which he is influenced will depend upon the strength, duration and nature of the judgmental stimulus" (p. 15)—and we would add, the quality and consistency of habilitative intervention.

As speech-language pathologists, we have a very special role to play, as it is only through communication, be it verbal, nonverbal, or augmentive, that the disabled individual can begin to establish the personal relationships necessary for continued growth and, indeed, survival.

Psychosocial Correlates

Surprisingly, there is not much literature on the adjustment problems and personality factors of the cerebral palsied child, perhaps because of the overriding concern by most caregivers for the child's other seemingly insurmountable handicaps.

Sigelman, Vengroff, and Spanhel (1984) performed a Life-Function Analysis on fourteen major impaired populations. Through a comprehensive literature search they gathered statements concerning limitations in functioning related to the fourteen conditions of impairment. Among the 1222 statements of limitation found for cerebral palsy, the following percentages for each of the major life functions were determined: mobility, 44 percent; communication, 30 percent; health, 14 percent; social-attitudinal, 6 percent; and cognitive-intellectual, 6 percent. Interestingly, among all fourteen major impairment groups, social-attitudinal statements were represented least in the literature surveyed in cerebral palsy, whereas communication problems were among the most frequent. Thus is we add social-attitudinal statements to communication statements, together they represent more than a third of all statements made about cerebral palsy.

The results of the Sigelman-Vengroff-Spanhel study should be viewed cautiously in that their findings are based on literature covering all age groups with cerebral palsy and, further, may represent more the academic interest of the writers rather than of the actual reality of the cerebral palsied person. Nonetheless, we cannot ignore the major concern about combined social-attitudinal communication factors.

Richardson (1969) insists that cerebral palsy cannot be defined in a unitary fashion. Impairment in motor functioning will affect and also be affected by sensory, behavioral, intellectual, and social elements. Because of these children's physiological limitations, they are hindered from participating in the active process of socialization. Thus the stage may be set for further alienation and negative reactions to their disability.

Gardner (1973) has described the profound psychological and physical frustrations of these children, particularly when at birth they are unable to have a normal interaction with their parents. Deprived of a satisfactory interaction, they develop feelings of low self-esteem and evolve into a social world with which they feel little relationhip. The range of reaction may extend from extreme rage to a self-imposed exile to an alienating world. Recognizing early that they are abnormal, they consider that their physically impaired body is perceived by others in terms of rejection.

Shontz (1984) has advanced contradictory propositions that, (1) the "psychological reactions to the onset or imposition of physical disability are not uniformly disturbing or distressing and do not necessarily result in maladjustment" and that (2) "reactions (favorable or unfavorable) to disabilities are not related in a simple way to the physical properties of the disabilities" (p. 128). He reports little systematic evidence to support the notion that psychiatric disturbance occurs any more frequently within the disabled population than within the population in general. Also lacking, according to Shontz, are any definitive studies relating degree of physical disability to personality. Among the four affirmative propositions put forth, Shontz suggests that there is no simple cause-effect relationship between the actual physical disability and a predictable adjustment reaction. He also suggests that environmental influences and the perceptions of others will have as great an effect upon the psychological reactions of the disabled person as that person's own internal perception. It is the interaction of these two major perceptions that must therefore demand our attention.

Perhaps the most controversial of Shontz's propositions is that the disability itself is only one factor affecting the individual's total life situation and that it may be minor relative to other influences. He goes on to suggest it is possible that "when a disability opens up opportunities for learning, challenges the persons to achieve successfully, in short promotes ego growth, it is a source of growth and ultimate maturity" (p. 130).

In the light of Shontz's constructs we must be cautious not to over-interpret, because he refers to physical disability in general. Certainly, the implications for other forms of disability discussed elsewhere in our text and for cerebral palsy must be considered. Shontz, in fact, stresses the importance of viewing and understanding the physically disabled person as a unique individual in the light of that person's particular life context.

Family Influences

It is obvious that the earliest familial reaction to the birth of a cerebral palsied child involves the response of the parents to the child. In a study involving thirty pairs of twins, one of which had cerebral palsy, Shere (1957) found that social and emotional maladjustment was not directly caused by the cerebral palsy itself but that the child's aberrant behavior pattern was related to the parental response to and attitude toward the child. Such findings appear to receive support in the postulates put forth by Shontz.

Unfortunately, there appear to be few definitive studies about the mother–child interaction immediately following birth or in the infant's early stages of life. No mother, even one who has successfully reared previous children, is prepared to cope with a child who has difficulty sucking, feeding, and swallowing. Not only must she deal with these problems but she must cope with the child's overall bodily reflexive patterns, which are foreign to her. Richardson (1969) discusses the parents' preoccupation with the child's overall bodily appearance and function, which becomes intensified the more the focus is on the child. This may be the parents' way of attempting to cope with the situation or perhaps to convince themselves of the actual reality.

In chapter 5 we discussed the significance of the complex interpersonal relationship in the development of speech and language and socialization in the normal child. Because the mechanisms of feeding and sucking are related to the earliest vocal cries of the infant, and because the mother may never become proficient in feeding her cerebral palsied child, there is some reason to believe that normal speech and language will be hindered. A further confounding influence may be the mother's or father's negative responses, either covert or overt, to the child's behaviors, as has been suggested by Shere and Kastenbaum (1966). Contributing to the disruption in the developmental process are the hospitalizations for complicated illnesses, resulting in separation from the mother and father.

Support systems for parents of cerebral palsied children are not always adequate for several reasons. Medical necessities often preclude attention to family adjustment reactions. Friends and extended family members not living in the home frequently distance themselves from the "birth tragedy," projecting their own fears and unresolved conflicts concerning life's traumatic events or physical disabilities. Thus the family is left to cope in whatever way is possible. A strong marital bond would certainly have a very positive influence on the overall adjustment process, which in turn would contribute to the child's overall well-being. A weak marital bond could, on the other hand, be fraught with reciprocal recrimination and blame, adversely affecting directly and indirectly the child's development.

The stress created by the birth of a cerebral palsied child can be better tolerated by a family that is essentially functional—that is, one in which all present members have established a sense of their own individual identities and, in Maslow's words, have "self-actualized." They are individuals who, in Hill's description (1958), can cope with the crisis by temporarily limiting their own personal ambitions and working cooperatively to develop positive goals.

In being able to separate themselves from the child, they are better able to see their child as a unique person who, although requiring considerable special attention from them, has the potential to achieve some degree of independence. They are able to relate to the child without overprotecting him or her, thereby reducing the common likelihood of helplessness and dependency. This is not to suggest that the child will not suffer the "slings and arrows of outrageous misfortune." All of the unselfish caring, love, and concern for the child will not alleviate the ever-present multihandicapping nature of the disability, but they can help to prevent many of the secondary disabling effects of poor physical and mental adjustment patterns. Most important is that a functional family can inspire the autonomous development and creative potential of the child, notwithstanding the permanent disabling features.

In terms of family systems theory, the cerebral palsied child should not become the identified symptom to represent a family pattern of conflict avoidance. In dysfunctional families, and inordinate amount of attention devoted to the child can be used as an excuse by the parents to avoid quality time with each other and allow the family energy to be dissipated. As Versluys (1984) has pointed out, although secondary gains for the patient such as attention, love, and care, may be apparent, the child is also, unfortunately, taught avoidance of responsibility and dependency. In this way the child gains an inordinate amount of power over the family.

Whatever speech and language difficulties directly related to the initial disability are present, these may be readily exacerbated by the ever-present dysfunctional family process, as we have discussed in Chapter 5, on language disorders.

Featherstone (1980) offers a complete description of marital stress resulting from sadness, anger, fear, and fatigue. She describes both the undermining and the strengthening of faith in the marital union that can occur as a result of the stress experienced. The disabled child can thus threaten the fabric of even the relatively solid marriage, by provoking powerful feelings, by representing the uneasy symbol of shared failure, by requiring changes in the family structure or system, and by fostering the basis for ongoing conflict.

Probably the most profound effect on the child and the overall family system are the grief reactions experienced in particular by the mother and father. Among the many theories advocated to explain the shock, disbelief, and denial of parents faced with the crisis of having a disabled child, Solnit and Stark (1961) advance the idea that the mother is mourning the loss of the expected healthy child and realizes the fear of having a damaged child. For mothers experiencing guilt, sorrow, mourning, anger, and apprehension, the warm nurturing relationship with the child may be disrupted or perhaps never initiated.

Because we have already described the mourning process elsewhere in the text, we need not repeat ourselves here except to suggest that the denial stage may have the most intense influence. Denial in and of itself should not be viewed negatively, however, because, as we have seen, it may serve to aid the family in coping with their new reality and in time help propel them to a more productive stage. Only when the disability, regardless of its severity, is seen as a family and not an individual dilemma can family members begin the process of adaptation and growth. Positive parental self-perception as well as positive perception of the child will undoubtedly enhance the child's own self-perception and in turn contribute to the future well-being of all.

Counseling the Family

Previously we discussed the importance and significance of providing the family information about the nature of disabling events that, among other results, affects the communicative functioning of the individual. The birth of a cerebral palsied child demands no less.

Typically, it is the pediatrician or the neurologist whose task it is to explain the nature of the child's disability and the profundity of its implications. Such a responsibility places a great burden on the physician, who is generally looked up to as the expert who will be able to predict the ultimate outcome of such a devastating event. Naturally, too many intrinsic and extrinsic factors make such a determination impossible, yet the family, particularly the parents of the child, are justified in expecting some explanation. Either callous, unfeeling, and glib input or unrealistic, overoptimistic, and vague explications are equally ineffectual in satisfying the immediate concerns of the parents. What they want and need is the caring, understanding, and honest support of their physician who is willing to listen and also to answer as many of their concerns as is professionally and humanly possible. Physicians need not burden themselves with perpetuating their "deity" image and can do themselves and the parents a great favor by referral to appropriate counseling professionals.

Mitchell (1981), who studied 152 families in New Zealand, drew up a composite statement based on their major concerns:

> As the parents of a handicapped child we want all those various professionals who deal with us to treat us with openness, honesty and sensitivity. While the pressures of a handicapped child in our family is never easy to come to terms with, please recognize that we have good support from our family and friends and that we are not emotionally incapacitated by our problems. Some of us, however, do need counseling, especially when we first find out about our child. Meeting other parents helps us to adjust, so please put us in touch with each other.
> Above all, perhaps, what we want is information—up to date information on

how we can help our child. Information on the services that are available to us, and information on the benefits to which we are entitled.

The professionals we find most helpful are those who see us often and offer us practical advice. Although we may find some problems in attending parent training courses, don't underestimate our willingness to take part—especially if they are based in our local community and provide us with ideas relevant to our child.

When it comes to school, please remember that we would like our child to attend a regular school—provided special help is available.

Finally we are articulate parents. Not all of us are able or willing to share our concerns with others. Some of us feel that we have a long-term problem that other people don't really understand. (pp. 65–66)

Most provocative about Mitchell's statement is that it reminds the professional that parents of cerebral palsied children can be remarkably resilient in their period of crisis and stress and that as long as they know that some support is forthcoming they and their children not only can survive but thrive.

Although the cerebral palsied child is a family issue, we support the contention made by Thurer (1984) that it is also a "woman's issue." As Thurer states in her provocative essay about the mothers of these children:

These women often struggle with a relentless grind of caring for an individual who may require feeding, dressing, toileting, frequent medical supervision, and constant supervision. Of course men may be involved in these tasks, but typically it is the female parent who is in charge of vigilantly overseeing the child's care. Sometimes these mothers have no respite. (p. 293)

Family counseling can be most effective when it also focuses on the issues that relate directly to the feelings and attitudes of the caregivers as well as the practical problems with which they must cope. They include the following:

1. Assisting the parents in working through their grief reaction, feelings of anxiety, guilt, depression, and hopelessness. Support must be given for their own psychological needs and their communication and parenting skills. It includes helping them to recognize that their feelings are normal and acceptable.
2. Enhancing their self-esteem in order to help them feel that they have control over their lives and in assisting them to become more assertive in their interaction with professionals.
3. Concentrating on strategies to assist their involvement in the education and treatment of their child and in establishing goals that are consistent with the child's potential as well as with their own family values and expectations.
4. Helping the parents to cope with unexpected stressful or crisis situations involving the child, such as serious illness and hospitalization, orthopedic surgery, or behavior problems.
5. Assisting the parents in dealing with their own marital relationship, particularly when it is being affected either directly or indirectly by the child.

Family counseling is not necessarily the only method of choice and may in fact be more productive when combined with parent support groups. The latter can serve to alleviate the family isolation and remind the parents that they are not alone in their struggles. In addition, families can give aid and comfort to each other, sharing their common problems. It is not unusual for such families to discover their own strategies and management procedures. Even the most expert professional cannot possible know all that would benefit the family. The common sharing of even the most minute details of daily problems and of "things that work" can add immeasurably to the overall functioning and adjustment of the family.

Although family therapy as a treatment choice for the cerebral palsy family has received scant attention in the literature, it may be most appropriate for those families with nonhandicapped siblings. Even so, families with no siblings would also benefit from a therapeutic approach that includes the participation of the parents and the child. We believe it is extremely important for the child to feel a vital part of the family regardless of the verbal communication deficit and physical disability. Although active participation may be negligible, the child nonetheless has the opportunity to communicate nonverbally; heretofore, that may have been inappropriate or impossible. Family therapy may in fact be the most effective means of encouraging "individuation" in all family members, particularly the child, as described variously by Minuchin, Jung, and others. We would define *individuation* as a life process in which the individual moves toward establishing a sense of personal uniqueness, distinction, and individuality apart from others. For the cerebral palsied child, it also means the growing self-concept of feeling important in and having a role in life.

Individual Counseling

Whereas counseling procedures for children described elsewhere in this book may be applicable to cerebral palsied children, the special physical and emotional circumstances of these children demand a somewhat modified approach. Too often these children are ignored psychotherapeutically, with emphasis being directed at the educational and therapeutic aspects of habilitation. Although educational and therapeutic approaches contain strands of psychotherapeutic elements, we believe it is important to identify the latter and maximize their use either independently or in conjunction with other strategies.

We have seen how play therapy can be used to facilitate speech and language development as well as enhance the emotional and interpersonal development of the child. For the cerebral palsied child, it is an opportunity to explore physically in the prone or sitting-up position the immediate environment, unencumbered by the restrictions of a wheelchair. It allows the child to develop physical, communicative, and educational skills by providing an opportunity to modify that environment. Such a process is consistent with the goals of the physical therapist, who, according to Anthony (1980), is concerned with restructuring the child's impaired skills, teaching new physical skills, and modifying the immediate environment to conform more appropriately to the child's level of physical skill. Most important, we believe, is the opportunity for the child to develop a sense of autonomy, personal integrity, and physical control (within limits, of course). The speech-language pathologist who is skilled in the use of speech-related physical therapy techniques advocated by Bobath and Bobath (1972) or Rood (cited by Gillette 1969) can add further to the child's overall development.

We recognize that cerebral palsied children who manifest the most severe features of their athetotic, spastic, rigid, or ataxic involvement would be hampered in their quest for physical control. We maintain, however, that speech-language pathologists can adjust their strategies to conform to the physical realities of their young clients and yet enhance whatever potential does exist. Again, it may be that the nature of the interpersonal relationship itself, regardless of severe physical disability, or even treatment mode, is perhaps one of the more crucial elements in fostering positive changes in most aspects of the child's development.

Speech-language pathologists can be successful only insofar as they have the support and can operate in conjunction with the parents, psychiatrist, physical therapist, psychologist, or rehabilitation counselor, among others. To function otherwise in the capacity we advocate could breach the boundaries of our ethical and professional responsibilities. Yet it is nonetheless important for us to be and feel secure in our request for cooperation and remain steadfast in our therapeutic convictions.

We need to recognize these same considerations in counseling with the older cerebral palsied child. Regardless of mainstreaming in the classroom, speech-language pathologists in the schools are often given the major responsibility for responding not only to the speech-language needs but to the psychosocial needs as well. In fact, it is not unusual for the latter to be part of the child's IEP (Individual Educational Plan). How responsive the speech-language pathologist must be to these needs is perhaps a moot question, as cerebral palsied children may make little distinction in the material they wish to share or in the behaviors they manifest in speech-language therapy. What is important is that the therapist be prepared to cope with whatever emerges. To focus on the child's speech and language needs only while the child is expressing other needs as well would be to invalidate the child's most crucial concerns. After all, there may be no other professional who is so often available to respond holistically to the child.

The challenge, as we see it, is to be as totally responsive to the child as possible while not abrogating our major responsibility as agents of communicative habilitation. We believe it is possible to integrate our traditional strategies with counseling strategies in such a way that the child's overriding needs, namely, interpersonal communication and adjustment, are met.

One important way to accomplish this is to bring the child to a certain degree of body relaxation through inhibition of reflex activity and normalization of body tone, as advocated by the Bobaths. The resistance techniques of brushing and icing as advocated by Rood or the use of progressive relaxation techniques may not only facilitate more intelligible articulation but also help to alleviate exacerbated body tension brought on secondarily by anxiety and psychological stressors. For extensive discussion of these and other techniques, the reader is referred to the writings of Payton, Hirt, and Newton (1977). Our major concern is that these physically manipulative exercises are carried out not in terms of doing something *to* the child but in terms of doing something *with* the child. Implicit, then, is the development of a therapeutic relationship involving mutual trust, empathy, critical listening, and nonjudging that we have described elsewhere. Such an approach encourages the child to devleop a greater degree of personal control while extending the limits of the physical disability.

Providing opportunities for the child to express personal concerns about and reactions to perceptions of him or her by others in the child's immediate environment could well be conducive to removing some of the barriers to more effective personal and interpersonal communication.

If we are to be significant caregivers in the cerebral palsied child's life, it is our responsibility to help alleviate the inner turmoil and suffering borne by such a child. If, on the other hand, we believe that we cannot assume such a role, then it behooves us to help obtain the assistance needed by the child.

CEREBRAL PALSY IN ADOLESCENTS AND ADULTS

The plight of the cerebral palsied adult attempting to become part of the mainstream, although significantly reduced, has not yet been fully acknowledged and dealt with even during this enlightened period of the 1980s. Unlike the assistance provided when they were younger, adults often do not have the benefit of professional assistance to aid them in developing the social skills and opportunities to relate successfully with nondisabled or even with other disabled persons in their environment.

Livneh (1984), based on a comprehensive review of the literature on the origins of negative attitudes toward people with disabilities, has developed a classification system that encompasses several sources of these attitudes. We shall outline them here, but, we recommend that the reader refer to the Livneh article and the extensive list of references cited for more definitive discussion.

There are twelve major categories, which we summarize as follows:

1. Negative attitudes, based on social and cultural conditioning and expectations, toward disabled individuals
2. The effects of early childhood influences on the development of adult stereotypic attitudes and standards

3. Complex psychodynamic systems that are responsible for creating unrealistic expectations and conflicts when relating to disabled persons
4. The igniting of unconscious anxiety in the nondisabled person, as the result of perceiving the disability as God's punishment for committing sin or as an excuse for committing a future evil act
5. Confusion and anxiety in nondisabled persons, brought about by being unprepared for the unstructured social, emotional, and intellectual relationship with the disabled person
6. The development of negative attitudes exemplified by a fundamental aesthetic-sexual antipathy toward visible disfigurement
7. The threat to the nondisabled person's own conscious and unconscious body image or concept kindled by the presence of the physically disabled person
8. The stereotypic and inferior status associated with being part of a minority group, thereby triggering discrimination and prejudice in the nondisabled person
9. The anxiety associated with death is identified with disability, thereby reminding the nondisabled person of his or her transient existence
10. Discriminatory practices against the disabled person as a result of prejudice-provoking behaviors, such as being dependent, fearful, and insecure
11. Specific negative attitudes are related to the visibility, severity, and functional ability of the disabled person
12. Negative attitudes are fostered by such demographic factors as sex, age, socioeconomic status, and educational level, as well as personality-connected factors in the nondisabled person, such as ethnocentrism, authoritarianism, self-concept, aggression, ego strength, and degree of self-insight

Psychosocial Correlates

Thus it is not unusual for cerebral palsied children to progress into adulthood, with continuing difficulties in their overall communicative functioning, as well as with problems of social-emotional adjustment, as long as negative attitudes toward them prevail. Among the more profound problems for these disabled adults are those of sexual dysfunction and adjustment and the relationship of these factors to self-concept. Although it would be inappropriate to discuss this issue at length, the reader is referred to more extensive coverage by Diamond and others (1984) and in the quarterly journal *Sexuality and Disabiity* published by Human Sciences Press in New York City.

Regardless of even the most diligent habilitative efforts earlier in their lives, the cerebral palsied adult continues in the struggle with problems of self-identity, body image, and feelings of inadequacy, frustration, and resentment. The limits of their tolerance are often taxed to the extreme in their attempts to become independent and self-sufficient—and many do, despite all of the socioeconomic barriers they still must confront.

We have said before that the personalities of individuals with cerebral palsy do not differ from the personalities of nondisabled individuals except for the consequences of the family system of which they are part. Should the individual have been overprotected by the parents as a child, it might be difficult for that individual, as an adult, to practice independence and self-sufficiency. Yet it is also conceivable for the individual reared in such a manner to respond conversely, that is to strive desperately for independent action and to be convinced of becoming self-sufficient.

Some cerebral palsied adults have been reared in families in which the disability had been denied and where, as a child, the individual was expected not only to learn self-sufficiency but also required to take on responsibilities unrealistic for even a nondisabled child.

Seth was such a child. From the earliest age, his father refused to accept the reality of his son's combined athetotic and spastic physical involvement. He could not tolerate having a son, an only one at that, who would not be able to do everything a nondisabled child could do. Seth's mother, a passive, morose, and often sickly person, could do little directly to counter her husband's dominating and dictatorial attitudes and actions. Seth's ambulatory ability was all the more reason for his father to exact from him complete obedience and to expect him not only to care for himself at the earliest age but to take on major household chores. Tearful protestations were met with physical and mental abuse characterized by strap whippings and ridicule about his "laziness."

School was a welcome respite for Seth, who was bright and, although severely dysarthric, was highly communicative and ingratiated himself with his teachers and a succession of school speech-language pathologists. His thirst for learning was unquenchable but he resented his father's authoritarian control over when to study and how much to study. Performance of the necessary household chores had to come first, always.

Family vacations, which generally consisted of long backpacking treks in the Sierra Mountains of California, offered Seth little relief from the demands of his father, who expected him to be able to keep up with the pace of his parents. Torturous as these physical exertions were for him, Seth, despite his quadraparesis, rarely protested but deeply resented his father's demands. His mother, because of her own physical malaise, never accompanied them.

At fifteen years of age, Seth was also expected to work after school and during weekends in order, in his father's words, to "pay for his own keep" and help support the family. (It should be noted that Seth's father was a gainfully employed commercial artist who earned a salary sufficient to support the family.) Seth's life was essentially prioritized in the following order: go to school; clean the house; do two hours of homework every weekday; and work at least sixteen hours a week. Whatever little time remained for play and recreation was spent breaking into car lots at night, hot wiring the cars, and driving them around. These were often solitary ventures because Seth had few friends to join him in his nightly escapades.

Upon graduation from high school, Seth left home to take a one-room flat and continued to work part-time while he attended a junior college. His meager earnings and social security payments, although barely enough to help support him, were sufficient to help him sustain his independence. The once weekly dinner visits to his parents soon ceased because he no longer wanted to wash all of the dinner dishes as condition for invitation to dinner.

Seth, having no friends and no essential support system to help give him guidance for the future, felt generally lonely and found solace only in caring for younger wheelchair-confined cerebral palsied children while ingratiating himself with their parents. In a very real sense he was soon treated as a member of the family without the demands previously made upon him by his own family.

One with which he was particularly close moved to a small rural community, which gave Seth the impetus to move there as well, since the city in which he had lived offered little for him. By now Seth was twenty-one years of age and obtained part-time employment in a plumbing supply business while continuing to attend a junior college. He soon entered into a homosexual relationship with his fifteen-year-old friend, apparently with the knowledge of the child's single parent.

Troubled by guilt, confusion, and uncertainty about his life, he sought psychotherapeutic assistance by a clinical psychologist to whom he revealed the extent of his homosexual relationship and his personal torment. Bound by what he perceived as an infringement of state law concerning sexual encounters with minors, the clinical psychologist reported Seth to legal authorities, who quickly arrested him. Despite the protestations of the child's mother and her son, Seth was forbidden to see either her or the child again and ordered to participate in group therapy sessions with abusive parents.

Initially, Seth felt alienated from the group and resentful that he was being perceived as a child molester, but because of a compassionate and understanding group therapist, Seth became an active participant in the group. He finally found a forum in which he could share himself and at the same time receive the support for which he had hungered all of his life. As Seth noted in a personal communication with the author: "They're the first people in my life who really understand what I must go through being palsied."

This anecdote is a poignant illustration of the dilemma in which some cerebral palsied individuals might find themselves. While not totally physically incapacitated, Seth strove to enter the mainstream of life of the non-disabled but found rejection or little support. Conversely, neither could he identify fully with those who were more severely disabled, except as a caregiver or protector. Ironically, he was labeled a child molester instead. Sexually rebuffed by nondisabled women and unable to establish relationships with women who were more physically disabled than he, few options remained open to him.

His own father's dogmatic, authoritarian, and excessive expectations must certainly be considered an influential factor in Seth's overall psychosocial development. Though one might argue that by such parenting, Seth learned independence at an early age, we would add, but at what cost?

Obviously, any expression of his own free will was stifled early by an abusive father who could never accept Seth's disability. Such denial contributed further to his inability to establish his own self-identity and was a factor in preventing him from belonging anywhere. In perpetual desperation Seth reached out to those to whom he felt he would be accepted, with little consciousness of his actions.

Seth's legal punishment for the "crime" he committed might be questioned by many of us, and although he appeared to derive substantial rewards from the group therapy experience, it raises serious ethical, legal, and moral issues about society's understanding and treatment of the cerebral palsied adult.

Individual Counseling

Too frequently, as in the case of Seth, cerebral palsied persons also fall within the proverbial cracks of the best intentioned habilitative programs. Seth had never received any substantial counseling except by his last high school speech pathologist, who was skilled in psychotherapeutic management and who had the support of her special education supervisor. Unfortunately, her contact with Seth was too brief and limited to help him make substantial changes in his attitudes and behavior.

We need not reiterate the counseling methods and techniques already discussed throughout this book, as many of those would be applicable with the cerebral palsied adult. We believe that particular emphasis must be given, however, to the person's conceptual body and communicative behavior image, vocational adjustment and stability and overall role in society.

Shontz (1970) has revealed the profound effects of the disabled individual's denial of deep-rooted feelings concerning the self in relation to body image. Because our perception of how we communicate is intrinsic to our overall concept of self, it is necessary for the counseling therapist to encourage the client gently to identify objectively both the acoustical and physical reality. Assuming that a trusting interpersonal relationship has been established, the client is more likely to be willing and motivated to explore ways in which communicative behavior can be improved or enhanced and the physical involvement that can be best adapted to daily functioning. To ignore the latter would, in our opinion, detract from maximizing the potential of the former, as communication is a manifestation of the totality of the individual. We would further emphasize that direct work on the dysarthria and dysarthrophonia will help develop a more positive body image attitude.

Kolb and Woldt (1976) recommend Gestalt counseling techniques in which fantasy and psychodrama are used to help the individual attend to parts of the body where sensation in blocked. They also believe that the disabled individual can best enhance interpersonal relationships through mutual body exploration with another individual in order to communicate on a purely sensory level.

Frequently, the fostering of extreme dependency in childhood will result in a lack of motivation and sense of alienation in adulthood, according to McDowell, Coven, and Eash (1984). They cite numerous references in the literature to support their contention. We have seen in the case of Seth, however, that forcing independence can have similar effects. We must refrain, then, from making rigid generalizations in our predictions of future outcomes, as each individual responds differently to early parenting influences. It is possible that Seth, for one, actually hungered for dependency precisely because he was *denied* opportunities for it in childhood. It appears to us that Seth needed to have early nurturing, loving, and caring, which would have allowed for some degree of dependency at first, and then gradually weaned in the direction of total independence.

Counseling should include the following toward helping the individual:

1. Establish realistic goals personally and vocationally in response to the present reality and ways in which the individual may effect changes in the environment to facilitate those goals.
2. Help the individual to formulate his or her sexual identity consistent with who that person *is* regardless of the physical disability and to explore ways in which positive relationships may be developed with others.
3. Help the individual to recognize and confront the many obstacles society has placed in front of cerebral palsied persons and ways in which these barriers may be circumvented. Awareness of the few positive changes society has made to ease the burdens of the handicapped person should also be brought to light.
4. Help the individual to discover the personal meaning of his or her life with due consideration to the positive role that may be played in relationship to the rest of society, and how changes on the latter may be effected.

CONCLUSION

We have only touched the surface of the complex psychodynamics operating in cerebral palsied individuals and of the counseling intervention that may facilitate positive change and growth. We do not wish to imply that the speech-language pathologist should necessarily be assigned or expected to assume the major role in such an intercession, but we do believe that it may be difficult to make the separation between the speech disorder itself and its effects on the individual. For this reason we must be prepared to function appropriately according to the reality with which we are confronted.

One final note that demands reiteration is the recognition that cerebral palsied persons are not characterized by distinctive psychological types. The family serves as the major source for our investigating the direction and quality of the developing personality and growth pattern. But only through the aid of ongoing interdisciplinary management can cerebral palsied persons find their proper place in society.

REFERENCES

ANTHONY, W. A. A rehabilitation model for rehabilitating the psychiatrically disabled. *Rehabilitation Counseling Bulletin*, 24 (1980), 6−21.

BOBATH, K., and BOBATH, B. Cerebral palsy, Pt. I: Diagnosis and assessment of cerebral palsy; Pt. II: The neuro-developmental approach to treatment. In P. H. Pearson and C. E. Williams (Eds.), *Physical Therapy Services in the Developmental Disabilities*. Springfield, Ill.: Chas. C Thomas, 1972.

BRADLEY, D. P. A study of parental counseling regarding cleft palate problems. *Cleft Palate Bulletin*, 10, (1960) 71−72.

BRANTLEY, H. T., and CLIFFORD, E. When my child was born: Maternal reactions to the birth of a child. *Journal of Personality Assessment*, 44 (1980), 620−623.

BUSCAGLIA, L. *The Disabled and Their Parents: A Counseling Challenge*. Thorofare, N. J.: Charles B. Slack, 1975.

DIAMOND, M. Sexuality and disability. In R. P. Marinelli and A. E. Dell Orto (Eds.), *The Psychological and Social Impact of Physical Disability*, 2nd ed. New York: Springer-Verlag, 1984.

DROTAR, D., BASKIEWICZ, A. IRVIN, N., KENNEL, J., and KLANS, M. The adaptation of parents to the birth of an infant with a congenital malformation: A hypothetical model. *Pediatrics*, 56 (1975), 710−717.

FEATHERSTONE, H. *A Difference in the Family: Life with a Disabled Child*. New York: Basic Books, 1980.

GARDNER, R. W. Evolution of brain injury: The impact of deprivation in cognitive-affective structures. In S. G. Sapir and A. C. Nitzburg (Eds.), *Children with Learning Problems: Readings in a Developmental-Interaction Approach*. New York: Brunner/Mazel, 1973.

GILLETTE, H. E. *Systems of Therapy in Cerebral Palsy*. Springfield, Ill.: Chas. C Thomas, 1969.

GOODSTEIN, L. D. Psychosocial aspects of cleft palate. In D. C. Spriesterbach and D. Sherman (Eds.), *Cleft Palate and Communication*. New York: Academic Press, 1968.

HARPER, D. C., RICHMAN, L. C., and SNIDER, B. C. School adjustment and degree of physical impairment. *Journal of Pediatric Psychology*, (1980), 377−383.

HILL, R. Social stresses on the family: Generic features under stress. *Social Casework*, 39 (1958), 139−150.

KOLB, C. L., and WOLDT, A. L. The rehabilitation potential of a gestalt approach to counseling severely impaired clients. In W. A. McDowell, S. A. Meadows, R. Crabtree, and R. Sakata (Eds.), *Rehabilitation Counseling with Persons Who are Severely Disabled*, p. 449. Huntington, W.V.: Marshall University Press, 1976.

LANGLOIS, J. H., and STEPHEN, C. The effects of physical attractiveness and ethnicity on children's behavioral attributions and peer preferences. *Child Development*, 48 (1977), 1694−1698.

LEFEBVRE, A. The child with physical handicaps. In P. D. Steinhauer and Z. Rae-Grant (Eds.), *Psychological Problems of the Child in the Family*, 2nd ed. New York: Basic Books, 1983.

LIVNEH, H. On the origins of negative attitudes toward people with disabilities. In R. P. Marinelli and A. E. Dell Orto (Eds.), *The Psychological and Social Impact of Physical Disability*, 2nd ed. New York: Springer-Verlag, 1984.

LUTZ, K. Counseling when there is a cleft palate. In R. E. Hartbaner (Ed.), *Counseling in Communicative Disorders*. Springfield, Ill.: Chas. C Thomas, 1978.

MCDOWELL, W. A., COVEN, A. B., and EASH, V. C. Special needs and strategies for counseling. In R. P. Marinelli and A. E. Dell Orto (Eds.), *The Psychological and Social Impact of Physical Disability*, 2nd Ed. New York: Springer-Verlag, 1984.

MCWILLIAMS, B. J. Cleft palate. In G. H. Shames and E. H. Wiig, *Communication Disorders: An Introduction*. Columbus, Ohio: Chas. E. Merrill, 1982.

———. Psychological development and modification. *ASHA Reports No. 5*. Washington, D.C.: American Speech and Hearing Association, 1970.

MCWILLIAMS, B. J., and SMITH, R. M. Psychosocial considerations. In B. J. McWilliams (Ed.), *ASHA Reports No. 9* Washington, D.C.: American Speech and Hearing Association, 1973.

MITCHELL, D. R. "Other people don't really understand": A survey of parents of young children with special needs. *Occasional Paper No. 2*. Project PATH, University of Waikato, Hamilton, New Zealand, 1981.

MUSGRAVE, R. H. MCWILLIAMS, B. J., and MATTHEWS H. P. A review of the results of two different surgical procedures for the repair of clefts of the soft palate only. *Cleft Palate Journal*, 12 (1975), 281–290.

PAYTON, O. D., HIRT, S., and NEWTON, R. A. (Eds.) *Scientific Bases for Neurophysiologic Approaches to Therapeutic Exercise: An Anthology.* Philadelphia: Davis, 1977.

RICHARDSON, S. A. The effect of physical disability on the socialization of a child. In D. A. Goslin (Ed.), *Handbook of Socialization Theory and Research.* Chicago: Rand McNally, 1969.

RICHMAN, L. C. The effects of facial disfigurement on teachers' perception of ability in cleft palate children. *Cleft Palate Journal*, 15 (1978), 155–160.

RUTTER, M., GRAHAM, P., and YULE, W. A neuropsychiatric study in childhood. *Clinics in Developmental Medicine*, 35/36 (1970).

SEIDEL, V. P., CHADWICK, O. F. D., and RUTTER, M. Psychological disorders in crippled children: A comparative study with and without brain damage. *Developmental Medicine and Child Neurology*, (1975), 563–573.

SHERE, E., and KASTENBAUM, R. Mother–child interaction in cerebral palsy: Environmental and psychosocial obstacles to cognitive development. *Genetic Psychology Monographs*, 73 (May 1966), 255–335.

SHERE, M. D. The socio-emotional development of the twin who has cerebral palsy. *Cerebral Palsy Review*, 18 (1957), 16–18.

SCHONTZ, F. C. Six principles relating disability and psychological adjustment. In R. P. Marinelli and A. E. Dell Orto (Eds.), *The Psychological and Social Impact of Physical Disability*, 2nd ed. New York: Springer-Verlag, 1984.

———. Physical disability and personality: Theory and recent research. *Rehabilitation Psychology*, 17 (1970), 51–59.

SIGELMAN, C. K., VENGROFF, L. P., and SPANHEL, C. L. Disability and the concept of life functions. In R. P. Marinelli and A. E. Dell Orto (Eds.), *Psychological and Social Impact of Physical Disability*, 2nd ed. New York: Springer-Verlag, 1984.

SOLNIT, A. J., and STARK, M. H. Mourning and the birth of a defective child. In *Psychoanalytic Study of the Child*, Vol. 16. New York: International Universities Press, 1961.

SPRIESTERSBACH, D. C. Counseling parents of children with cleft lips and palates. *Journal of Chronic Diseases*, 13 (1961), 244–252.

STARR, P. Physical attractiveness and self-esteem ratings of young adults with cleft lip and/or palate. *Psychological Reports.* Vol. 50 (2) (April 1982) 467–70.

———. Facial attractiveness and behaviors of patients with cleft lip and/or palate. *Psychological Reports*, 46 (April 1980), 579–582.

THURER, S. L. Women and rehabilitation. In R. P. Marinelli and A. E. Dell Orto (Eds.), *The Psychological and Social Impact of Physical Disability*, 2nd ed. New York: Springer-Verlag, 1984.

TIZA, V., and GUMPERTZ, E. The parents' reaction to the birth and early care of children with cleft palate. *Pediatrics*, 30 (1962), 86–90.

VERSLUYS, H. P. Physical rehabilitation and family dynamics. In R. P. Marinelli and A. E. Dell Orto (Eds.), *The Psychological and Social Impact of Physical Disability*, 2nd ed. New York: Springer-Verlag, 1984.

WEACHTER, E. H. Concerns of parents related to the birth of a child with a cleft of the lip and palate with implications for nurses. M. A. thesis, University of Chicago, 1959.

8

PSYCHOLOGICAL CONSIDERATIONS OF HEARING-IMPAIRED PEOPLE AND THEIR FAMILIES

Part I: The Psychology of Hearing-Impaired Children

THE PSYCHOSOCIAL DYNAMICS OF HEARING IMPAIRMENT IN CHILDREN

The medical, educational, communicative, and audiological implications of hearing impairment in children are well known. The psychosocial factors that characterize hearing disorders in children have received little attention in the literature, particularly with respect to the services noted above. As recently as 1982, Blair and Berg reported the insufficiency of supportive educational, social, and emotional services for these children and presented a strong case for the training of educational audiologists to serve them. Blair and Berg refute directly the contention "that the solution to hearing loss among children is simply wearing a hearing aid" (p. 541).

Children with hearing loss differ significantly among themselves in terms of many elements, including degree of loss, onset, etiology, intelligence, presence of other physical problems, personal coping mechanisms, response by the family, and quality of habilitative management. In this chapter our major attention will focus on the child's perception of self in relation to the hearing impairment and the influence of the family. We will also consider how counseling strategies can be applied most effectively to aid the child and family in the overall adjustment to the problem.

Etiology

Although organicity is predominantly associated with causes of hearing impairment, it should also be acknowledged that some children have what has been described as a "functional impairment" in which no organicity can be determined to explain discrepancies between audiometric results and observable behavior (Ventry and Chaiklin 1962). Both congenital and acquired hearing loss are associated with heredity, toxins, disease, injuries, or varying combinations of any of these. The psychosocial ramifications cannot be differentiated, however, on the basis of cause, as many individual factors will account for the way in which the child adapts to the problem. It seems more fruitful to distinguish psychosocial factors on the basis of congenital and acquired hearing loss.

Congenital hearing loss By congenital, we mean that hearing loss is incurred either while the embryo is in utero or immediately at birth. Thus the infant is, to some varying degree, cut off from the major sensory avenue necessary for speech and language development. Among the probable causes might be a toxic reaction to a drug ingested by the mother during pregnancy, familial genetic pattern, viral infection such as rubella during the first trimester of pregnancy, or birth delivery complications. Although such factors serve as ready explanations, we cannot ignore the possibility that emotional stressors may trigger a physiological intolerance in the mother during pregnancy, consequently affecting the fetus. Presently, there is no empirical evidence to support such a hypothesis, but it could be a fruitful area for research. More important for us is an understanding of the psychological effects of genetic or other congenital hearing anomalies on the child and the family.

Acquired hearing loss In acquired hearing loss, it is generally implied that the child already had had normal hearing at birth but because of subsequent disease, physical, or (less often) psychological trauma, has lost the ability to hear. Conceivably, hereditary factors related to constitutional predisposition may play a role either directly or indirectly in the susceptibility to the hearing loss. There are wider quantitative variations in degree of acquired hearing loss, and although psychological ramifications are present with congenital hearing loss, they are more complex and varied with the former, particularly if speech and language have already developed. The likelihood of combined congenital and adventitious factors, though less frequent, should also be considered.

Regardless of idiopathic origin, the effects upon the child and the family are cause for particular concern.

Adjustive Reponses of the Child

It is impossible to generalize about the adjustive responses of the child to hearing loss, whether congenitally or adventitiously acquired, as they would include a complex interplay of many factors. Among them are severity of hearing loss, time of acquisition, familial and social influence and effects, nature and quality of educational and habilitative efforts, and the unique personality and coping characteristics of the child. To present even a prototype example would force us to make generalizations that might distort our understanding of the problem. We prefer instead to discuss each of the major effects in terms of their special characteristics and allow the reader to formulate and apply his or her own perspective.

Effects on speech and language acquisition   Time of onset of hearing impairment and loss is likely the major variable that determines the acquisition of speech and language. The child who has never had the benefit of sufficient auditory exposure to speech and language is unlikely, except under the most extraordinary circumstances, to develop these sufficiently in order to communicate normally in a hearing world. The child who is in the process of developing speech or language, or who has already developed the skill, is likely to retain the ability except under the most dire conditions, such as total loss. Even then, the possibility exists for retention of what has already been gained.

Of greater significance is that the child who has already acquired speech and language has had the benefit of developing ideational or cognitive processes appropriate to the living environment, whereas the child who is born deafened or hearing impaired is deprived of the opportunity to relate to the world cognitively. In the former case a communicative relationship has already been established between parent and child, tapping at cognitive resources. When speech and language has not been learned, a crucial ingredient necessary for the parent–child relationship is lacking. Only through gesture and use of body language is it possible to establish a relationship, but in the case of profound hearing loss it is mired in what Ramsdell (1960) has described as the "primitive level" of hearing. Only through the earliest and most intensive intervention efforts is it possible to ensure that the child will be in the mainstream of the communication world of the hearing, but even then other variables will influence the outcome.

Effects on psychosocial development   In Chapter 5 we discussed the complex interactive relationship between psychosocial and speech-language development in normal hearing children. The ramifications of such a relationship in the case of deafened and hearing-impaired children are more extraordinary.

The child who is born deaf and deprived of the full verbal communicative interaction with the parents is prone to internalize thoughts and feelings, lacking the opportunities to experience the full range of sensory experiences necessary to relate to the parent and the environment. The deaf child is usually impulsive and socially immature, struggling to adapt in any way possible to the deficit. As Boothroyd (1982) has noted: "They perceive themselves as being acted upon more than acting and may compensate by developing rigid and manipulative behaviors" (p. 61). Hess (1960) has written of the tendency for these children to have a fantasy life that excludes awareness of the individuality of others and being unable to approach new situations in a flexible manner.

Because normal cognitive and speech-language development is likely to suffer in these children, it seems remarkable that many are able to adapt at all despite their isolation from a hearing environment. Perhaps a good number of them learn to cope with their loss by utilizing other cues within their environment along with their own unique defense mechanisms. Appropriate and early professional intervention and support from knowledgeable parents will certainly contribute further to the adjustment.

Children with a lesser degree of hearing impairment, although having the advantage of greater sensory exposure to others and their environment, may also suffer psychosocially. Those who incur hearing loss after having learned speech and language have to adjust to their changed circumstances, but they do so with varying degrees of frustration, anxiety, guilt, and inappropriate behaviors. They, too, are struggling to adapt and, depending on the nature and degree of parental support and profesional intervention, will learn to cope accordingly.

Consistent with the theme of this book, we hesitate to generalize how children will respond to their loss and to the efforts employed to help them. The many complex variables inherent in the interpersonal communicative process and the unique constitutional coping process of the child will often determine the outcome. We should, therefore, not be surprised when we encounter profoundly deaf children who actually adjust significantly better to their loss than those children who are less impaired or who have already established speech and language. Indeed, "it may be easier to live with what one has never had than to live with what one has lost."

For adolescents, deafness or acquired hearing impairment have very special implications. Because the peer group often becomes the determining factor defining social competence, the hearing-impaired adolescent is vulnerable to social rejection, precipitating depression, withdrawal, or regression to a less mature emotional state. For the individual who was born deaf, and depending on earlier educational and habilitative intervention, adolescence is the crossroads for embarking on a path toward the world of the deaf, the world of the hearing, or a compromised adaptation to both. Regardless of degree of impairment, the entire adjustment is shaped by intellectual, family, and unique individual character factors as well as by the quality of previous educational and habilitative efforts.

Effects on learning   The special educational needs of and minimal sup-portive services for school-age hearing-impaired children have been well documented (Blair and Berg 1982). The effects of hearing loss on learning from birth to five years have received less attention and, as Culross (1985) has noted, there are virtually no assessment instruments that can adequately measure the educational potential and psychological abilities of preschool hearing-impaired children.

Lacking the necessary sensory avenue for learning speech and lan-guage, the deafened infant appears to seek out alternative ways of relating to the environment in order to learn. This shifting to other sensory channels, which has been described fully by Studdert-Kennedy (1976), is necessary in order for the child to integrate whatever information can be received. How deaf and hearing-impaired children handle this information is unclear, but it would seem logical that with even minimal access to the auditory channel, a child has a greater potential for learning normally. We are certain of one thing: even profoundly deaf children are capable of developing a symbolic system necessary for learning, but how well these children learn depends on inherent intellectual and external familial conditions.

On the high school level, learning takes on special significance for the deafened and hearing-impaired adolescent. Peer pressures, sexual urges, emotional lability, and self-esteem are often hooked into the person's per-ception of the hearing impairment. Too often the disability may be used as an excuse to become reclusive, deficient in studying, antagonistic to others, or to drop out. Unfortunately, such behaviors are often interpreted by others not in terms of the implications of hearing impairment but as the acting-out behavior of a nonconforming teenager. What is misinterpreted is the young person's cry for equilibrium, emotional support, and practical assistance.

Reaction of the Family and Others

Like the parents of children born with cerebral palsy, cleft palate, or some other major physical impairment, parents of children born deaf go through a similar grief process. How they move through the process is dependent on several conditons, including the unique coping mechanisms of the family, the quality and degree of outside professional assistance, and the child's own adaptability to the blockage of the auditory channel. If deafness or impairment of hearing develops adventitiously, grief may also be experienced but in a more varied or subtle manner. Again, much will depend on other variables. The reader will find a succinct and useful discussion of mourning as it applies to deafness in children in Boothroyd (1982). It will also be helpful to review the process as it is discussed in other chapters, and in particular the adaptive process to child disability as identi-fied by Shontz (1975).

More important and significant from our perspective are the specific effects of any degree of hearing impairment on individual family members, the marital relationship, and the overall family equilibrium.

Effects on individual family members   Feelings of anger, bitterness, disappointment, frustration, and anger experienced by the parents in particular will vary greatly, depending on each parent's own unique association with the child and own personal emotional stability. To some extent, the degree to which each parent has fulfilled or is fulfilling his or her own life's goals will determine how well he or she will adjust to the child's disability.

Much, too, will depend, certainly, on whether or not one parent or parents of deaf children are hearing impaired or deaf themselves. We hesitate to generalize outcomes of such circumstances because of the uniqueness of all parents. Conceivably, it is as possible for deaf parents to provide the most educationally and habilitatively as it is possible for normal hearing parents to provide the least for theirs. Generally, though, the deaf child of normal hearing parents starts out with one major advantage—a potentially auditorily rich and stimulating linguistic environment.

We are more familiar with adventitiously hearing-impaired youngsters in normal hearing families. The variety of effects of individual family members here are probably more infinite. Let us look at one such family.

Some time ago, the author counseled a family in which the eleven-year-old son had incurred a severe hearing loss three years previous following a succession of serious middle ear infections and questionable medical management. Though very intelligent and sophisticated, the mother blamed herself for not having prevented the ultimate condition. Although her marriage was relatively stable, she had felt unfulfilled as a woman and had always considered her three children a burden despite the fact that there had never been any previous serious physical problems. Projecting her own guilt onto her severely deafened son, she felt compelled to dote on him and protect him from all life's stressors. She shopped for the best professional help she could possibly find but "never could find the right hearing aid for him." Her life had become a crusade that left little opportunity for her son to deal personally with his own struggles. Instead, the author was confronted with a fearful, dependent, noncommunicative youngster who had few friends and who was barely getting by in school.

This description is just one of the many possible illustrations of the effects of a child's hearing impairment on one family member. But it is also meant to illustrate a dynamic interplay between parent and child. Most important for us to understand is that parents do not necessarily pass through the various stages of the grief process in an orderly fashion or at any one time. As Boothroyd (1982) has clearly indicated, "The mourning sequence can be replayed several times in the parents' lives" (p. 64). We would add that any one stage may appear out of its classical sequence and may be manifest subtly or in combination with other stages. Thus an attitude such as denial by the parent may be expressed as a refusal to accept the hearing loss, the fitting of a hearing aid, modifying firmly entrenched behaviors, or combinations thereof.

In any case, the child is affected either through overt or covert attitudes and actions by the parent. How readily the child falls victim to the unresolved anguish, rejection, and helplessness of the parent may be due in part, as indicated earlier, to the child's own unique mode of coping or constitutional tolerance. It is our task as caregivers to assess these various interplays of feelings, actions, and events in order to provide the best we have to offer professionally.

The way in which the family relates to the hearing impaired adolescent will have a profound influence on high school adjustment, 'passage through puberty,' individual self-esteem, and career or vocational choice. Regardless of time of onset of the hearing loss, the family will need to continue to nurture and enhance their child through all of the struggles typically associated with adolescence and those directly or indirectly associated with hearing impairment. To either reject or to overprotect at this time will only make their child more rebellious or dependent, and will maintain the parental-infant bond. What needs to happen is a gradual separation whereby the adolescent must begin the process of functioning autonomously as an adult.

Effects on the marital relationship   The reality of hearing loss in the child is not the cause of marital dysfunction, but can be the catalytic factor to disrupt what may have been a shaky marriage. Like the arrival of any child with either a physical or psychological disability, one or both partners may use the circumstance to inflict on the other blame, resentment, accusation, or recriminations that ostensibly may appear to be related to their reaction to their child's disability but in fact is tied to their own unresolved marital problems.

Ironically, in some cases, although the traumatic occasion may be an excuse for both parents to inflict abuse on each other, it could also serve to bring to the surface issues with which they previously had not been forced to cope. They may seek professional help for themselves, which ultimately will benefit their afflicted child. Unfortunately, this sequence of events is not the case generally. They are more likely to get further immersed in their own marital difficulty, which in turn can have a devastating effect on the child and the rest of the family.

Effects on family homeostasis   A psychologically healthy family can meet the multiple needs of a hearing-impaired child and at the same time cope with their own individual reactions. They are not absolved from suffering stress or experiencing the various stages of the grief process. Family members can deal with the crisis by temporarily minimizing their own personal ambitions, modifying their own role responsibilities to meet the needs of the hearing-impaired child, and cooperatively working together to minimize the effects of hearing impairment on the entire family (Hill 1958). These are families that are adaptable to change, genuinely affectionate with one another, and able to solve problems through congruent communications. At the core is a dynamic, creative, and loving marital relationship. We do not wish to imply that a functional family can satisfy all of these requirements or even that such an ideal family actually exists. But as long as a family strives in the manner that is suggested, a hearing-impaired child will be a much more fortunate recipient.

In a more dysfunctional family, the equilibrium is disturbed in that the hearing-impaired child may serve to deflect attention away from other conflicts. The child may displace the "identified" symptom in another family member from a previous familial conflict, thereby creating a situation in which the emotionality between the child and parent may become highly charged. If marital dysfunction has been present, the hearing impairment in the child may serve to submerge the conflict further by getting enmeshed in it. Parental attitudes and behaviors such as overprotection and overinvolvement are projected onto the child, who is now viewed as incompetent and made to feel "different." Thus the true perspective of the hearing impairment is either lost or distorted.

The reader will recall from the earlier anecdote how the eleven-year-old hearing-impaired child became the recipient of the mother's unresolved struggles. In that family, attention was first drawn away from the other children, one of whom became asthmatic, withdrawn, and uncommunicative. These behaviors however served to draw attention now to what the asthmatic child needed, thus becoming the identified patient. In this case the father took on the major role of caregiver while the mother continued to dote on the hearing-impaired child. What originally was one family had in a sense become two families living in the same physical environment but in reality emotionally draining each other. The third child, striving to maintain some semblance of family equilibrium, began to act out his resentment from being excluded from parental attention by reverting to infantile behaviors such as enuresis and tantrums.

The parents, realizing that all seemed to be collapsing around them, jeopardizing the entire family, sought counseling assistance in order to reestablish a healthy equilibrium.

Murphy (1979), in his introductory chapter to an excellent monograph on families of hearing-impaired children, alludes to the importance of family relationships in terms of family functioning and growth. Murphy implies that hearing impairment in the child cannot be separated from the entire interpersonal process that distinguishes the life of the family. He cites pertinent research concerning the father's role in assisting the hearing-impaired child and the need for more research relative to the father's as well as the mother's role.

Based on research and clinical work. Schlesinger and Meadow (1972) in their seminal text "illuminate the relation between family patterns and social-intellectual-linguistic development in deaf children" (p. xi). They have applied the Eriksonian model of the eight stages of development toward our understanding of the psychosocial development of the deaf from birth to death. For them, the chief handicap of early profound deafness is not bound only to the auditory deficiency but also to the communicative process within the family. In our view it is no less important to view the lesser hearing-impaired child in a similar manner.

COUNSELING STRATEGIES

Only in recent years have writers in the field of audiology stressed the need for counseling intervention for parents of hearing-impaired children (Stream and Stream 1978; Murphy 1979; Luterman 1979; Sweetow and Barrager 1980; Clark 1982). Although these writers recognized that the role of the audiologist must be enlarged beyond the identification and assessment of hearing loss, hearing aid dispensing, and aural rehabilitation, they say little regarding the need for the child to be counseled as well. Also, in the otherwise excellent guidelines for counseling the family or parents there has been little written about the use of family therapy. We, therefore, need to examine all of these procedures.

Family Counseling

Clark (1982) provides us with several excellent guidelines to assist in counseling parents of hearing-impaired children. We summarize them as follows:

1. *The intake procedure*: An opportunity for the audiologist to obtain a case history and determine the exact need of the parents. An interpersonal relationship is established.
2. *The diagnostic interview*: Confirmation of the degree and quality of the hearing loss and providing only general information so that the family will not be overwhelmed. They are given an opportunity to express their reactions.
3. *Subsequent counseling*: Providing more in-depth counseling so that the family can have a more complete understanding of the problem and of the habilitative-educational process. The counseling audiologist must provide enough time for the family to assimilate what they have learned and what they are experiencing.
4. *Fostering an interpersonal relationship*: The necessity for the counseling audiologist to be open to the continuing concerns, feelings, and attitudes of the family. Nonjudgmental listening should be practiced by paying attention to what the family needs and less of what the audiologist wants to discuss.
5. *Three major questions asked*: Following Luterman (1976, 1979) the parents are asked three types of questions: (a) The request for further information; (b) confirmation from parents of the educational and habilitative procedure proposed by the audiologist; and (c) content questions with affectual components.
6. *Facilitating questioning by parents*: Providing an open atmosphere so that parents will not feel intimidated but free to ask anything they wish. An empathic and authentic attitude by the counselor is a must.

7. *Dealing with the grief process*: Being prepared to cope with the wide range of feelings inherent in mourning and helping the family understand that what they are experiencing is not abnormal.

8. *Shaping expectations*: Providing an honest picture of the implications of the hearing loss and a realistic assessment of what can be expected in the future.

9. *Ongoing opportunities for counseling*: Continued counseling may be necessary so that parents may work through their feelings and be given the opportunity to have more of their questions and concerns answered.

Providing information   A study by Sweetow and Barrager (1982), who surveyed 154 parents of hearing-impaired children, draws our attention to the need for these parents to have much more information about hearing loss than they are typically given. Among the specific needs determined were

1. Translating "technical terminology into laymen's language."
2. Means of communicating more effectively with their hearing-impaired child.
3. The desire for "contact with other parents of hearing impaired children."
4. The desire for more written literature on the subject of hearing loss.
5. The desire for "more specific information on educational sources."
6. "More frequent referrals to external sources for assistance in emotional and financial support."
7. The desire for "audiologists to take parents' observations and comments more seriously" (p. 847).

The comprehensive parent education program suggested by Dee (1981) is a practical and straightforward approach to helping these parents realize that their feelings are no different from those of others caught in a crisis.

Probably one of the most important considerations for the counseling audiologist to keep in mind when providing information is timing. It is necessary to be sensitive to the quantity and quality of information the parents can handle during the ongoing counseling relationship. The extent of their emotional reactions to the crisis will determine, in part, how much information they can process at a particular time. One effective way for the counselor to judge this is to check out with their clients on an ongoing basis how much they feel they need to know. If the parents are helped to realize that they are free to ask questions at any time, the counselor will have a better sense of how much and what they will need to know.

Means of coping   The counseling audiologist cannot solve the family's problems surrounding the hearing impairment of the child but he or she can provide the family the necessary guidelines they will need in order to cope. It is the writer's belief that the counselor's prime task is to help the parents become as fully aware as possible of their own personal attitudes, beliefs, needs, and expectations before they can be in a position to help their child. They need to see themselves not as owning the hearing loss personally but viewing it as belonging essentially to the child. In this way they will be better able to objectify the child's problem, gather a clear perspective of what *they* can do, and follow through with whatever educational and habilitative strategies are necessary.

This is no easy duty because parents tend to want to assimilate their children's problems, the process of which in our view is likely a projection of their own unresolved feelings of guilt, resentment, and need for a perfect child and an absence of conflict. The counselor may find considerable resistance to exploring these aspects of parent–child relationships and must temper empathic understanding with gentle persuasion if parents are to change their firmly entrenched belief system. A judgmental know-it-all or condescending approach would certainly be detrimental not only to the therapeutic process but to the eventual educational and habilitative outcome. However, if we as counselors can be conscious of these occasional professional slips in ourselves, then we are unlikely to do any irreparable harm.

Parents who are helped to relate to their hearing-impaired children in the way we are suggesting can better aid in developing the emotional and intellectual resources that are naturally available to children and thus ensure the most positive results.

One other task that is particularly important for the counselor is to be certain that the family knows exactly how to follow through with their own responsibilities toward the child and with the various other professional resources available to them. It is one thing to recommend that a hearing aid be fitted and another thing to make certain that it is appropriately used by the child. If recurring ear infections are the problem, the counseling audiologist may need to make certain that the child is checked out otologically.

We are not suggesting that the audiologist alone should be the prime caregiving coordinator. There may in fact be others, like the otologist, the speech-language pathologist, and the teacher, who might also play a guiding role in helping the parents follow through with their responsibilities.

One of the most revealing results of the study by Sweetow and Barrager (1980) are the major concerns of the parents. When they were asked, "In general how would you like to see the role of the audiologist expanded or improved?" the three most common answers were

1. The audiologist should handle the hearing aids.
2. The audiologist should work more closely with the schools.
3. More information on educational programs and emotional support should be provided. (pp. 846–847).

From our perspective the chief concern is that parents also know exactly where to go for assistance, know what to do, and do it. As professional caregivers, we must demand no less from ourselves.

Family Therapy

Family therapy is a particularly relevant counseling procedure because it helps maintain the communicative interaction, which can readily be lost if the child is severely hearing impaired or deaf. Although typically the child may have difficulty in following the verbal interchanges, all attempts should be made to involve the child. If language has already been learned, amplification will certainly enhance the communication process.

Family therapy is educational as well as therapeutic and helps remove the stigma of the "identified symptom or patient."

As an educational and therapeutic process   Consistent with the theme of this text, we believe family therapy to be a more thorough means of assisting the family to cope with many of the difficulties confronting it, and no less so for the hearing-impaired family. Although it could be argued that the affected child should not be subjected to one more situation in which he or she will feel cut off from communication, and that traditional parent counseling will conveniently protect the child from being exposed to material that could be emotionally harmful, we suggest a different point of view.

The child, depending on the nature and degree of the hearing loss itself, is likely already to feel thwarted in understanding what is ocurring in the immediate perceptual environment. Confused and bewildered, children may feel detached, isolated, and in some cases alienated from those around them, but the family therapy situation need not exacerbate these feelings. On the contrary, it could well enhance positive attitudes of belonging, self-identity, and self-worth merely by including the child in the process that will at least provide visual and perhaps some auditory input.

We would also question the notion of shielding children from material to which they had already been exposed during daily family interactions. It is better that these elements be brought out into the open in the nurturing atmosphere of family therapy rather than allowing them to fester in a milieu where communication is either closed or incongruent.

Family therapy is family counseling, but more. It gives all family members an opportunity to learn, on differing levels, how to discover specific ways, with each other's assistance, to best contend with the reality of hearing loss. It also provides the right set of circumstances in which family members can assist themselves and each other to feel better, mature emotionally, and most important, to make the best of what previously may have appeared to be an impossible situation.

Diminishing the impact of the identified symptom   We have already discussed how the hearing impairment becomes the identified symptom in terms of family systems theory. Although hearing loss is a symptom in the ordinary sense of the word, it should not be used to represent aspects of underlying family dysfunction. That is, it must not be allowed to take on a meaning that is not inherent in the hearing loss itself. To do this, the family may be guided in several ways. Of overriding importance, though, is that the family be involved in the beginning of the rehabilitation process.

1. Help them to discover whatever areas of conflict interfere with healthy family functioning.
2. Help them to understand the effects of hearing impairment as a family issue and not beonging to only one person per se.
3. Foster congruent communication among all family members, making certain that the hearing-impaired child has access to whatever communication aids are available.
4. Help each family member to understand his or her own unique role within the family and individual relationships with one another.
5. Help family members plan future goals for themselves as well as for the entire family.
6. Recognize differences in families regarding members' attitudes toward either a total, oral, or manual approach to speech and language.

These guidelines are not necessarily exclusive to the hearing-impaired family, but they must be used in the context of how the hearing impairment impinges on all family members. Moreover, because hearing-impaired families differ among themselves, the counselor needs to be careful not to formulate generalizations about the effects of hearing impairment, habilitative and educational goals, and prognostic signs unless they are relevant to the particular family being treated.

Individual Counseling

It seems remarkable that although the literature has given considerable attention to the value of parent counseling, virtually no emphasis has been placed on counseling the child individually. Can we assume that only parent counseling or family therapy will assist hearing-impaired children to use all of their emotional resources to enhance their educational, social, and habilitative goals? We doubt it. Besides, there have been no definitive experimental studies to determine outcomes based on parent counseling or family therapy intervention.

We believe that individual counseling, either separate from or in conjunction with other strategies, can enhance the emotional, social, and educational life of the child. The particular procedure used will be determined by the age of the child, degree of impairment, communicative competence, and cooperation of the parents. The procedures can include play therapy, client-centered aural rehabilitation, or direct counseling.

Play therapy   Play therapy for the hearing-impaired child is similar in many ways to play therapy with other communicatively disordered children, as discussed in previous chapters. To avoid redundancy, we describe only those aspects that are particularly pertinent to the hearing-impaired child.

1. Depending on the degree of hearing impairment, rapport may be established through basic signing, nonverbal body expression, amplification, or any combination thereof. Use of puppets can be helpful here.

2. The free expression of feelings and verbal speech and language is encouraged, with the child encouraged to pay direct attention to the facial appearance of the therapist. Here the therapist will need to be highly animated, so that the recognition and reflection of feeling by the therapist will be communicated.

3. Extensive use should be made of sound toys as a means of communication, toward developing cognitive skills, and of enhancing whatever residual auditory acuity is present.

4. The parents should be encouraged to observe the sessions, preferably through a one-way mirror, in order to carry over into the home several of the skills being taught in therapy.

We have to realize that although play therapy may serve to stimulate the expression of emotional material, to foster interpersonal communication, and to enhance learning, it is not a panacea for habilitation, It is a procedure, however, that may be used in conjunction with the total management program. The therapist will need to determine its relevance, depending on the emotional needs of the child, cooperation of the family, and availability of other caregiving services.

Client-centered aural rehabilitation   It is difficult to imagine the use of aural rehabilitation outside the process of client-centered counseling because they are both part of the interpersonal communicative process and are mutually complementary. For instance, if one of the goals in therapy is to maximize the efficiency with which a child uses a hearing aid, it will be necessary not only to reinforce a positive attitude about its use but also to help the child break down barriers to its acceptance. The obstacles may include emotional conflict, poor self-esteem, embarrassment, denial, withdrawal from relationships with peers, unconsciously motivated destruction of the aid, or any combination of these. The reader can obviously add several more of these resistances based on individual clinical experience.

The effectiveness with which the hearing-impaired child learns to speech-read will also be determined not only by perhaps an intuitive ability to use available cues within a communicative situation but also by the desire to learn from the environment. For the professional caregiver to rely only on the use of speech-reading techniques detached from the child's attitude or emotional state is neither realistic nor efficient. Here, too, it will be necessary to establish the optimum conditions under which the child can learn to speech-read regardless of the severity of the hearing impairment, and this includes the counseling process.

The problems for the deaf child are somewhat similar yet also quite different. Much has already been written concerning the integration of the deaf child within the community of the nonhearing impaired and about the controversy surrounding the more than one-hundred-year-old war over the oral versus manual approach. Although these are issues that go beyond the scope of this chapter, they are relevant to professionals who must counsel the deafened child.

Probably one of the chief challenges to professional counselors is to separate their own personal biases from the reality of the child's unique life circumstances and intellectual and educational potential. Counseling here becomes a process in which the counselor needs to learn what expectations are realistic for the child while the child must learn to develop maximum efficiency in communicating, regardless of the community within which the child may ultimately function. The counselor may frequently be faced with the dilemma of recognizing objectively that a vast potential for the child exists, and should be acutely aware of the child's environmental circumstances that may impede that potential. Only then can some resoltuion be achieved.

Although we have no standards to assist us in case-by-case intervention, there are generic guidelines that may be useful regardless of degree and quality of hearing impairment:

1. *Assessing the hearing along with the psychosocial status of the child.* It may be useful, or necessary, to have access to the services of a psychologist or psychometrist who is acquainted with the hearing problems of children.

2. *Educating the child about the hearing loss.* Too frequently we educate the parents and assume somehow that the child will get the information through osmosis. Informative data need to be given to the child geared to that child's age and intellectual level.

3. *Orientng the child to the use of a hearing aid.* Fitting the aid is not enough. Teaching its use and care is meaningful only if we (a) allow the child to express his or her personal reactions to wearing it and respond empathically to possible resistances or concerns, and (b) allow for possible resistance as an expression of real difficulties the child may be having with a particular aid and consider refitting if necessary.

4. *Having the child teach us what is needed in order to function more adequately.* We cannot assume that the age or naivete of the child precludes awareness of obstacles to maximal use of residual hearing. We need to be open to whatever information is forthcoming from the child and place it in proper perspective to data we have objectively gathered.

5. *Distinguishing emotional issues that are associated with hearing loss from those that are unrelated.* This is no easy task for the counseling audiologist because none of us behaves in a linear manner but instead responds behaviorally to the sum total of our experiences. What is necessary is that we discover those negative influences in the child's environment that at least appear to be unrelated to the hearing loss. These may include (a) possible problems in being raised by one parent; (b) effects of divorce; (c) extreme poverty; or (d) an emotionally disturbed family.

6. *Dealing with emotional disturbance in the child.* Somewhat related to guideline 5, it may be necessary to refer the severely emotionally disturbed child for more extensive psychotherapeutic assistance, and preferably to a professional who is well acquainted with the problems of hearing loss in children.

7. *Providing a supportive, empathic, and trusting therapeutic environment.* An environment in which the child feels free to express concerns regarding the loss of

hearing and its many implications provides a valuable opportunity in which to apply our audiological knowledge effectively. Too often children view us as adversaries, united with parents against them, regardless of our best intentioned efforts. It is, therefore, of considerable importance that we relate to the child in the most genuine way possible rather than pose as individuals who "know what's best" for the child. This does not imply that we act the role of "buddy," but that we appear to the child, and the child appears to us, as distinct persons in our own right.

8. *Use of special counseling techniques.* Consistent with the philosophy expressed throughout this text, we need to feel free to use whatever strategies with which we feel competent and that appear appropriate to a particular child. Among them are confrontation, self-disclosure, and contracting. In most instances these will need to be connected to aural rehabilitation strategies, but always bear in mind that it is the child who matters and not the technique.

Counseling or family therapy is usually thought necessary when hearing loss is first determined and during habilitative and educational planning. But as the following anecdotal accounts illustrate, it may be important a considerable time after the onset of hearing loss and initial intervention. It may, in fact, be important on an intermittent basis throughout the child's early and pubescent years. Tsappis (1985) summarizes the psychological experiences of two congenitally hearing-impaired adolescents.

The first incident addresses the adolescent's increasing sexual awareness and various behaviors defining male and female social roles. During an annual visit to the Speech and Hearing Center, the mother of a sixteen-year-old male reported that her son had recently discontinued hearing aid use, and strenuously resisted and rejected parental efforts to encourage his continued use of amplification. The young man was experiencing a moderate to severe, congenital, sensorineural hearing loss. He had been successfully using binaural amplification since approximately age two. His speech and language and academic performance were excellent. He obviously had used two hearing aids consistently for fourteen years with good results, and no complaint. Consequently, his sudden rejection of amplification and resistance to parental support represented an important issue requiring resolution.

When I questioned the young man in the clinic about his rejection of hearing aids, my effort to obtain information was received with a shrug of the shoulders and a mumbled, "I don't know." Electro-acoustic evaluation of the hearing aids indicated that they were functioning according to factory specifications, and audiologic evaluation indicated no change in hearing when compared with prior test results. Following the structured hearing and hearing aid evaluations, I invited the young man to the hospital for a coke. Conversation drifted from school, recreation activities and girls to automobiles. During this informal discussion I learned the young man recently had obtained his driver's license. He reported that during the course of the evening on his first driving date, his companion laid her head on his shoulder. The young lady's head provided a reflective barrier at the pinna, which resulted in generating considerable acoustic feedback at his right hearing aid. The young lady did not know her escort wore hearing aids. Consequently, when the feedback occurred she was quite startled. The young man reported that when the incident occurred she practically jumped out the passenger door while the car was moving. She apparently huddled as close to the passenger door as she could and with a look of concern and confusion asked, "Did I hurt you?" In view of this report, it is not surprising that a young man who had just obtained the greatest symbol of American independence and mobility, and who was struggling to behave in a way that would identify and establish his masculinity, discontinued hearing aid use. The instruments were obviously directly responsible for causing considerable embarrassment during one of the most important evenings of his life. His attempt to explain what had occurred apparently did little to resolve his companion's concern at the time. We jointly agreed that anticipation of future events might dictate whether he should wear binaural or either monaural right or left instruments, depending upon his social circumstances.

The thought that possibly such an event could be responsible for a male adolescent's reluctance to continue to use required amplification was remote. Typically considerable attention is directed to the adolescent female's attitudes regarding physical characteristics, glasses and hearing aids; however, as illustrated by the present event, little effort is directed toward dealing with male adolescent attitudes.

The second incident involves a 13-year-old male experiencing a severe to profound, congenital, sensorineural hearing loss. He also had been successfully wearing amplification since approximately age two. Over the years, in typical fashion, he occasionally expressed his curiosity regarding the etiology of the hearing loss to his parents, and his need to use hearing aids that were not required by his close friends. His parents had previously informed him that the loss was the result of maternal rubella occurring during the first trimester of pregnancy. Their descriptions were accurate and appropriate to his age at the time of the question. Over the years, the explanations offered were accepted with little or no ongoing dialogue, and family life proceeded as usual. At aproximately age 13, following detailed discussion of the etiology of his hearing loss, his behavior toward his mother changed considerably. Responses to comments and questions regarding various family matters were abrupt and succinct. He generally began to avoid any verbal or social interaction with his mother, while generally maintaining his usual social routine with other family members. During a heated discussion, he confided to his parents that he "hated his mother" because she and the illness she contracted while she was carrying him were directly responsible for his permanent affliction. The report obviously resulted in considerable parental concern.

I referred the family to a local psychiatrist with an excellent reputation. My immediate opinion was that since such feelings of parental hostility are known in the psychiatric community, therapy would be extremely beneficial. I expected that the youngster's speech and language level would present no communication difficulties for the psychiatrist. Unfortunately, one and one-half years of therapy and counseling did little to help the young man with his feelings of rage. In frustration, during that time, the parents sought help from various psychiatric and psychological professionals to no avail. At the end of the one and one-half years, the family terminated therapy. The family problem and young man's attitude toward his mother continued for approximately one year following conclusion of therapy. Outward hostility toward his mother then diminished, and eventually resolved. The family now enjoys the open, interactive relationships that existed prior to the overt onset and demonstration of anger. The problem apparently resolved as quickly as it began; however, the family was frustrated through the lack of assistance available that might have resolved the problem more quickly and avoided approximately three years of family disharmony.

These reports do not differ necessarily from those of normal hearing individuals whose anger is directed toward parents or who are coping with their adolescence. They do illustrate the value of psychotherapeutic intervention even when it is resisted. Apparently, a child and family may "get better" despite it. The difficulties that can be expected in children with more profound hearing losses and limited oral language may be presumed to create even greater concerns for us.

Group Counseling

Whether a hearing-impaired child is being educationally mainstreamed or in a self-contained classroom, group therapy can be a valuable adjunctive aid toward habilitation. Its value is probably greatest when it can be integrated along with aural rehabilitation that includes group amplification, auditory training, and speech reading. Among the psychological benefits to be gained are the following:

1. Helping these children to recognize and understand that they are not alone as they experience their hearing loss.
2. Learning to discover their own unique ways to cope with their loss.
3. Sharing with each other methods that have been useful and those that have not.
4. Depending on their age, learning how to adjust more effectively to special problems associated with adolescence, relationships with normal hearing peers, family relationships, and school studies.
5. Developing positive attitudes about themselves by learning how to maximize their potentials and minimize their liabilities.

Although it may not be possible to establish a set of guidelines that will determine the efficacy of having a particular child in group therapy, it would be more useful for the counseling audiologist to make a case-by-case decision, either independently or in consultation with other professionals. Most important is that the decision made must be based on what the child needs, the cooperation of the family, and the availability of resources. Furthermore, group therapy should not be viewed as a substitute for other management practices, and every effort must be made to provide those that will benefit the child most.

One final note should be added. Regardless of the group therapy counseling model used, every effort should be made by the counselor to establish a therapeutic process whereby the children learn to assist each other rather than become individually passive agents in a group. Though the counselor may at various times lead, educate, reflect, clarify, and possibly even judge, the children themselves should be given the responsibility to work through with each other whatever problems are present and those that may arise.

CONCLUSION

Although children with hearing loss share many of the psychosocial concomitants associated with children having other communicative disorders, and in fact may be afflicted with those disorders also, many factors are unique to hearing impairment itself. We need to be cautious, however, not to generalize these elements to all hearing-impaired children, nor neglect to recognize the possibility of phenomena untypical of these children.

Clinically, audiologists are familiar with the psychodynamic challenges these children present, but are also frustrated by the absence of solid experimental research to help them better understand the processes and to facilitate the delivery of their services. Audiologists are faced with no less a challenge when intervening with the hearing-impaired adult.

Part II: The Psychology of Hearing-Impaired Adults

THE PSYCHOSOCIAL DYNAMICS OF HEARING IMPAIRED ADULTS

A major distinction between the psychosocial dynamics of hearing-impaired children and hearing-impaired adults is that the adult population generally has had no hearing impairment for most of their lives. Although an individualistic approach is necessary to our understanding of their problems, they present, as Orlans (1985) has indicated, a singular combination typical to those whose hearing has been unimpaired during the substantial portion of their lifetime. More than that, however, they also present us with the common problems of adults who must adjust to any radical change in their lives, regardless of the nature, quality, and degree of the disability or the event.

The central focus of this section is on age and etiological correlates and how the hearing-impaired adult is affected personally, socially, and vocationally. A further concern is the adjustment process that relates to the marital relationship, family functioning, and the effects on the children of hearing-impaired adults.

Etiology and Age

Among adults who become hearing impaired, it is important that we make several distinctions regarding age and etiology so that we can better understand their adjustment to the loss and the counseling management that may follow. It should be further understood that we cannot always generalize adjustive responses nor the remediation needs on the basis of etiology or age alone, as many individual variations will dictate the course and progression of the overall rehabilitative process. The following anecdotes will illustrate what we mean.

Mr. P, an auto mechanic, began losing his hearing in his late twenties and wore a hearing aid until he went totally deaf at age fifty-five. Over the years he had learned speech reading, but most of it was self-taught. Although he and his family, a wife and a grown son and daughter, were unprepared for a total loss, their essential mutual love, caring, and trust sustained them all during the traumatic final year of hearing. Family therapy was initiated to help them through their adjustment process, but was discontinued after three sessions because they were capable of letting go of their previous hope for arrest of the gradual hearing loss. Mr. and Mrs. P were also able to begin plans for making other changes in their lives. These consisted of preparations for Mr. P's early retirement, an intensive program of aural rehabilitation, and an extended motor home tour throughout the United States.

We are not suggesting that the family did not suffer the anguish typifying the trauma of total hearing loss, but the mental health that characterized the family was a key factor to their overall adjustment and positive planning for the future. Although the year-long program of aural rehabilitation helped him to understand only 30 percent of normal speech, he felt ready to "move on to other things in my life."

Recently, after twelve years following his traumatic loss of hearing, Mr. P volunteered for the most highly developed electronic cochlear implant, which even without speech-reading cues helps him to understand about 40 percent of normal speech. Using both, he now hears well enough to carry on normal conversations.

It should be understood that Mr. P's decision to volunteer for the research project involving cochlear implantation was not based on a personal search for the proverbial Golden Fleece, but a willingness to help otologic and audiologic researchers in their quest to enable thousands of other totally deaf people to hear normal speech.

Our other anecdotal account concerns Madge T, a single, attractive, well-groomed thirty-five-year-old practicing courtroom attorney who, as a result of otosclerosis, ultimately acquired a moderate bilateral hearing loss. Resisting efforts to be fitted wth a hearing aid, she denied that her loss warranted aiding and continued courtroom work despite admonitions by trial judges to pay more attention to what was being said during trial proceedings. Curiously, even without aiding, she should have been able to function at least adequately in the courtroom, albeit with concentrated attention, but her high degree of anxiety prevented even that. Rather than confronting the reality of her life situation, she took fewer and fewer cases, depleting whatever savings she had in order to maintain the style of living to which she had been accustomed. Almost prepared to give up practicing entirely and getting more and more depressed, she sought psychiatric assistance.

Although psychotherapy was instrumental in uncovering deep-seated struggles related to her self-concept and adequacy as a woman trying to function in an essentially male-oriented profession, she continued to resist her psychiatrist's advice to purchase the aid with which she had been adequately fitted.

After several months she terminated psychotherapy and sought further otologic-audiologic assistance. Soon she relinquished the notion that further surgery would be of any benefit to her and was now open to further counseling from her audiologist. Although he had recommended that it would be useful for her to return for further psychiatric assistance, she preferred instead to work through her "blocks," as she put it, with her audiologist.

During the first few months of counseling she agreed to wear intermittently the aid she had finally purchased, and with continued therapeutic support, empathy, and at times, confrontation was wearing the aid consistently after one year.

These two illustrations are examples of etiological, psychological, environmental, and individual factors that constitute adjustment to hearing loss by adults. It is useful, however, to consider how together age and etiology play a significant role in the adjustment process, and to be aware that the premorbid attitudes and affectual state of the individual will also determine the reactive response to the hearing loss.

Traumatic hearing loss and age   Generally speaking, the occurrence of traumatic hearing loss at any age during adulthood is likely to cause far more upheaval in that person's life than we would expect with gradual impairment, regardless of age. This is not to suggest that the psychosocial consequences for the latter would necessarily be any less profound in specific cases.

It can readily be understood that any drastic change brought about by external forces will test the unique adjustment resources of any individual afflicted with sudden loss of hearing. If the trauma occurs in conjunction with other disabling conditions associated with such events as a gunshot wound to the head, automobile accident, fall, or toxic poisoning, we would expect the adjustment process to be far greater and more complex.

For the young adult who is typically entering the stage of developing a career, establishing primary relationships, and becoming a self-directed individual, the reaction to a traumatic loss of hearing may stalemate him or her from achieving any one or combination of these goals. What the audiologist must differentiate are the effects of the individual's reaction to the loss from the direct effects of the loss itself on the wide range of possibilities in that person's life. Obviously, the combined effects will also require a considerable degree of counseling expertise if the impaired individual is to embark in a new or modified direction.

In middle adulthood, traumatic hearing loss produces somewhat different consequences. Here the individual is already practicing a particular profession or occupation, has likely established a family, and has already adopted a particular self-identity role. Depending on the strength and the quality of these, the individual may be able either to find a way to cope with the loss or lose personal perspective in the form of self-doubt, self-recriminations, resentment, and anger. Although the latter may also characterize the younger adult, the older adult may be experiencing a midlife crisis that in no way is related to the traumatic loss of hearing but could certainly influence it now.

Here the combined effects may influence and distort either the real implications of the loss itself and/or the individual's personal response to it. The task for the audiologist will be to help the individual sort out all of the personal issues that either directly or indirectly relate to the hearing loss.

In older adulthood, depression frequently appears, and with the occurrence of traumatic hearing loss, is likely to be intensified, particularly if the individual is also suffering from other physical or psychological incapacities or if it occurs in conjunction with other physical problems. The adjustment of the individual to the many problems associated with aging in general has been well documented (Breslau and Haug 1983). Any drastic alteration of physical capabilities like traumatic hearing loss, however, is likely also to magnify such issues as dependency on children, fear of death, general helplessness, loss of self-esteem, and lack of purpose and meaning in life. Perhaps already feeling alienated from the environment, as similarly aged friends and family members die, the individual is cut off further, dramatically, from the world.

The overwhelming effects of traumatic hearing loss in the aged population probably present to the counseling audiologist the greatest challenge of all. It will be necessary to sort out all of the effects of the loss and the circumstances with which the client must struggle.

Hearing loss with gradual onset The counseling audiologist is more likely to be confronted with hearing loss as it develops gradually in the adult. Here, too, however, the variables of etiology and age play a significant role, although the process of progressive hearing loss presents with somewhat different implications. That is, the process allows the individual to adjust more slowly and perhaps more thoroughly to the overall loss, but the psychosocial effects may not necessarily be any less profound in individual cases.

Young adults whose hearing losses are due to middle ear, cochlear, retrocochlear, or brainstem dysfunction may not necessarily differ affectually in terms of the pathology itself, but more likely in terms of the degree of loss. Like the young adult whose loss has been precipitous, the individual is apt to feel some degree of self-imposed alienation from normal hearing peers. That person will perhaps resist wearing a mechanical device that may call attention to itself. Whereas a precipitous loss of hearing may be cause for the individual to take immediate remediation measures, the individual whose loss is gradual may adapt a wait and see attitude in hopes the loss will either remit or disappear.

Rousey (1971) has suggested that occasionally the grief response to a hearing loss may unconsciously characterize feelings of sexual inadequacy. Such feelings should not be interpreted literally but rather be conceptualized in terms of interpersonal relationships, particularly in the case of hearing-impaired young adults.

In middle adulthood, personal and life responsibilities typically become more numerous and complex. The individual is certainly not immune to the effects discussed above, but if family, professional, and social conditions have already been stabilized, the person is more likely to adapt to hearing loss. No longer striving like the younger person to achieve a sense of identity, place, and position in life, the older person is apt to have the advantage of an environmental support system that may mollify the effects of hearing loss. Obviously, not all hearing-impaired older adults will fit such categorization; thus the counseling audiologist must be wary of overgeneralizing.

Older adults with gradual onset of hearing loss characterize the largest population with whom the audiologist is likely to deal. The effects of presbycusis, resulting in gradually decreased acuity for pure tone signals speech recognition, have been well documented (Hayes 1984). Less is known of the presbycusic effects on the psychosocial aspects of the population, although Alpiner (1979) and Orlans (1985) give us a comprehensive picture of the current knowledge on the subject. It cannot be assumed that because the hearing impairment is gradual that the effects are any less profound for the person. It is important, then, that we look at the specific adjustive responses that are made.

Adjustive Responses of the Adult

Although the adjustive responses of adults with hearing impairment may vary, depending on age and etiological factors, there are specific effects that relate to self-esteem, emotional stress, and adjustment in the work environment. The adjustive responses of the older adult are particularly noteworthy.

Effects related to self-esteem and emotional stress   We recognize that the individual response to hearing impairment is dependent on a number of variables, including the environmental, social, and psychological characteristics of the person. To discuss these within the context of specific psychological theories would take us beyond the scope of this text. We believe it is useful to describe the effects within a generic framework instead.

To begin with, the prior emotional status and coping capabilities of the individual determine, in part, how the hearing loss will be experienced and how adjustment will occur. One further significant factor is the degree to which and the quality with which the individual has already shaped his or her personal life. Thus the individual who has been functioning in a healthy and productive manner is better prepared to cope with the distress caused by hearing impairment and more likely to take constructive steps toward rehabilitative management. Also, the individual who copes realistically with the loss and is future oriented is less likely to suffer the extreme of grief that is characteristic of those whose lives have been unfulfilled and wrought with emotional conflicts. Thus we should not be surprised when we encounter some individuals who are devastated emotionally by their even mild or moderate loss while others with more severe losses appear to adapt quite well.

Effects in the work environment   Related to our discussion, the individual who suffers hearing impairment may need to make certain adjustments within the work environment in order to maintain a lifestyle to which he or she is accustomed. In rare cases it means transferring to a new environment or vocation.

In our anecdote given earlier, Mr. P never considered a change of occupation, though as he began to lose his hearing, it was recommended that he wear ear defenders while working in the noisy environment of an auto repair shop. The degree to which such an environment contributed to the onset of his loss is irrelevant to our present discussion, but it should be noted that Mr. P was quite diligent in his efforts to protect his ears as often as practically possible.

More significant was the fact that even with the virtually complete loss of hearing, Mr. P continued in his same occupation with the same firm. Although he certainly needed to make some adjustments, such as relying more on auto repair manuals than on fellow worker input, he also, in his own personal way, educated his work supervisor and other workers in means by which they could help him. These included having them speak directly to him, but naturally, and expecting them to treat him not as disabled, but as different.

In the case of Madge T, the adjustment in the work environment was not so simple. Even while wearing her aid in the courtroom and during client consultation, she continued for some time to be self-conscious, anxious, and preoccupied. Viewing herself as disabled, she felt insecure in taking on the difficult cases by which she had always felt delightfully challenged. Instead, she relied more on legal matters that involved less face-to-face interaction and courtroom work. Frustrated by what she considered uninteresting and dull cases, she seriously contemplated giving up her profession, although her aided hearing in no way interfered with her ability to function as she had previously. It was only her negative self-perception that was creating a self-fulfilling prophecy of a failure. Fortunately, after a year and a half of counseling from her audiologist, she began to take on the kinds of cases she had always enjoyed, and ironically became interested in the legal problems of the disabled.

What is most important to understand from these case illustrations is that it is necessary to distinguish between the objective realities and requirements of any particular work environment and the perceptual attitudes of the hearing individuals toward self in relation to that work environment. In a very real sense, hearing loss to some degree may be as severe as we choose to make it.

Special problems of the older adult   The adjustive reponses of older adults to their hearing loss may be quite similar to those of the younger adult, but there are differences. Some we have discussed earlier. Older adults who have not reconciled themselves to the aging process or who have not adjusted to the many upheavals associated with old age, like the death of a spouse or friends, forced retirement, or frequent illnesses, may be less apt to accept the hearing impairment, aural rehabilitation management, and the wearing of a hearing aid. This is not to infer that they are necessarily emotionally disturbed or have not lived creative, useful, and productive lives. What may be evident is that their life patterns have become essentially fixed and rather than seek to make any changes, even if these apparently are for "their own good," they would rather "make the best of it" without external assistance.

These adjustive reponses might be clinically described as defense mechanisms, which serve to protect the person from the effects of what is being experienced and may also be a means by which conflict is handled. They can be useful or counterproductive for the person; which can be determined only by the overall psychosocial assessment of the individual.

Probably the greatest influence on the adjustive responses of older adults are elements associated with family relationships.

Reaction of the Family

Hearing impairment in adulthood affects not only the individual but also those with whom that person relates daily. Surprisingly scant research is available to describe the effects on the marital relationship, overall family functioning, and the children and other family members. Little is known of how the stress brought on by hearing impairment affects everyone and interpersonal relationships. Oyer and Oyer (1985) have made a considerable contribution to our understanding of adult hearing loss and the family, but as they point out, few scientific experiments have studied the relationship between the two.

In terms of family systems theory, we are certain of at least one thing:

the adventitious development of hearing impairment in an adult family member will disrupt the functioning of the family. The degree and quality of the dysfunctioning are dependent, though, on previous family functioning and emotional stability of each member.

Effects on the marital relationship We cannot assume that acquired hearing impairment in one person will automatically affect a marriage even if marital problems existed prior to onset. If a healthy and creative marriage has existed, the hearing impairment may actually help bring both parties even closer together. Should marital difficulties increase, timed with the onset of hearing impairment, it is likely that a preexisting marital conflict may have been present but concealed. The hearing impairment may serve to activate the original conflict, not to necessarily reveal it but to obscure it further under pretense of the hearing loss. Let us illustrate this.

Les and Diane had been married thirty years and had a relationship that was barely tolerable. Childless, they had used each other to inflict their own personal, unresolved inner turmoils without ever coming to terms with the true essence of a relationship requiring love and trust.

Les, an avid hunter and disdainful of any ear protection, sustained a moderate to severe bilateral hearing impairment due to acoustic trauma. Refusing to wear the hearing aid that was fitted and would likely have helped him, his relationship with Diane deteriorated further in the form of mutual recriminations. Diane ridiculed him for being childish about refusing to wear the aid and felt angry and frustrated whenever he did not hear her. Her sarcasm, which had always been present, did not abate but became more volatile. Les, on the other hand, was infuriated with the increased intensity of her voice and her "bitchiness." Although previously they both had done many things separately, they now spent even less time together. Whatever time they did spend together often consisted of arguments surrounding his stubbornness and her judgments about his hearing impairment. Neither person was able to relinquish the projections and the defenses that had built up over the lifetime of the marriage, nor did they desire a divorce.

This anecdote illustrates how extreme marital dysfunction may sometimes distort the incidence of hearing impairment. Based on a model by Jacobson and Bussod (1983), we would say that the way in which a couple copes with hearing impairment in one partner will be determined by the distortions in each person's perception of the other. The degree to which these perceptions are based on the perceiver's own unresolved conflicts rather than on the actual qualities of the other person will determine the wideness of the discrepancy and the amount of distress over the hearing impairment.

Effects on family equilibrium Recalled from our discussion of family systems theory that although a communication disorder symptomatizes one individual, it does not imply that individual to be the actual "identified patient" who serves a scapegoat function for the family as a whole. For example, if the mother acquires a hearing impairment and is unable to cope adequately with it, and if there are preexisting unresolved family or marital conflicts, the stage may be set for another family member to take the burden of the problem or the attention away from the hearing impairment. This person now represents the true "identified patient."

We have said that family patterns of interaction are directed toward maintaining the status quo, or the equilibrium, with which the family is familiar. Thus if family anxiety is aroused with the advent of a hearing impairment to unbalance the scale, at least one family member becomes "identified" as the person instrumental in regaining homeostasis for the entire family.

Ideally, if the wife and mother is able to manage constructively the consequences of her hearing impairment with open support from the rest of her family, in particular from her husband, no other family member will need to assume the burden or become an identified patient. Thus she becomes reponsible for maintaining family equilibrium by the nature of her positive efforts. Most important is the necessity to separate the issue of hearing impairment from other, unrelated family issues. Only when the former is submerged by the latter do the real problems begin to surface.

Effects on adult children   Grown-up children of older adults with hearing impairment may play a significant role in assisting their parents to cope with their loss. A significant variable in this interaction is the quality of the parent–child relationship. A relationship in which mutual respect and support have been present will be the most effective in helping the hearing-impaired older person to adjust to the hearing loss. The implied assumption is that an open communication system has existed in which each person has been able to relate to the other as individuals in his or her own right. Age differences are of no consequence because they can at least acknowledge each other's intelligence, capabilities, knowledge, emotional attitudes, and points of view.

They are not individuals who are enmeshed in unresolved parent–child struggles or caught up in parent–child role reversals. Should the parent resist efforts either to wear an aid or participate in an aural rehabilitation group, it does not mean that the son or daughter should adopt a hands-off attitude but rather should communicate his or her personal feelings of opposition to the parent's stance. At the least, a dialogue can be initiated in which mutual attitudes and feelings can be expressed, acknowledged, and respected, even if some judgments are made. Most important is the mutual agreement that the parent must make the ultimate choice regardless of the consequences.

More frequently, the children of older or elderly parents with impaired hearing feel they must assume the burden of their parents' problem. The guilt they often experience when the parent is disinterested in receiving professional help is not so much related to the fact that they have failed to convince the parent of the necessity but more likely related to having failed the parent previously in other matters. An example of this might be the elderly mother who feels that her son has made too little effort to visit her more often since her husband died. Indeed, she may resent his intrusion now because "he's never been there for me when I've needed him anyway." Certainly her own present negative attitude toward him and professional assistance or the wearing of an aid is connected to unresolved parent–child issues that probably belong to earlier times.

There are some children, also, who are essentially disinterested in their parents' hearing impairment and feel that anything asked of them, like arranging for transportation to an aural rehabilitation group, is an impositon. Here, too, the issue is not the present negative response to the parent but a manifestation perhaps of long-standing resentments, anger, and bitterness characteristic of their essential relationship.

Such reactive responses by children are frequently evident when the parents are confined to a convalescent hospital or nursing home. Audiologists who consult in such institutions are quite familiar with families who do not follow through with recommendations regarding a change of ear mold, keeping fresh batteries on hand, or visiting more frequently.

Clearly, children of elder parents with hearing impairment are affected in various ways, and although we might be tempted to categorize their behavioral responses, we must view them selectively and individually. In doing so, we are in a better position to determine how we can intervene psychotherapeutically, if necessary.

COUNSELING STRATEGIES

We believe that in order for any aural rehabilitation program for hearing-impaired adults to succeed, some form of counseling intervention must be included. This seems obvious, as aural rehabilitation, like counseling, is a communicative process in which the individual is assisted to relate more effectively with others by enhancing whatever hearing abilities are present. Besides, it seems unlikely for a person who has not adjusted emotionally to the impairment to derive much from an aural rehabilitation program that relies merely on a curriculum or on specific techniques only.

The professional caregiver must decide first, however, which overall counseling strategy is appropriate, realistic, and potentially meaningful for the client. Second, it must be determined if counseling is to be used within the aural rehabilitation session itself or as an adjunctive procedure. Unfortunately, there is no objective or empirical evidence to assist us in that decision; thus the counseling professional must rely on whatever data the audiological evaluation has revealed and on information gathered during initial interviews with the client and/or the family.

Each of the major counseling strategies described has its own intrinsic value and, although they could be suitably combined with some clients, we address each separately.

Family Therapy

Generally, family therapy is an appropriate procedure if the hearing impairment has induced a crisis in the family. Either the actual patient, another member who has become the "identified patient," or both may provide the justification for such intervention. If family therapy is to have any chance of success, however, the family must be motivated at least to participate in the process. Participation does not necessarily ensure success because typically family members will resist the therapist's attempts at change. It is necessary, however, for the therapist to help the family stay focused on how the hearing impairment has activated other dysfunctional elements within the family and to deal with these as they surface.

Hearing loss as a family issue   In family therapy, the hearing loss is treated as a symptom that has affected the entire family. In this sense family therapy is quite different from traditional therapy models. The hearing-impaired individual is thus urged to share deeply held feelings with other family members and they are encouraged to do likewise. The importance of this approach is highlighted by the fact that the hearing impairment itself may be interfering with normal family communication, and it will be necessary for individual or collective attempts to be found in order to modify or eliminate that interference.

The father who shuts himself off from other family members, however, may be doing so not because of his hearing impairment but for different reasons. The hearing loss could be used as an unknowing excuse to conceal other unresolved personal or family issues. Such issues need to surface if the hearing impairment is to be placed in its proper perspective.

Similarly, if another family member is having more difficulty in adjusting to the hearing impairment than the father, it must be determined what the underlying feelings and attitudes are. These in fact have less to do with the actual impairment than they do with that person's essential relationship with the father. It does not mean that the person necessarily becomes the "identified patient" because of symptoms serving the family as a whole, unless the person's actions are used to protect other family members or conceal other other family issues. The family therapist may have to work separately with that person and the father to determine what the essence of their relationship is.

If the person's behavior or attitude is used to obscure other family issues, the family therapist will need to promote a more functional family structure in which the hearing impairment is placed in a realistic and objective perspective. The hearing-impaired family will need to discover, with the assistance of the family therapist, its own mode for coping with hearing loss in one member and for dealing with contaminating family issues.

Special therapeutic problems of aged parents We have said that defensive attitudes on the part of older hearing-impaired individuals are a means of self-protection and a way of coping with hearing loss. In families where these individuals live with their grown children, these attitudes get enmeshed in other issues concerning not only their relationships with their children but also in matters concerning their self-concept, adjustment to old age, and loss of other functions.

More often than not, unfortunately, older parents have little choice in living with their adult children. Either because of other physical disabilities, loss of a spouse, or severe economic conditions, the older parent may feel guilty about disrupting his or her children's lives or being a burden and simultaneously feel resentful about dependency on them.

It becomes the therapist's task in such family circumstances first to help the hearing-impaired person to separate out feelings regarding the loss and its appropriate management from other emotional issues, and second, to help the children understand that their well-intentioned judgments about what should be done to help can be counterproductive. Although we still consider the problem of hearing loss a family one, it must be the affected parent's reponsibility to take charge of the predicament and do what is personally deemed best.

It is important too, however, that the children be given the opportunity to ventilate their own feelings and for the hearing-impaired parent to acknowledge the validity of their children's attitudes even if they should differ from his or her own. Regardless of differing opinions or attitudes, the loss should remain the major focus of attention. Of course, if other underlying emotional issues or conflicts are observed to be operating, they must be distinguished from the hearing-impairment issue and dealt with independently if necessary.

The value of family therapy in these circumstances is that a valuable opportunity is provided for each family member to understand and appreciate each other differently and to enhance interpersonal relationships in a way that may never have been possible without the occurrence of the hearing impairment. Family therapy may not be the solution to all the relevant issues. It at least allows, however, for the maintenance or the establishment of the personal integrity of each individual, regardless of other rehabilitative services deemed important or appropriate.

It is the hearing-impaired adult who must make the ultimate decison regarding further remediation for the impairment. To deny that person the power to do so would, in Schlesinger's view (1985), imply that the individual does not have "the cognitive competence, psychological skills, instrumental resources and support systems needed to influence his or her environment successfully" (p. 105).

Individual Counseling

Of all the counseling strategies, individual counseling is likely to be the most appropriate for adults with hearing impairment. Its relevance is determined by the degree to which the individual is adjusting to the loss and motivated toward being helped by amplification (if deemed necessary) and aural rehabilitation. In fact, it is best employed within the context of the audiological evaluation, the hearing aid fitting, and the aural rehabilitation process.

It is particularly important, however, that the audiologist be sensitive to the emergence of emotional attitudes or issues that do not relate directly to the hearing impairment. The individual can be gently encouraged to seek more intensive psychotherapeutic assistance if the problems cannot be dealt with professionally by the audiologist. Such referral, however, could also be self-defeating, if the "helper" is uninformed about the consequences of hearing impairment and practices the "medical model," which, according to Schlesinger (1985), sees the hearing-impaired person as "ill or incapacitated" (p. 111).

We tend to agree somewhat with Schlesinger's view, based on the research of Coates, Renzaglia, and Embree (1983), that considerable evidence exists to suggest "that well meaning helpers may often do more harm than good" (p. 110). Silbergeld's examination of the negative effects of psychotherapy (1983) is also pertinent. We believe, however, that the potential benefits of counseling far outweigh its negative effects. (Further discussion of this issue is found in Chapter 9.)

Above all, the hearing-impaired client's attitude toward counseling must be respected even if it means rejection of the process. The audiologist may have to be satisfied with providing information, even if it should only fulfill basic technical purposes such as accommodation to amplification or care and use of the aid. Speech reading, too, in such cases, may have to be treated solely as an educational process.

Moreover, it must be understood that many hearing-impaired adults learn to adapt to their loss without the client-centered counseling we would advocate for other hearing-impaired individuals. Thus we need to examine what our criteria should be and several counseling intervention guidelines.

Criteria for intervention   The individual who has been traumatized emotionally by the hearing loss and who has no external support from others is likely to welcome the input of an empathic, understanding, and caring audiologist. Likewise, the individual who is struggling to reconcile the known benefits from amplification with preconceived notions of the stigma attached to hearing aid use might be motivated to "talk out" the conflict if unable to make a decision.

There are some hearing-impaired individuals who initially are not willing to discuss their feelings of depression or explore the implications of their loss but, because they derive nonjudgmental support from their audiologist, may in time risk revealing very personal feelings they have been concealing. Oftentimes the aural rehabilitation process itself arouses feelings of frustration, struggle, or despair, and clients welcome the opportunity to ventilate their concerns, particularly if the modified approach is not identified as counseling per se.

Sometimes it is the spouse or other family member who seeks counseling assistance because he or she is unable to cope effectively with the hearing-impaired individual's continual self-pity, withdrawal, and depression and who has also refused counseling assistance. Although family therapy might be the treatment of choice in such instances, it is of little value without the participation of the hearing-impaired person. Nonetheless, counseling can at least assist the spouse in coping more effectively at home and may in fact indirectly help the other person as well.

Any decision by the audiologist to intervene psychotherapeutically must be based on the unique situational circumstances of the client with careful attention to individual client needs. It is impossible to generalize the effect of hearing loss on any one individual; thus the audiologist must view each case separately and be flexible enough to vary the therapeutic or educational approach as deemed appropriate.

Guidelines for client-centered intervention   Counseling begins once the individual has been informed of the degree and nature of the hearing loss following otological and audiological examination. Depending on the adaptive capabilities of the client, it may continue throughout the entire aural rehabilitation process, which includes learning to live with amplification. For the most part, counseling here is nothing more than effective communication therapy.

1. *Learning the facts about the loss.* Knowledge is enlightening but also painful. Once the reality has been objectified by means of the differential assessment, the worst fears are either realized or reduced. As information is provided, the client must have the opportunity to respond both affectively and cognitively. It may be difficult for the client to process all the information at once; thus care should be taken to impart information gradually and if necessary to repeat it in subsequent interviews, in order to avoid overloading.

2. *Providing a therapeutic environment for the interpersonal relationship.* Such an environment is one in which the audiologist can admit to the client that some questions like "How long will it take me to adjust to my aid?," "Will my hearing get worse?," "What if speech reading doesn't help me?," or "Will others get used to me and my hearing loss?" cannot be readily answered. But every attempt is made to be supportive of the client's concerns and understanding of even irrationally expressed attitudes. Being defensive or provid-

ing the client a false sense of security should be avoided so that the individual can gradually learn to adopt a realistic attitude toward the hearing impairment.

3. *Helping the client to become his or her own change agent.* A major goal in therapy is to encourage clients to take control of their own life relative to the hearing loss, use of amplification, and the maximizing of the opportunities to use the environment in the fullest way possible. The client is helped to recognize that there is a choice between wallowing in self-pity and depression or learning to live with the hearing impairment. The therapist must also realize that resistance to such a choice is natural and that vacillation is likely. Thus a confrontative approach should be used gently and caringly.

4. *Facilitating hearing aid use.* Orientation to the most effective use of amplification should be individualized so that the client will know what it can or cannot do for him or her. The frustrations and the delights associated with its use in varying situations should be reported and mutually analyzed. Modifications of settings, change of ear molds, internal adjustments, or even substitution of another aid may be necessary to maximize use. Any resistance expressed to wearing the aid requires continued therapeutic attention. The user, nevertheless, will have to make the ultimate decision, even if that decision is contrary to the wishes of the rest of the family.

5. *Integrating counseling with speech reading.* Frequently the attempts at learning to speech-read are fraught with frustration and intermittent failure. Conceivably, the client may be preoccupied with other matters that interfere with concentration. These other concerns will need to be aired and resolved so that the client will stay focused on the primary task at hand. Should the speech-reading process itself be difficult to master, the client must learn to realize that it is natural for some comprehension in speaking situations to be lost. Sometimes speech reading can be formally structured as part of the counseling dialogue itself and thereby serve comprehension and affective needs simultaneously. Most important for the client to realize is that speech reading can be learned but that it requires considerable diligence and effort to develop the skill.

6. *Dealing with depression and withdrawal from social interaction.* During the adjustment period, the client will experience wide shifts of mood and tend to feel cut off from others. He or she may in fact isolate himself or herself either as a means of coping or as a defense to fend off further anxiety. The client should recognize that such behavior is not unnatural and even that his or her wish not to discuss feelings is also acceptable. Indeed, some clients feel that they must reconcile their feelings with their loss through independent self-searching in spite of the "rescue" efforts by the therapist. It is better that clients feel free to engage the therapist at their own discretion rather than be prodded to disclose everything being experienced. If the client's depression should encompass all daily life situations, the therapist can at least indicate what he or she personally is perceiving and experiencing from the client and thereby indirectly motivate the person to share more.

7. *Making the environment more conducive to listening.* Sometimes clients must be helped to assert themselves more so as to create an environment whereby listening is better facilitated. It may include such things as requesting an amplified telephone for the office, educating fellow workers about the importance of speaking directly to him or her, or transferring to another job activity within the firm. At home, it means that the client will modify the listening environment by urging reduction in ambient noise from varying sources or improving the acoustics of the home. Generally, it means mastering control of the environment rather than becoming a victim of it.

Kaplan (1985) cites several references that should be helpful to the reader and discusses intervention strategies that can be used, particularly for the elderly client.

8. *Treating hearing loss when it is used or exaggerated as an expression of underlying psychological conflicts.* Occasionally, clients ostensibly will commit themselves to a regimen of aural rehabilitation, but at the same time sabotage efforts to make substantial gains. The following anecdote describes one such case:

Mia, a thirty-year-old Vietnamese woman with a severe to profound bilateral hearing loss acquired during her childhood in Vietnam, was making only minimal progress in an intensive aural rehabilitation program that included speech reading, auditory training, and speech and language training (for her foreign dialect and for speech conservation). She was also enrolled in an ESL (English as a Second Language) class. During actual clinical work, she was very cooperative and usually met the criteria for all of the tasks undertaken. Bilateral amplification was apparently also quite beneficial. The problem was little carryover from session to session so that her therapist was unable to increase the complexity of the tasks.

Mia lived with Victor, an American-born Caucasian two years younger than herself, who apparently had taken on a "Pygmalion" or "Henry Higgins" role in their living-together relationship. Only after several months of therapy was it learned that Mia had been living under considerable pressure from Victor to conform to his own expectations and practice her clinical assignments beyond any reasonable presumptions. Sensitive to Mia's need to talk about her relationship with Victor, the therapist provided clinical time for Mia to ventilate feelings of resentment, anger, and hostility toward Victor. He had been adamant in refusing joint counseling, viewing Mia's overall problems as her own, but he did make a modest attempt to reduce the pressure at home. Most revealing, after several weeks of counseling, was that Mia had been unwittingly fixating clinically in order to strike back at Victor and his paternalistic and dictatorial authority. Only through continual counseling did Mia arrive at a point where she could assert her independence and separate her hearing, speech, and language needs from her emotional relationship with Victor.

9. *Learning to accept a different self-image.* The degree to which a hearing-impaired adult is able to adjust his or her perception of self in relationship to the loss is determined in part by the quality of that individual's previous

emotional health and stability. In order for a client to move toward a more realistic attitude, it is necessary first for the therapist to help the person separate the objective reality of the loss from other issues that had been unresolved prior to the loss.

The therapist can also aid the client to have positive and realistic expectations that he or she can perform successfully with a hearing loss, which in turn will lead to a positive outcome. Bandura (1977) has described this treatment concept as self-efficacy, which is quite different from the concept of outcome expectancy whereby the individual only *believes* that a particular behavior will result in a particular outcome. Self-image is related to self-efficacy in the sense that if the client's perception of self as a hearing-impaired person is negative, then there is a greater likelihood that he or she will have lower expectations about communicating with others. Thus a positive outcome is less likely because of the implied self-fulfilling prophecy, which says that what a person expects will often happen.

The guidelines we have presented are not meant to characterize any one counseling approach but should reflect the personal and professional position of the therapist. They should also be followed within the context of the client's unique circumstances and personal needs. Above all, if the client resists what the therapist is attempting to accomplish, then it is important that other goals, strategies, or theories be generated in the hope that they may be better accepted.

Group Counseling

Among the elderly in particular, group counseling as part of the aural rehabilitation process appears to be the treatment of choice. Throughout the United States more and more senior citizen centers, often in conjunction with university or hospital speech-language and hearing programs, are offering space and personnel toward developing ongoing rehabilitation services. These are not meant to replace traditional therapeutic services but to augment them in very practical ways for the senior citizen with a hearing impairment. They are intended to serve as social support networks, self-help opportunities, and citizen participation possibilities to help reduce the alienation, depression, and worries older people experience in relation to their hearing loss and other physical ailments.

Although group counseling can certainly be beneficial for any age group, we have chosen to concentrate on its practicality for older clients. We outline several major advantages:

1. *Peer support.* There is nothing more lonely for an individual with a hearing impairment than to feel that he or she is the only person suffering from the effects of hearing impairment. The opportunity to share with one

another experiences, troubling concerns, and fears can help reduce feelings of vulnerability, incompetence, and helplessness. The peer counselor needs to allow for the greatest latitude in the communicative interpersonal relationships as they develop, but also serve as an information provider and feeling clarifier. The counselor must also be sensitive to the differing coping strategies each of the group members use and allow for the confrontations each makes on the others. The individual who refuses to wear an aid because of its intermittent discomfort is likely to be more responsive to another member who also has had the experience than to the counseling audiologist "who really doesn't understand what I'm going through."

2. *Enhancement of speech-reading skills.* There is no better situation in which to practice speech-reading skills than one that closely approximates the real world of the clients. Regardless of the difference between the safe, protective, and supportive milieu of group counseling and a noncaring, unconcerned, or rejecting environment outside of therapy, the counselor can readily simulate situations or communicative interactions that are similar and that have created difficulties for the members.

3. *Opportunities for coping with other issues.* A frequent concomitant benefit of group counseling is the opportunity for the members to explore with one another concerns that are separate from the hearing loss or that are only indirectly related. It is difficult to imagine, however, that the hearing impairment does not impinge on every aspect of the individual's life, to some degree at least. Consider, for example, relationships with grown children, managing retirement, loss of a spouse, getting older, other physical problems, and living out the remaining years creatively and productively. For the counselor, the task may appear formidable, but need not be so as long as he or she does not attempt to carry the burden of clients' concerns or act as rescuer.

4. *Cost-effectiveness.* Considering the drastic increases in the cost of medical and ancillary health services during the last twenty years, and the inability of the older population to afford such services, group counseling can be a welcomed opportunity to minimize the costs somewhat. Besides, local and state governments or charitable agencies are more likely to give financial support for such cost-efficient services, but only through public and professional lobbying and educational efforts.

5. *Citizen participation.* Group counseling may also serve to motivate its members to take a more active role in their community as they begin to recognize more clearly that their loss of hearing can become an opportunity for self-growth and for helping others. An excellent example of this is the founding of the Self-Help for Hard of Hearing People (SHHH) organization in 1979 by Stone (1985). This organization has given many hearing-impaired adults a new meaning for their lives as well as having become the advocate for hearing-impaired people in industry and government.

CONCLUSION

The psychological ramifications of hearing impairment in adults of all ages present the audiologist a challenge that cannot always be met by virtue of his or her previous traditional training. Although others in the psychotherapeutic helping professions serve an important and often significant role in caregiving for the hearing-impaired adult, it is the audiologist in particular who most frquently shares center stage with the client. Consequently, it is imperative that the audiologist develop the counseling skills that can be facilitated by his or her own natural intuitive abilities, interpersonal communication and clinical competence, and professional commitment.

REFERENCES

ALPINER, J. Psychological and social aspects of aging as related to hearing rehabilitation of elderly clients. In M. A. Henoch (Ed.), *Aural Rehabilitation for the Elderly*. New York: Grune & Stratton, 1979.

BANDURA, A. Self-efficacy: Toward a unifying theory of behavioral change. *Psychological Review*, 84 (1977), 191–215.

BLAIR, J. C., and BERG, F. S. Problems and needs of hard-of-hearing students and a model for the delivery of services to the schools. *Asha*, 24 (1982), 541–546.

BOOTHROYD, A. *Hearing Impairments in Young Children*. Englewood Cliffs, N.J.: Prentice-Hall, 1982.

BRESLAU, L. D., and HAUG, M. R. (Eds.), *Depression and Aging—Causes, Care and Consequences*. New York: Springer-Verlag, 1983.

CLARK, J. G. Counseling in a pediatric audiologic practice. *ASHA*, 24 (1982), 521–526.

COATES, D., RENZAGLIA, G., and EMBREE, M. When helping backfires: Help and helplessness. In J. D. Fisher and A. Nadler (Eds.), *New Directions in Helping*, Vol. I: *Recipient Reactions to Aid*. New York: Academic Press, 1983.

CULROSS, R. R. Adaptations of the pictorial self-concept scale to measure self-concept in young hearing-impaired children. *Language Speech and Hearing Services in the Schools*, 16 (April 1985), 132–134.

DEE, A. D. Meeting the needs of the hearing parents of deaf infants: A comprehensive parent-education program. *Lanugage, Speech and Hearing Services in the Schools*, 12 (1981), 13–19.

HAYES, D. Hearing problems in aging. In J. Jerger (Ed.), *Hearing Disorders in Adults*. San Diego, Calif.: College Hill Press, 1984.

HESS, D. W. Evaluation of personality and adjustment in deaf children using a modification of the make-a-picture story (MAPS) test. Ph.D. dissertation. University of Rochester, 1960.

HILL, R. Social stresses on the family: Generic features of families under stress. *Social Casework*, 39 (1958), 139–150.

JACOBSON, N. S., and BUSSOD, N. Marital and family therapy. In M. Henson, A. E. Kasdin, and A. S. Bellack (Eds.), *The Clinical Psychology Handbook*. New York: Pergamon Press, 1983.

JONGKEES, L. B. W. Psychological problems of the deaf. *Annals of Otology, Rhinology and Laryngology*, 92 (1983), 8–13.

KAPLAN, H. Benefits and limitations of amplification and speech reading for the elderly. In H. Orlans (Ed.), *Adjustment to Adult Hearing Loss*. San Diego, Calif.: College Hill Press, 1985.

LUTERMAN, D. *Counseling Parents of Hearing-Impaired Children*. Boston: Little, Brown, 1979.

———. The counseling experience. *Journal of the Academy of Rehabilitative Audiology*, 9 (1976), 62–66.

MURPHY, A. T. The families of handicapped children: Context for disability. In A. T. Murphy (Ed.), *The Families of Hearing Impaired Children*. *Volta Review*, 81 (1979), 265–278.

ORLANS, H. (Ed.). *Adjustment to Adult Hearing Loss*. San Diego, Calif.: College-Hill Press, 1985.

OYER, H. J., and OYER, E. J. Adult hearing loss and the family. In H. Orlans (Ed.), *Adjustment to Adult Hearing Loss*. San Diego, Calif.: College-Hill Press, 1985.

RAMSDELL, D. The psychology of the hard of hearing and the deafened adult. In H. Davis and S. R. Silverman (Eds.), *Hearing and Deafness*, Rev. ed. New York: Holt, Rinehart & Winston, 1960.

ROUSEY, C. Psychological reactions to hearing loss. *Journal of Speech and Hearing Disorders*, 36 (1971), 382–389.

SCHLESINGER, H. S. The psychology of hearing loss. In H. Orlans (Ed.), *Adjustment to Adult Hearing Loss*. San Diego, Calif.: College-Hill Press, 1985.

SCHLESINGER, H. S., and MEADOW, K. P. *Sound and Sign*. Berkeley: University of California Press, 1972.

SHONTZ, F. C. *The Psychological Aspects of Physical Illness and Disability*. New York: MacMillan, 1975.

SILBERGELD, B. *The Shrinking of America: Myths of Psychological Change*. Boston: Little, Brown, 1983.

STONE, H. E. Developing SHHH, a self-help organization. In H. Orlans (Ed.), *Adjustment to Adult Hearing Loss*. San Diego, Calif.: College-Hill Press, 1985.

STREAM, R. W., and STREAM, K. S., Counseling the parents of the hearing impaired child. In F. N. Martin (Ed.), *Pediatric Audiology*. Englewood Cliffs, N.J.: Prentice-Hall, 1978.

STUDDERT-KENNEDY, M. Speech perception. In N. J. Lass (Ed.), *Contemporary Issues in Experimental Phonetics*. New York: Academic Press, 1976.

SWEETOW, R. W., and BARRAGER, D. Quality of comprehensive audiologic care: A survey of parents of hearing-impaired children. *Asha* , 22 (1980), 841–847.

TSAPPIS, A. Personal communication. 1985.

VENTRY, I. M., and CHAIKLIN, J. B. Functional hearing loss: A problem in terminology. *Asha*, 4 (1962), 251–254.

9

THE USE OF POWER
IN THE THERAPEUTIC
RELATIONSHIP

ANALYSIS AND UNDERSTANDING OF THE CONCEPT
OF POWER

If we are to take Webster's definition of "power" as an "ability to act; capacity for action or being acted upon; capability of producing or undergoing an effect; . . . the possession of sway or controlling influence over others; also a person . . . invested with authority or influence or exercising control," then it is readily apparent we are applying the broadest perspective to the use of power in the therapeutic relationship in speech-language therapy.

Backus (1960), in her provocative study of psychological processes occurring in the client–therapist relationship in speech-language therapy, reminds us that we have placed so much emphasis on rational thinking that we have neglected our feelings and intuition, and are insufficiently aware of the creative power within us. She goes on to state:

> We have thought so largely of the "rescuing power" for our lives as coming from events, things and persons in the outside world. Thus when we *are* aware of feelings welling up from levels deeper than consciousness they are more often the negative ones. Moreover, what is unconscious in us is unknown

and we usually fear what is unknown. Psychic energy is indeed power to be respected and under certain conditions even to be feared. To be feared, however, should mean to be reckoned with creatively rather than to be ignored through further repression (p. 507).

Implicitly, then, we can view power as operating along a continuum representing both positive and negative aspects. Unfortunately, we cannot always be certain, or in agreement as to *what* is positive or negative, as that will depend on *who* makes the inference. Take, for example, the phrase "the use of power for the greatest good of the client." We are immediately confronted with the task of defining the nature of power as it may be used for a particular purpose. We must also define what is meant by "good" because that depends on the value judgments of who is *doing* and who is *receiving*. We can perhaps answer this dilemma by exploring first the motives behind the use of power.

Motives in "Helping"

On the surface, it would appear that the helping relationship is one in which the helper, the speech-language pathologist or audiologist, initiates a process whereby the client will be relieved of his or her communication impairment. Beneath this desirable altruistic aim, however, lies the very complex hidden agenda of the therapist, who may on one level enter the profession of speech-language pathology or audiology for money, satisfaction with the substantive nature of the field, or the pleasure derived from helping someone else, and on a deeper level for satisfying ego needs of power, validating oneself, or solving one's own problems. No value judgment should be implied here because our own human nature and uniqueness determine the course we follow in our professional and personal lives. That our motives indeed have hidden meanings urges us to explore these factors so that we can enhance our own personal and professional growth as well as that of our clients.

Guggenbuhl-Craig (1971), a Jungian psychiatrist, has introduced the thesis that in their desire to help, members of the helping professions can also psychologically damage their patients or clients. Although he refers in his writings more specifically to the physician, priest, teacher, psychotherapist, and social worker, speech-language pathologists and audiologists could be included in this group. He suggests that negative and positive motives get activated in helping. In one sense the helper is highly motivated to do all that is possible for the client, but at the same time may be imbued with a sense of self-importance and reflect an attitude of professional omnipotence. The helper then gets caught up in what Guggenbuhl-Craig describes as a "lust for power" over the client. This becomes most evident when the helper recognizes behavior by the client to be self-defeating or perhaps destructive. In attempting directly to change the behavior and overcome the client's resistance to change, the helper's power is demonstrated. The helper rationalizes its use in order to enforce what is "right and good for the client." This is not to suggest that the helper is harming the client per se. These actions, in fact, might be quite beneficial to the client. But there is the reality that the helper is unwittingly pretending to act selflessly. The more imbued the helper becomes with the ability to "know what's best," particularly when the client's behavior is positively changed, the greater the likelihood of making uncritical and questionable decisions later.

Nothing, however, can deaden our professional sense more than the sweet smell of therapeutic success. It lulls us into a state of complacency, and if we are later confronted with unexpected and difficult challenges from our clients, we are apt to rely on what has worked before. This is particularly evident if the new material is threatening to our own egos. When caught unaware we may tend to defend ourselves with the one arsenal we know is at our disposal—our professional power—and thereby possibly obscure the issues. Heller (1985), in his extensive study of the power relationship between the client and therapist, describes in great detail how power can enhance the therapeutic relationship, client confidence and hope, or how it can be used to induce client powerlessness and the imposition of the therapist's values. Heller is careful not to condemn dynamics of power but to analyze and unravel its elements as it is used in psychotherapy.

Applying a Transactional Analysis (TA) model as developed by Eric Berne, Hornyak (1980) describes how "games" are used in the interpersonal relationship in speech-language therapy, as a manifestation of "hidden agendas," which result in ulterior transactions between people. On the social level, the person may be doing or seeking one thing but on the inner or psychological level, the person may be doing or looking for something else. Because two persons are involved, the transaction first takes on the aspect of a "con" that is fed by the other person, who is also operating with a hidden agenda, referred to as a "gimmick." As Hornyak states:

> The two players now transact with each other until a crisis point or climactic moment occurs in which the relationship between the two players suddenly changes. This is called the switch and is followed by a state of confusion, called the crossup, in which both players try to figure out what has happened and determine why their relationship has changed. This is followed by a payoff for each player. Payoffs are familiar feelings such as despair, anger, hopelessness, or elation (p. 86).

We would agree that the communicative interaction between therapist and client is obscured and further contaminated by hidden motives, as implied by Hornyak's analysis. Yet we must also take into account the fact that the therapist and client do not start out on the same level as assumed by a TA interpretation. The client, from the onset, is in the inferior position, whereas the helper is in the position of authority or power. Thus it is the *helper's* major responsibility to initiate and maintain a constructive transactional process.

In our view, the helper uses power as a means for self-protecton. Carl Jung (1968) has explained this self-protection to be within all of us and related to the "shadow side of our unconscious." That is, we are not always aware, or do not always have a conception, of why we behave the way we do. This unknowing part of ourselves is characterized by our unrealized potentialities, undiscovered fears and conflicts, and the aspects of ourselves we resist looking at. That is, the "shadow" represents thoughts, feelings, and attitudes that, although unknown to us, characterize much of our daily behaviors and interactions with others. For example, if the client, during the early phase of the therapeutic relationship, asks for justification of the fee being charged, the therapist may either deal with this issue in an objective, mature, way, fully conscious of personal attitudes toward money, or may react in a subjective, defensive manner, unaware of the deep-rooted attitude stirred. Unwittingly, the therapist may be concealing personal material that is threatening, and this behavior is subsequently characterized by a need to dominate the relationship as a means of self-protection. This gets translated into a demonstration of power over the client in which the therapist is in a safe, superior position to maintain control over the client and the therapeutic situation.

Projection and the "Shadow Side"

Certainly, we would be loathe to admit that we actually derive pleasure or comfort from feeling superior to our clients and that we are egotistical or self-serving. The fact that we have chosen a humanitarian profession, often characterized by frustration, nebulous outcomes, and sadness, suggests that the choice may derive from our own unresolved or even resolved struggles. We are not always in complete control of our psyches, conscious of all our motivations and needs, or immune to the pain and struggles of our clients. We are indeed affected by our clients.

In our attempts to help we could actually be resisting our own negative impulses that may in some way be associated with attitudes and behaviors of our clients. These resistances are generally connected to projections that we define as the casting out on another person the ideas and impulses that belong to us, oblivious to the real person with whom we are relating. This is where power may get negatively expressed. Our unawareness of many of our inner struggles distorts the possibility of a completely objective appraisal of our clients. Judgments, therefore, may be made not in accordance with what the client truly needs but in terms of what the helper is needing. The more material our clients evoke, the greater the possibility for our "shadow side" to be activated in conjunction with our increased use of negative power.

We are not questioning our conscious intention here but only the ramifications of our own unrealized expectations and attitudes that may be connected to our personal inner struggles. As Guggenbuhl-Craig describes it, "There is a perpetual split between conscious values and the power of the shadow which would like to destroy those values." According to Jung, it takes considerable moral effort to become conscious of our "shadow" because it means looking at those parts of ourselves we do not like. Although this is essential for self-knowledge, we resist because of the painstaking work involved. Although it is possible for us to assimilate aspects of our shadow into our conscious personalities, there are certain features that defy assimilation because they are too frightening to acknowledge and therefore are usually connected to projections.

The author recalls a graduate student who admittedly could not work effectively with her client because "he is so hard to like." This in effect isolated the therapist from her client. To objectify who that client really was meant that the therapist had to be willing to explore deeply within herself what she was projecting onto her client. Obviously, this client represented some things the therapist could not face within herself. Fortunately, in this case, the student was determined to discover what was so disturbing to her about her client and ultimately was able to admit to herself that he reminded her of certain things she "detested" in herself. Interestingly, once she brought this revelation to consciousness, she not only began to relate more positively to her client but also began to feel better about herself as a person and as a therapist. The student, unsurprisingly, has since developed into a highly competent and mature speech-language pathologist.

This example not withstanding, we should be leery of making the generalization that one instant of self-revelation is all that it takes to become an objective therapist. The student now saw the opportunity and the need to learn more about herself, albeit with considerable effort and courage.

ONSET OF THE THERAPEUTIC RELATIONSHIP

The initial sessions in speech-language therapy are critical in that they determine, in part, how the client–therapist relationship will evolve and the direction the therapy process will take. We must bear in mind that the course of therapy will be determined in part not so much by what the therapist *does* but who that person *is*. Jung's theory of personality type is relevant to our discussion here (Campbell 1971).

Jung believed that though there are basic differences in the way people use their perception and judgment, it does not mean that people are necessarily right or wrong, bad or good. It does mean, however, according to Myers (1962), that "people differ systematically in what they perceive and the conclusions they come to . . ." and "as a result (they) show corresponding differences in their reactions, in their interests, values, needs, and motivations, in what they do best and in what they like best to do" (p. 1).

Jung's theory is particularly important when we consider the effects of power as it emerges in the therapeutic relationship. That is, we must understand that the way power is used by the therapist is on the basis of how that person judges and perceives the client within the reality of the therapeutic situation. The use of negative or positive power is not to be viewed as good or bad, right or wrong, but merely as the manifestation of complex interpersonal dynamics within the therapeutic environment.

The Purpose of Therapy

Crucial to the development of the relationship and the progression of therapy are the conscious purposes first established by both the client and the therapist. The client desires to improve the ability to communicate. The therapist is viewed as the expert who will remove the problem so that the client will be able to communicate like everyone else. The therapist, too, has a conscious purpose—to help the client develop a more normal way of communicating. On the surface at least, there appears to be congruence between the client's and therapist's goals, but the reality is quite different, as we shall see.

Purpose of the client Beneath the overt expectation or intention to communicate more effectively are unconscious motives that contain expectations of which neither the client nor the therapist may be aware. Unwittingly, the client also desires to be free of all other of life's problems as well. Thus the therapist could easily be assigned the role of "savior" by the client. For example, the aphasic adult, aside from desiring full language recovery, may unconsciously seek resolution of premorbid marital difficulties through the empathic therapist. In doing so, the client tends to relinquish control over personal choice-making possibilities, putting the therapist in the position of making a choice to either welcome or reject the opportunity. If the therapist chooses the former, the "savior" role expectation of the client is strengthened and perhaps guaranteed. If, however, the therapist chooses to deal only with language issues, the client's purpose is incompletely satisfied. We shall discuss the implication of this later.

Purpose of the therapist Meanwhile, the therapist has the conscious purpose of helping the client to develop a more normal way of communicating. Conducive to this goal is the conscious aim to use predetermined strategies that are believed by the therapist to be appropriate to the presented problem. The way in which these strategies are employed also depends on the philosophical orientation of the therapist, be it behavioral, humanistic, directive, or nondirective, or combinations of these. Consciously or unconsciously, the therapist may also wish to help the client resolve other personal issues related directly or indirectly to the main problem. Regardless of the goals, the therapist attempts to enlist the client's help in improving or modifying the communication disorder.

On a conscious level at least, we might say that the therapist is using power appropriately. But as we have already noted, the unconscious shadow side may also be operating. On one level the therapist may be caught between the desire to be the expert who will help this "poor fellow" and the realistic unwillingness to take on the perhaps frustrating burden of helping the client make changes in other aspects of living. On the deeper level, though, the decision is influenced by the therapist's own unconscious needs that may emerge at the onset of therapy as projections, which in turn will determine the nature of the therapeutic alliance.

The Therapeutic Alliance

We have seen that the therapist's initial conscious intention may be to enlist the client's help in improving the latter's communicative ability. The client's conscious intention is to have the therapist solve the communication problem. The two intentions are not necessarily incompatible as long as it is made clear from the outset what is expected of the client, why practice is important, and what the focus of therapy will be. If these are acceptable to the client, there appears little likelihood of an ensuing power struggle. If, on the other hand, these intentions are not first clarified by the therapist, a power struggle could emerge. The client may find it very frustrating and believe it unimportant to practice outside of formal therapy. Meanwhile, the therapist believes outside practice to be crucial in order for any change to take place and cajoles the client into practicing. Not only is the stage set for the development of a parent–child relationship, as described by Berne (1964), which can interfere with client growth, but also for activation of unconscious elements in the client that can sabotage the therapeutic process.

The relationship takes on greater complexity if the client expects and hopes to rely on the therapist to find solutions to all of his or her problems. Here the therapist would be taking on the projections of the client and may find it difficult not to be affected by them. The therapist may, in fact, enforce power and prominence as a result of having his or her own unconscious tapped.

Guggenbuhl-Craig describes the intensification of the power struggle between therapist and client as a "game of sorcerer-and-apprentice." The client expects and hopes to find the all-powerful sorcerer who will answer everything. How much "magic" or power the therapist exerts on the client depends of course on the degree to which the therapist has recognized and acknowledged the "shadow" personally and the projections that emanate from it.

But even the "magical alliance" cannot tolerate the effects of other underlying issues. For example, the client may resist the home assignments because they interfere with other urgent needs. The client's wife may be an impatient person who will resist taking on the role of "therapy aide." She could do so, but grudgingly, and the client recognizes it. Here, again, the therapist's projections intrude into the therapeutic relationship. Puzzled by the client's apparent uncooperativeness and stubbornness, the therapist readily generalizes that the client is essentially negative toward his rehabilitation. If the therapist has had previous experiences with negative clients, personal preconceived attitudes now appear. The situation is made more complicated by the spouse's psychological processes, and the struggle between client and therapist becomes acute. It can become so powerful that it may obstruct therapeutic success and destroy the entire therapeutic process before it can begin.

THE POWER STRUGGLE
IN ONGOING THERAPY

We now need to look more closely at how the complex interpersonal relationship manifests itself in ongoing therapy and in the communication process.

The Conflict Between Conscious
and Unconscious Intentions

It has been seen that in a clinical relationship the client's and the therapist's conflicting intended goals may be obscured or distorted by unconscious motives, which in turn may create a power struggle. This may not be apparent at first, but through the ongoing relationship the conflict between conscious and unconscious intentions begins to emerge.

Hood (1974) has described the difficulty with which the client faces change and growth, because of fear of the unknown and defense to challenge or threat. The therapist, according to Hood, must be in tune personally in order to be sensitive to the client's needs. If not, an incongruence will develop between the parties, resulting in friction, denial, and defensiveness. The therapist must now deal not only with client's hidden agenda but with his or her own as well so that the interpersonal interaction can be relatively free of contamination.

It is the therapist's task, nonetheless, to establish a hierarchy of procedures that the client must follow in order to achieve success in ameliorating the identified speech-language disorder. The therapist is now in the seat of power. As long as the client cooperates (making the clinician feel successful), all will be well. This is not to imply that the client will not benefit. The client, obviously, also wants to eliminate the speech-language problem, but at what cost? The client must put oneself at the "mercy" of the therapist, which could trigger elements associated with the shadow, thereby making him or her vulnerable in terms of self-concept. In this way, the client loses power as new patterns of behavior are adopted that may appear very foreign.

The client thus must put complete faith in the therapist, but is that possible? Not if there are more powerful unconscious forces that contribute to the client's vulnerability. Not if it means the client can no longer use the disorder, such as stuttering, to define or justify a current mode of personal existence. Moreover, if the client has become overly dependent on the therapist, the opportunity to take greater responsibility for the problem and its solution will be hindered. Hood reminds us too of "the inability of the client to accept present and changing roles, status and relationship conflicts, and to give up using [the disorder] as an ego-protecting mechanism" (p. 51).

The Therapist's Role

Defining the therapist's role in the therapeutic relationship is probably the most complex, challenging, and deceptive aspect of speech-language therapy procedures, in that it assumes we can objectively decide what that role should be. As Perkins (1974) has noted: " The intervention of one person, the therapist, in the life of another, the client, is sufficiently sanctified when done in the name of therapy that motives, reasons, and effects are rarely examined" (p. 369). Alluding to the therapist's hidden agenda, Perkins asks us to consider our values, motives, therapeutic orientation, professional responsibilities, and training with respect to our clinical intervention. Most relevant in our view is the choice, conscious or unconscious, that the therapist makes in the pursuit of improving defective communication. Let us examine several of these possible choices.

As benign dictator   At one extreme, the therapist may choose to assume the role of "benign dictator," legislating every step the client must take in order to communicate more effectively, discounting "extraneous" material (elements such as the client's unconscious connection between sexual and communicative adequacy) and charismatically intimidating the client into accepting what the therapist believes is best. The therapist justifies this approach by reason of education, ability, and previous successes. Not only is the therapist the "expert," but the judge and jury as well, who will insist that the client conform to the therapeutic regimen established.

Here the therapist's use of negative power comes into full play. The more the client conforms to the therapist's prescription, the more impressed the therapist becomes with a personal image as healer and the less likely to recognize personal underlying motives. If the client questions or resists certain intervention strategies, the therapist views this as childlike and asserts power as a parent. In either case, the therapist deprives the client of responsibility for the problem and may destroy the very process that would ensure communicative success, that is, the develpment of a process through which the client must learn to take charge and to cope when the therapist is no longer present.

The client's realization of success in speaking and independence is not a threat to the therapist's conscious goal but to the unconscious motives that characterize the therapist's shadow side and represent individual life struggles. These may consist of needs for control and dominance that compensate for feelings of self-doubt and inferiority and that placate strivings for self-worth. The client also responds on the conscious level, unaware of the dominant unconscious motives that characterize his or her own shadow side. These may consist of a need to always be in control, for total independence, and for complete self-sufficiency, perhaps compensating for more deeply rooted feelings of low self-esteem. What results is a dual intra-interpsychic conflict represented as a struggle for power.

It would be difficult for the therapist we are describing to acknowledge, in response to the client, that "there, but for the grace of God, go I." Certainly, such an admission would not be permissible for that person, and moreover would serve no purpose. What is of chief importance to the benign dictator is that as long as the communication disorder is improved, nothing else is relevant as far as speech-language therapy is concerned. If that is so, then perhaps we are only technicians who should limit ourselves to the surface aspects of communication and refrain from involvement in meaningful interpersonal relationships in therapy.

As benign supertherapist   At a different point on the continuum there is the therapist who feels qualified (though may not be) to cope with all of the client's conflicts and problems that are associated directly, indirectly, or not all with the speech-language problem. This person is the "benign supertherapist," who, being in the power position as helper, attempts to intrude into the client's unconscious world and takes on the responsibility of facilitating not only effective use of speech and language but also changes in all aspects of the client's life. For this therapist, it is not enough to deal only with symptomatic features of, let us say, a functional voice disorder. The therapist is interested in making the client aware not only of etiological factors associated with vocal dysfunction but of other dysfunctional aspects of that person's life. Here is a situation where the client's conscious intention to "correct my voice problem" is given secondary importance by the clinician, who believes that permanent vocal change can come about only through the analysis of the client's personality and emotional attitudes.

We characterize this approach as negative use of power by the therapist. Even if the client accedes to the therapeutic desires of the therapist, the unconscious motives of each are activated. And if there is an immediate conflict between the client's and therapist's conscious motives, the conflict is further intensified. The therapist interprets the client's appropriately realistic resistance as a refusal to face the facts. The therapist cannot recognize that perhaps irritation felt toward the client is related to deep-seated insecurities about personal therapeutic competence, or deeper yet, related to unresolved conflicts over strict parental controls in the therapist's own childhood. The client, in turn, is threatened by possible exposure of personal material with which she or he has not dealt with or of which that person is unaware. For the client, the therapist may also represent a parental figure to whom the client may still be bonded.

The ensuing power struggle may result in any one of several possibilities. The therapist ultimately dominates, coercing the client to accept "what is good for her." The client then acquiesces, discounting the validity of her early conscious intention. Or the client resists, her lack of cooperation interpreted as unwillingness to work on her voice problem. Or the client chooses to terminate therapy, labeling the therapist as "one of those Freudian kooks" and blocking off any desire to change her vocal behavior or look beyond the vocal symptoms. Any subsequent encounter with another therapist is likely to be viewed with perhaps natural overcautious concern, which could inhibit therapy based on a different orientation.

The therapist, too, is ultimately affected by whatever course therapy takes. Forced to confront the many challenges, inner and outer, to personal "expertise," a self-protective professional barrier is erected to fend off threats by other clients. In doing so, the therapist consolidates individual power, further abrogating objectively conceived conscious intentions.

As sophisticated therapist   Even the more sophisticated psychotherapeutically oriented therapist may be treading on territory well obscured by the client's major conscious intention and fall victim to personally established intellectualizations. Considering, as an example, the adult aphasic client, the therapist may lose sight of the more pressing functional linguistic needs of the client. Astute as the therapist's assessment of the client's psychosocial state may be, and competent in the subsequent psychological counseling of the patient and/or family, the risk is run of raising issues that may actually impede linguistic progress.

Several years ago, the author had created a therapeutic situation whereby his fifty-five-year-old female right hemiplegic, apraxic and aphasic client was provided the opportunity to ventilate long-repressed feelings of resentment toward her husband. Although unrelated to her stroke, her anger and depression replaced any desire to focus attention on her apraxic use of language. Nonetheless, after five months of psychotherapeutic counseling twice a week, she had achieved a level of better than minimal functional communication. During the fourth month of therapy, she expressed misgivings about not "working on language exercises." When these were introduced, however, she elected to continue talking about her "empty marriage" and "thoughtless husband." (It should be noted that both she and her husband had adamantly refused family therapy.) Also during the fourth month postonset, she began to have consistent attacks of diarrhea immediately prior to her therapy session. Toward the end of the fifth month of therapy, she confirmed her personal physician's and this author's private analyses by stating insightfully and linguistically perfectly, "I guess I don't want to let go of all my shit." Unsurprisingly, she chose to terminate therapy rather than delve further into the "emptiness of my thirty years of marriage." She refused, also, any therapy limited to traditional strategies, as these too she felt would "get my head working again."

This clinical anecdote illustrates that although the immediate functional linguistic needs of the patient were not necessarily neglected, the therapist was in a sense "seduced" by the clinical challenge of dealing with a classic dysfunctional marital realtionship. Disregarding the stirrings of his own shadow side, his negative power was constellated in his attempt to prove his hypothesis. An early decision was made to satisfy the author's own "professional expertise," thereby encouraging an ambivalent client to discuss long repressed issues for which no real solutions could be attained during speech-language therapy. Had she been able and willing to delve more deeply into her own shadow side, she perhaps could have achieved a more meaningful awareness of herself and begun to consider other options open to her. Had the author been fully in tune with his own shadow, regardless of his client's level of awareness, the employment of purely traditional speech-language treatment strategies might have been efficacious and justified.

It should not be presumed, however, that the client would still have continued therapy. Given this particular client and special environmental circumstances, it is conceivable that no therapeutic strategy would have been ultimately successful, despite the functional level of communicative competence actually achieved. The author, confronted with a moral dilemma, made a choice based on his experience and level of self-awareness. That the client too made a choice to terminate therapy suggests how tenuous therapeutic relationships are, and emphasizes again the significance of the human factor in all of us.

As benevolent therapist   Typically, we would be more familiar with the helper who can be described as the "benevolent therapist." Although use of undesirable power may not be expressed to the degree in the previous examples, it may be exercised in a more subtle manner and yet contain elements that can be manipulative.

Take, for example, the stuttering client whose conscious intention to become fluent is congruent with the therapist's conscious intention. A behavioral approach in conjunction with client-centered counseling has been initiated and mutually acceptable. Therapy may in fact proceed with the client carrying out successfully the fluency contracts that have been mutually agreed upon. The client may also feel free to reveal in therapy elements that heretofore had been hidden unconsciously. Because these elements relate to the stuttering behavior, the therapist listens and attempts to understand. The client, highly responsive to the therapist's empathic attitude, now feels freer to share more, or may use the occasion to avoid pertinent issues by discussing social niceties. But this is now intruding upon therapeutic time necessary for contract time directly related to fluency improvement.

What may be occurring is either the germination of resistance to more difficult contract work or else the emergence of a need to discuss anxieties concerning stuttering and/or other related issues. In any case, the therapist's previous attitude of composure is disrupted. The therapist may respond initially by gently persuading the client to stay with the contract or may allow the client to continue exploring other concerns. If the former is pursued, the therapist may meet with greater resistance by the client and then have to cope with personal feelings of guilt for having forced the issue. If, on the other hand, the therapist accedes to the client's wishes, the client may feel compromised and that he or she is not accomplishing "all that I should be doing."

Regardless of the choice made, the therapist's shadow side is evoked and the therapist may begin to feel frustrated, angry, or helpless. The therapist's projections are now manifested by the manner in which control over the client and therapist power are displayed. The therapist feels overwhelmed by the client's ambivalent attitudes, unable to separate his or her own feelings of powerlessness from the struggles of the client. If the therapist refrains from coercion, and continues to go along with the client, he or she may be denying a growing anger or frustration. If the therapist dictates the course therapy must follow, the initial agreement with the client has been nullified. In a sense, the therapist feels "damned if I do and damned if I don't." Either way power is used negatively. The client is no longer the subject of real concern because the therapist becomes bound up in personal psychic struggles. (Naturally such therapists would deny this preoccupation and appear to most observers to be in full control of the clinical situation and their clients.)

Even if we were to predict that the likelihood of a positive therapeutic outcome would depend on everything in therapy progressing by the book, we would have to ask the question: "Whose book?" And if a prescriptive therapy model is dictated initially, the further question arises: "Can it be followed?"

As powerless therapist   On the continuum where the therapist relinquishes all apparent power, there would certainly be little hope or reason for any improvement in the communicative impairment being treated. Hopefully, we might assign such a label as "powerless therapist" only to novice student therapists who would be receiving the best in professional supervision. (The delicate issue of supervisory power and its use is familiar to many students as well as former students, but we have chosen not to discuss it at this time. Perhaps the reader who is both therapist and supervisor may uncomfortably identify with several issues presented in this chapter. If so, let the shoe fit as it may!)

The client receiving therapy from a powerless therapist would be confused and bewildered by his or her lack of intention or power. In Transactional Analysis terms, the therapist may take on the role of "Child" in order to get approval from the client, who is projected upon as the "Parent." In doing so, the therapist wills all control of the therapeutic situation to the client. But this may be characterized as a form of manipulation that has evolved from the therapist's shadow side and could be considered an aspect of negative power unconsciously used. The end result would be therapeutic chaos, driving the client away to seek someone more competent. Should the client choose to remain in the therapeutic situation, satisfying client power needs, the therapeutic process is also unlikely to have a positive outcome.

Ridiculous and unimaginable as the powerless therapist example may seem, it may not be as infrequent as we would wish and does point up the inevitable interplay of unproductive unconscious intentions when conscious motives are allowed to be distorted.

USE OF POSITIVE POWER

The use of power in and of itself is not necessarily destructive, and the illustrative examples given are not meant to imply absolute and distinct therapeutic conditons or rigidly categorize therapists. As therapists, we not only vary our roles according to the clients with whom we work but also our clinical behavior for any one client. Thus it is likely that the distinction between the types of therapists we have described may begin to blur. Obviously, though we may always strive for perfection as therapists, we cannot expect to succeed all the time. It is not surprising, then, if we see a little bit of each type of therapist in all of us.

Ideally, what we hope to learn, however, is that the therapist who guides and yet is flexible to the client's needs will provide a therapeutic environment where the client can grow and change within his or her greatest potential. We refer to the therapist who does not take on personally every negative response by the client, but uses the response constructively to help the client. That is, the therapist is able to separate personal ego concerns from those of the client, uncontaminated by psychological projection. In so doing, the therapist must be able and willing to assume the challenge of the client's projections, fully aware of the power assigned as a natural consequence of the therapeutic role. The therapist must also be conscious of how dramatically the power element may change during the therapeutic process, aware of the subtle nuances that may sometimes challenge the therapist's therapeutic role and authority.

We are not suggesting that the ideal therapeutic relationship should be free of any power struggle. Such struggles are common and natural to all interpersonal relationships, particularly the therapeutic relationship. They could well serve as catalysts for positive change in the client, enabling the latter to confront issues that heretofore may have inhibited progress. They also provide opportunities for the therapist to change and grow personally and professionally with each client experienced. Simultaneously, power struggles provide opportunities for the client to assume more responsibility for change, taking power into his or her own hands and gradually weaning him- or herself away from dependency on the therapist.

In Chapter 1 on counseling, we discussed transference and countertransference and their effects on the therapeutic process. It is readily apparent that such dynamics are intrinsic to projection, but when viewed objectively by both client and therapist, they can be put to productive use for the mutual benefit of all, by raising self-awareness and contributing to personal growth.

THE CHALLENGE TO THE THERAPIST

Our therapeutic task is formidable. It entails, first of all, our willingness and action to search within ourselves to discover those unconscious elements that constitute personal anxieties, struggles, biases, and unresolved conflicts. This certainly can be difficult and emotionally painful; our natural tendency is to resist looking at those aspects of ourselves that threaten us. Nonetheless, it behooves us to attempt to understand what the personal shadow components mean and how they enter into and intrude upon the therapeutic relationship.

Perhaps the most difficult task of all is for us to be willing to maintain a constant vigil over our shadows. We cannot assume that once we have been enlightened by a new self-discovery that we can now "work it all out with the client" and be done with it. Our personal shadow world is in constant flux, always revealing newer and perhaps more threatening features as we move through life's experiences. This becomes more apparent to us with each new client interaction. It is all too easy for those of us with many years of professional experience to rest on the laurels of success and to discount opportunities to look within ourselves during the therapeutic process. In fact, the more comfortable we feel as therapists, the greater the danger of being intoxicated by our own power. As Guggenbuhl-Craig aptly puts it: "He cannot, like the biblical Isaac, spend just one night wrestling with the angel to win his blessing. His struggle for the blessing must last a lifetime." (p. 155).

Finally, we must recognize that as long as we are human as well as professionals, we can never be perfect in all of our behaviors and that we will always err, depending on certain circumstances. But we must realize that we also have within us the power to choose to continue to err or to change our actions so that our clients can derive the full benefit not only of our professional expertise but also our humanness as well.

RESEARCH CONSIDERATIONS

In this chapter several theoretical issues have been raised and a number of assumptions implied. To put these to experimental testing presents a prodigious task, one with which researchers of the Jungian orientation have had to struggle. We, nonetheless, believe that some attempt, difficult as it may be, can be initiated to support the conjectures made.

It appears to us that one of the most crucial questions we must answer is, How can we objectively analyze what occurs during the interactional therapy process? Collaterally, what is it that we wish to measure? A linguistic discourse analysis, alluded to in Chapter 1, would not provide us with the necessary objective analysis of the affectual and attitudinal features discussed here. Labov and Fanshel (1977) explored the goals and techniques of psychotherapy through precise analysis of linguistic forms used by the therapist and client during fifteen minutes of one session—hardly sufficient to generalize to other clients, therapists, and circumstances. Bandler and Grinder (1975) applied transformational grammar clinically in their analyses of psychotherapy, translating surface structures into deep ones systematically, but failed to provide any penetrating analysis of underlying motives, much less any sufficient understanding of the affectual interactional process. Weintraub (1981) demonstrated the possiblity of defining and measuring several speech characteristics apparently related to psychological defense mechanisms in the psychotherapeutic process. He developed a system of verbal behavior analysis that was highly sensitive to nuances of style among various groups of individuals sharing deviant styles of thinking and behavior. Flanagan (1954) developed the Critical Incident Technique (CIT), consisting of a series of procedures for making direct observations of human behavior. It has been demonstrated to be highly effective in measuring typical peformances in various occupational settings, in measuring proficiency, motivation, and leadership, and in counseling and psychotherapy.

Flanagan's and Weintraub's investigations would be fruitful avenues of research to follow in formulating objective analyses of the interactional process in speech-language therapy. With the aid of computer-based data collection, it would be possible to correlate many variables simultaneously in the analysis of syntactic, semantic structures. It should be understood, however, that at the present time computers will not solve all the inherent variables associated with measurable categories of verbal expressions. We would be naive, also, to hope that scoring systems on computers could be sensitive enough to lead toward validation of Jung's concept of shadow or of unconscious processes per se. It is hoped, however, that we could be provided with an effective base for understanding the complex dynamics of manipulative functions both positive and negative in speech-language therapy.

CONCLUSION

In this chapter we have attempted to describe the complexity of the interpersonal relationship in speech-language therapy relative to the way power becomes manifest in that relationship. We have seen that when elements of our psyches coincide with those of our clients there is the possiblity that deeply unconscious motives, represented by our shadow side, may dominate and perhaps endanger the therapeutic process. When this occurs in us, as therapists we may easily lose sight of what our clients genuinely need and in doing so may exert negative power over them. We illustrated several ways in which power is used by therapists with different psychological traits and how adult clients may affect and be affected by the helping process. Although child clients were not discussed, it should be readily apparent that they would be vulnerable to the clinician's power and thus a greater challenge to the therapist's struggle for objectvity.

As Pickering (1984) has suggested in a revealing study of interpersonal communication in speech-language pathology supervisory conferences, supervisors and students "appeared to lack knowledge about how to analyze the interpersonal dimension of therapeutic relationships." Pickering futher adds that "client change will need to be complemented by an emphasis on process-oriented, transactional, and existential-phenomenological issues" (p. 195). We would concur, and thereby encourage our profession to take steps toward facilitating and understanding the complex dynamics underlying the interpersonal relationships in speech-language pathology.

A final note is in order. Despite the necessity for being conscious of all of the psychological factors related to power that impinge on the therapeutic relationship, we need not be ashamed of the pride we feel when we do indeed help our clients communicate more effectively. The "good" we do in fact says much for the essential emotional health of speech-language-hearing professionals and the clinical competency with which we practice. We conclude with the question: "Why not enhance our skills and ourselves even further?"

REFERENCES

BACKUS, O. The study of psychological processes in speech therapists. In Barbara, D. A. (Ed.), *Psychological and Psychiatric Aspects of Speech and Hearing*. Springfield, Ill.: Chas. C Thomas, 1960.

BANDLER, R., and GRINDER, J. *The Structure of Magic I: A Book about Language and Therapy*. Palo Alto, Calif.: Science and Behavior Books, 1975.

BERNE, E. *Games People Play: The Psychology of Human Relationships*. New York: Grove Press, 1964.

CAMPBELL, J. (Ed.). *The Portable Jung*. New York: Viking, 1971.

FLANAGAN, J. C. The critical incident technique. *Psychological Bulletin*, 51 (1954), 327–358.

GUGGENBUHL-CRAIG, A. *Power in the Helping Professions*. Irving, Tex.: Spring, 1971.

HELLER, D. *Power in Therapeutic Practice*. New York: Human Sciences Press, 1985.

HOOD, S. B. Clients, Clinicians and Therapy. In L. L. Emerick and S. B. Hood, *The Client-Clinician Relationship*. Springfield, Ill.: Chas. C Thomas, 1974.

HORNYAK, A. J. The rescue game and the speech-language pathologist. *Asha*, 22 (1980), 86–89.

JUNG, C. G. *Analytical Psychology: Its Theory and Practice (The Tavistock Lectures)*. New York: Pantheon, 1968.

LABOV, W., and FANSHEL, D. *Therapeutic Discourse: Psychotherapy as Conversation*. New York: Academic Press, 1977.

MYERS, I. B. *Myers-Briggs Type Indicator Manual*. Palo Alto, Calif.: Consulting Psychologists Press, 1962.

PERKINS, W. H. *Speech Pathology: An Applied Behavioral Science*. St. Louis, Mo.: C. V. Mosby, 1974.

PICKERING, M. Interpersonal communication in speech-language pathology supervisory conferences: A qualitative study. *Journal of Speech Hearing Disorders*, 49 (May 1984), 184–195.

WEINTRAUB, W. *Verbal Behavior: Adaptation and Psychopathology*. New York: Springer-Verlag, 1981.

APPENDIX: RECOMMENDED TRAINING REQUIREMENTS

It should be obvious from the theme and substantive nature of this book that most traditionally trained speech-language pathologists and audiologists are generally unprepared academically and clinically to counsel effectively with the communicatively impaired or their families. Although the American Speech-Language-Hearing Association has professed the importance and desirability for counseling expertise in its members, there has been minimal evidence of university communication disorders curriculum support to satisfy that requirement. Despite the fact that some programs do offer courses in parent counseling, psychodynamics, and counseling theory and practice, and further recommend that electives be taken in psychology, counseling, and social work departments, most graduates feel ill-prepared to cope effectively with the psychological needs of their clients and families.

The dilemma for most programs is that they are already overburdened by professional demands for futher course offerings in such subject matter as dysphagia, head injury, linguistics, and specialized diagnostic test instruments. Academicians in the profession can certainly add several others to the list.

We do not wish to suggest that current programs need be drastically altered to fit the philosophical position presented in this text, although many programs throughout the country are continually being modified to satisfy new and unmet needs of the profession. We do recommend that the following suggestions and rationale be considered and that they at least be openly debated. It will be evident that several ideas are already implemented and should add greater validity to our proposal.

1. Undergraduate students in communicative disorders programs should be encouraged to take as many elective units as possible in such courses as introduction to psychology, abnormal psychology, personality theory, and learning theory. It is assumed that the student will be required to have a varied liberal arts background in general studies that would allow for inclusion of these courses.

2. It should be possible to include coverage of the psychology of the various communicative disorders discussed in introductory courses. Coverage should be limited to the most elementary psychological principles because the novice student is generally confounded sufficiently with the complexities surrounding the various communicative disorders.

3. Many programs provide clinical experiences for undergraduates that are essentially observational in nature. We consider it important for these students to have opportunities to observe master clinicians who are skilled in the techniques of counseling communicatively disordered individuals and/or their families. In those programs where undergraduates are expected to perform clinically, they can be introduced to counseling practices, but only under the most strict supervision by a master clinician skilled in psychotherapeutic techniques. (Unfortunately, at the present time there are probably few university or college instructors who feel comfortable or trained enough to take on this responsibility. This is all the more reason for intensive psychotherapeutic training at the doctoral level.)

4. Assuming undergraduate students will have experienced the above, the transition to more complex psychodynamic principles and practices can more readily be made, assuming, of course, that the graduate program in communicative disorders is prepared to make such offerings available. We realize that master-level programs in either speech language pathology or audiology are highly specialized and that faculty are often frustrated by the inability to cover everything they consider important. The feasibility, however, of including the psychodynamic features associated with the various disorders is strengthened by the fact that the disorders will be covered in a more highly specialized manner.

5. To complement any specialized course work that can be offered as electives in counseling itself, graduate students should now have frequent exposure to as many clinical opportunities as possible in order to practice counseling skills, when appropriate. Again, it must be presumed that the students will be supervised at least 50 percent of the time at first, depending on the counseling competence level of the student.

6. Graduate students should be encouraged to enhance their counseling skills by enrolling in courses outside the major department. These recommendations are not intended to delay graduation as long as the school or university allows an interdisciplinary policy whereby the student would be permitted to take a core of courses on a postmaster's level, without having to reenroll formally at the institution.

7. One of the key indicators that marks the successful counselor is a background that includes an extensive and intensive clinical practicum in counseling therapy. We hesitate to recommend a specific number of clinical practicum hours, but suggest instead that the student be allowed, following mutual agreement with the counseling supervisor, to take a practicum test after an externship of no less than 200 client contact hours. In California, the State Board of Behavioral Examiners requires that students must have a minimum of of 3000 supervised clock hours before they can be eligible for licensing as a marriage, family and child counselor. After January 1, 1986, at least 1500 of these must be at the postmaster level (similar to ASHA's requirement of the CFY) before they can be licensed. They must also take an oral and written examination.[1] We do not suggest that individuals who counsel their communicatively disordered clients should be required to be licensed as marriage, family and child counselors, as long as they do not breach the ethical boundaries of dealing only with the problems associated with the communicative disorder itself. We would urge, however, that they pass a competency exam in the use of counseling skills before they be allowed to counsel.

We recognize the complex philosophical and administrative problems inherent in such a recommendation and would therefore encourage the American Speech-Language-Hearing Association and state organizations to make a thorough study of the issue. Certainly there are those individuals who, having been certified and licensed as speech-language pathologists or audiologists, also qualify for licensing as marriage, family and child counselors. The author is acquainted with several such individuals who are duly licensed in the state of California.

8. Students enrolled in doctoral programs should have ready access to an elective core curriculum that provides sufficient learning in counseling theory and practice, particularly if these competencies have not been satisfied for their predoctoral degrees.

9. There are many opportunities for those already certified and licensed as speech-language pathologists or audiologists to gain access to counselor training in either universities, institutes, independent seminars

---

[1]Note: Except for a few additional course requirements and the 3000 hour clinical practicum, it would have been possible for those holding the master's degree or its equivalent to be eligible for licensing under a "grandfather" provision (Board of Behavioral Science Examiners, Regulation and Law Update, January 1984, State of California Department of Consumer Affairs).

and workshops, or professional conferences, in order that they be better prepared to serve a counseling role in their professional settings.

10. Speech-language pathologists and audiologists typically have already satisfied several competencies in counseling by virtue of their academic background. In fact, before 1978 the California State Board of Behavioral Examiners accepted a master's degree in communicative disorders as satisfying most academic requirements for the marriage, family and child counseling license. The board now requires that persons desiring licensing in marriage, family and child counseling shall hold a doctoral or a master's degree that contains "at least one course in each content area as set forth below and not less than thirty (30) semester or forty-five (45) quarter units of education courses as follows:

1. Human biological, psychological and social development
2. Human sexuality
3. Psychopathology
4. Cross-cultural mores and values
5. Theories of marriage, family and child counseling
6. Professional ethics and law
7. Human communication
8. Research methodology
9. Theories and applications of psychological testings, and
10. Not less than six (6) semester or nine (9) quarter units of supervised practicum in applied psychotherapuetic technique assessment, diagnosis, prognosis and treatment of pre-marital, marital, family and child relationship dysfunctions. (p. 21)

For a more complete description of licensing requirements, see Board of Behavioral Science Examiners Regulation and Law Update, January 1984, State of California Department of Consumer Affairs, pp. 1-39.

Although 125 hours in personal counseling may be credited toward the 3000 supervised clock hours, it is surprising that such counseling is not stipulated as a requirement for the license. In this author's opinion, it plainly raises serious ethical, moral, and professional questions that are addressed in the final chapter of this text.

INDEX

Ackerman, N. W., 130–131
Adler, R., 45–46
Ainsworth, M. D. S., 152
Albert, M. A., 68
Alpiner, J., 280
American Heart Association and stroke
 clubs, 55
Anaclitic depression, 152
Anderson, S., 17–18
Andrews, G., 116, 120, 122, 128–129
Annegers, J. F., 78
Annell, A. L., 160
Anthony, W. A., 248–249
Aphasia, 38–73 (*see also* Cerebral vascular
 disease, family therapy in)
Aphasia, counseling in:
 indicators and rationale for, 60
  concrete responses, modification of, 62
  denial, dealing with, 60 (*see also* Denial)
  depressed or frustrated non-verbal
   patient, counseling with, 65
  emotional lability, dealing with, 61
  extended care facility or nursing home,
   enhancing adjustment in, 62–63
  guilt, dealing with, 61–62
  linguistic error, patient response to,
   65–66

patient attitudes toward therapy and
  options for behavioral change, dealing
  with, 66–67
 premorbid psychological problems,
  dealing with, 64–65
 stress, dealing with, 64 (*see also* Stress)
 initial considerations, 52
 information, importance of providing,
  52–53
 premorbid from postmorbid issues,
  separation of, 53–54
 rehabilitation efforts, family involvement
  in, 54
 spouses and family, 54–56
Aphasia, family therapy in:
 criteria for, 57–58
 rationale and value, 56–57
 therapist guidelines, 58–59
Aphasia, research considerations in:
 family communication scale, 69–70
 personality type, 69
Approach-avoidance theory (*see* Stuttering)
Arnold, G. E., 160, 189
Aronson, A., 113, 189–190, 192–193,
 195–196, 198–199, 207, 209, 211, 213,
 216–219
Aronson, S. M., 40

319